T0293543

Nursing Care of Older Adults: Diagnosis, Interventions and Outcomes

Nursing Care of Older Adults: Diagnosis, Interventions and Outcomes

Editor: Ross Barbosa

hayle medical

New York

Hayle Medical,
750 Third Avenue, 9th Floor,
New York, NY 10017, USA

Visit us on the World Wide Web at:
www.haylemedical.com

ISBN 978-1-64647-582-7 (Hardback)

Cataloging-in-publication Data

Nursing care of older adults : diagnosis, interventions and outcomes / edited by Ross Barbosa.
p. cm.
Includes bibliographical references and index.
ISBN 978-1-64647-582-7
1. Geriatric nursing. 2. Older people--Diseases--Nursing. 3. Older people--Diseases--Diagnosis.
4. Older people--Diseases--Treatment. 5. Older people--Medical care. 6. Older people--Hospital care.
7. Nursing. I. Barbosa, Ross.
RC954 .N87 2023
610.736 5--dc23

Contents

Preface

Nursing includes the collaborative and independent care of people and involves preventing illness, supporting good health, and caring for the disabled, sick or dying people. The purpose of nursing care of older adults is intended to assist medical professionals in identifying signs and symptoms, assisting in diagnosis, and choosing relevant outcomes to monitor and evaluate the older adult's status. Nursing interventions are steps taken by the nurse to help the patient reach their goals and achieve the desired outcomes. Some of the examples of nursing interventions include monitoring the body vitals periodically, administering medications, educating the patient, and assessing the patient's pain levels. This book contains a detailed explanation of the diagnosis, interventions and outcomes associated with nursing care of older adults. It presents researches and studies performed by experts across the globe. Those in search of information to further their knowledge will be greatly assisted by this book.

After months of intensive research and writing, this book is the end result of all who devoted their time and efforts in the initiation and progress of this book. It will surely be a source of reference in enhancing the required knowledge of the new developments in the area. During the course of developing this book, certain measures such as accuracy, authenticity and research focused analytical studies were given preference in order to produce a comprehensive book in the area of study.

This book would not have been possible without the efforts of the authors and the publisher. I extend my sincere thanks to them. Secondly, I express my gratitude to my family and well-wishers. And most importantly, I thank my students for constantly expressing their willingness and curiosity in enhancing their knowledge in the field, which encourages me to take up further research projects for the advancement of the area.

Editor

Preface

Part 1

Care of the Elderly and Nutrition

1

Geriatrics and Orthogeriatrics: Providing Nutrition Care

Ólöf G. Geirsdóttir, Karen Hertz, Julie Santy-Tomlinson, Antony Johansen and Jack J. Bell

Abstract

Engaging older adults, and all those who care for them, is pivotal to providing high-value nutrition care for older adults. Nurses and other interdisciplinary team members are essential to this process. The aim of this chapter is to provide an overview of the rationale and evidence for interdisciplinary and systematised nutrition care as an effective nutrition care approach for older adults with or at risk of malnutrition. This chapter also serves as a guide to detailed chapters

Ó. G. Geirsdóttir (✉)
Faculty of Food Science and Nutrition, School of Health Science, University of Iceland, Reykjavík, Iceland
e-mail: ogg@hi.is

K. Hertz
Royal Stoke University Hospital, Stoke-on-Trent, UK
e-mail: karen.hertz@uhns.nhs.uk

J. Santy-Tomlinson
Orthopaedic Nursing, Odense University Hospitals/University of Southern Denmark, Odense, Denmark
e-mail: juliesanty@tomlinson15.karoo.co.uk

A. Johansen
Trauma Unit, University Hospital of Wales, Cardiff, UK

National Hip Fracture Database, Royal College of Physicians, London, UK
e-mail: antony.johansen@wales.nhs.uk

J. J. Bell
Allied Health, The Prince Charles Hospital, Chermside, Queensland, Australia

School of Human Movement and Nutrition Sciences, The University of Queensland, St Lucia, QLD, Australia
e-mail: jack.bell@health.qld.gov.au

across this book to provide focal points on different aspects of nutrition care that should be considered across primary prevention, acute care, rehabilitation, secondary prevention and community settings (Dreinhöfer et al., Injury 49(8):1393–1397, 2018).

Keywords
Fragility fracture · Malnutrition · Nutritional assessment · Nutrition care · Older Hip fracture · Sarcopenia · Nutrition care

Learning Outcomes
By the end of this chapter, you will be able to:

- Recognise the complexities of nutrition care for old people.
- Explain the rationale and benefit of shifting towards integrated, transdisciplinary nutrition care across healthcare and community settings.
- Apply key questions that will support timely, efficient and effective nutrition care for older persons across broad populations, conditions and settings.

1.1 Defining Malnutrition

Malnutrition broadly refers to deficiencies, excesses or imbalances in a person's intake of energy and/or nutrients. Undernutrition includes energy or macronutrient deficiencies (protein-energy malnutrition) and micronutrient deficiencies or insufficiencies, while overnutrition is routinely associated with overweight, obesity and diet-related noncommunicable diseases [1, 2]. This book will present a focus on malnutrition as undernutrition.

There is no definitive or 'gold standard' screening or diagnostic criteria for malnutrition [3]. Despite the availability of several validated nutritional assessments, malnutrition is often under- or misdiagnosed, overlooked and undervalued in multimorbid older adults, such as those with a fragility hip fracture [4–7].

Malnutrition diagnosis requires a thorough assessment and single-point diagnostic measures are unreliable. For example, malnutrition may be recognised in a chronically malnourished patient with normal albumin levels, but it can also be present in an acutely unwell older adult despite a high body mass index (BMI) of 50 kg/m^2 [4]. Conversely, an older adult with reduced handgrip strength resulting from motor-neurone disease should not immediately be considered malnourished without further investigation.

Muscle strength and function diminish as part of the normal ageing process, so a centenarian presenting with limited muscle reserves should not automatically be given a diagnosis of malnutrition, until it has been established whether loss of muscle mass, strength and function is in part attributable to malnutrition, for example, related to anorexia of ageing.

1.2 Nutrition Care in Older Adults: A Complex and Necessary Challenge

Malnutrition in older people is increasing in prevalence as the population ages [2, 8–10]. The prevalence of undernutrition in older people living in the community is about one in five [11–13]. Within clinical settings, malnutrition prevalence rates routinely approach half of older adults, although prevalence estimates vary substantially depending on the population, the healthcare setting and methods used for assessment [14–18].

Poor nutritional status is well established as a negative prognostic indicator among older adults, leading to functional decline, lower quality of life and increases in complications, morbidity and mortality, lengths of stay, unplanned readmissions, institutionalisation and costs [19–25]. It is worth noting that malnutrition can more than double the risk of dying for older adults [26, 27].

A practical case example is an older community-dwelling person admitted with fragility hip fracture. Although the surgical intervention and fracture union may have been successful, extended length of stay, residential care placement and early mortality can all still arise with sarcopenia, functional decline and multiple pressure injuries, all of which are attributable to hospital-acquired malnutrition.

A further dimension to the implications of malnutrition is the societal consequence of ageing. The increasing burden on the working age population is captured in the Old-Age Dependency Ratio [28, 29], and this emphasises the importance of good nutrition throughout the lifespan. Implications include:

- Society will need older adults to be independent for much longer in the future.
- Survival into old age is not going to be enough; quality of life is more important to older adults than longevity.
- Demographic change is going to be extremely rapid, increasing pressure on health and social care services; society must start adapting and adopting measures immediately.

The challenge of providing nutrition care for ageing populations is multifactorial. Urgent attention is required globally so that older adults and healthcare providers can understand the continuum of nutrition care across the lifecycle. 'Healthy eating' and optimal nutrition health during pre-older adult years must provide the groundwork for healthy ageing, but we need to re-evaluate what 'healthy eating' looks like in older adults.

The onset of frailty and other conditions of old age requires us to consider changing the focus of nutrition care away from lifestyle advise and the prevention of obesity and towards prevention of functional loss and the maintenance of muscle mass, bone integrity and quality of life.

This may at first appear counter-intuitive, for example, prescribing supplements in an obese inpatient at risk of malnutrition after hip fracture or deprescribing a long-standing 'low-cholesterol diet' for someone admitted to a cardiac unit with underlying malnutrition [30, 31]. It may simply mean accepting the risk of aspiration in an older adult with end-stage Parkinson's disease and allowing them unrestricted food and fluids for the comfort, enjoyment and social interactions that mealtimes offer. When and where such shifts in the focus of nutrition care should occur will depend on age-related changes, comorbidities, sociocultural factors and, most importantly, what matters to the older adult.

1.3 Malnutrition: A Truly Wicked Problem

Malnutrition is multifactorial and underlying factors that can lead to malnutrition are many and varied. In some cases, malnutrition cannot be resolved, although attentive management may improve outcomes for older adults and the systems that care for them. There are no single 'silver bullet' solutions; this is one of many reasons why malnutrition is considered to meet the definition of a 'wicked' problem as initially described by Rittel and Webber (Table 1.1) [32, 33].

1.4 Building the Rationale for Integrated Nutrition Care

It is important that healthcare providers are proactive in identifying individual causes, signs and symptoms of malnutrition. If identified early, malnutrition can be treated with individualised nutritional intervention plans which should be supported by effective systems and cohesive, integrated care processes [1]. While early recognition and treatment of malnutrition are recognised as beneficial for the health and wellbeing of the older person, nutritional diagnosis and a timely nutrition care can also reduce overall healthcare and community costs [34–36].

Table 1.1 Why malnutrition in older adults should be considered as a wicked problem [32, 33]

- Profession and scientific definitions and diagnostic criteria continually evolve over time
- Shared and overlapping boundaries between ageing, cachexia, frailty, obesity, sarcopenia and other conditions
- Unique individual presentations in ageing limit the usefulness of clinical algorithms and the accuracy of tools
- The diagnosis and related underlying problems cannot be routinely reduced to single-base variables
- The aetiology of malnutrition is multifactorial; underlying factors that can contribute to malnutrition are many and varied
- There are unfixed, iterative and adaptive solutions that require tailoring across settings
- There are no 'right' or 'wrong' solutions; and in many cases management, rather than resolution, may be appropriate
- There are no 'silver bullets' providing all the solutions
- Clinician actions are constrained by a lack of or contradictory evidence, resource limitations, the balance between food as a right to life and food as a medicine and older adult preferences and beliefs
- Intervention and outcome evaluations are routinely confounded by other factors
- Every older adult and setting should be considered essentially unique

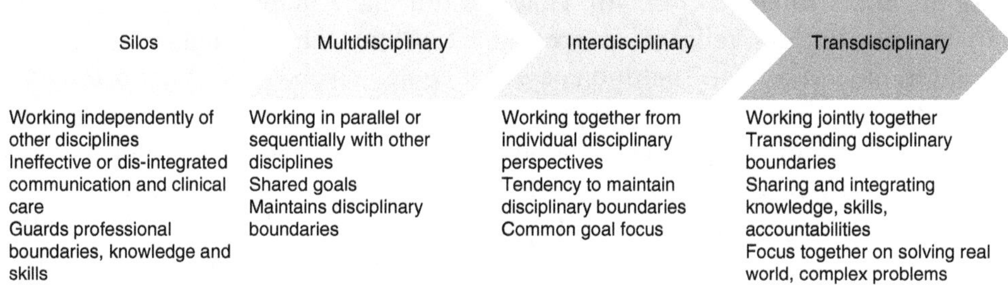

Fig. 1.1 Moving from silos to transdisciplinary care [41, 42]

The nature of nutrition care, and geriatric practice more generally, predicates a comprehensive approach delivered by multiple healthcare providers across the continuum of care [37, 38]. Appropriate nutrition care for older adults is not something that will occur organically, but requires cultivating towards integrated, transdisciplinary approaches to deliver efficient, effective and sustainable nutrition care across acute, rehabilitation and community settings [7, 27, 39, 40]. Multi-agency collaboration; integrated organisational and administrative structures; shared skills, tasks and goals across all relevant actors; collaborative leadership; and, most importantly, a focus on what matters to the older adult are all key components of transdisciplinary care. These are also the necessary ingredients to manage the wicked problem of malnutrition. Consequently, continual progression along the continuum from siloed, single-discipline approaches to transdisciplinary care (Fig. 1.1) is most likely to impact positively on nutrition care.

1.5 Managing the Wicked Nutrition Problems with a SIMPLE Approach (or Other Tailored Models)

The sheer volume of older adults with or at risk of malnutrition or other nutrition-related diagnoses, combined with increasing health expenditure and competing demands for resources, have resulted in demand outstripping supply of individual access to nutrition specialists [22]. Internationally, there are several models available that support interdisciplinary healthcare teams to deliver timely and appropriate nutrition care, for example, the Systematised, Interdisciplinary Malnutrition Program for impLementation and Evaluation (SIMPLE), the More-2-Eat implementation programme targeting improving nutrition culture within hospitals and Malnutrition Universal Screening Tool (MUST) [27, 43, 44].

These models usually triage those screened into one of three groups: those 'not at risk' and appropriate for standard care, those who are at risk or malnourished who are appropriate for interdisciplinary or 'supportive' nutrition care and those who are likely to benefit from the intervention of a nutrition care specialist, or 'specialist nutrition care'. Specialised nutritional interventions tailored to individual requirements have demonstrated positive influence on outcomes in the acute and rehabilitation settings [27, 45, 46]. However, for many individuals across diverse geriatric care settings, reliance on 'specialist' nutrition care may not add additional benefit to the fundamental nutrition care that could and should be provided by the rest of the team as 'supportive' nutrition care. Specialised nutrition care may be delayed because of many diverse reasons, varying from inadequate availability of specialists, no weekend cover or clinical prioritisation requirements, and, in many locations, it may simply not be available because of either lack of funding or the availability of clinicians to fill advertised positions, particularly in rural and remote settings.

1.5.1 Keep It SIMPLE When Appropriate

While recognising that nutrition care in older adults is often complex, in a high proportion of cases and settings, supportive SIMPLE nutrition care is appropriate.

Figure 1.2 provides an illustrative summary of how healthcare professionals can contribute to systematised, interdisciplinary supportive nutrition care for individual older adults with, or at risk of, a nutrition-related diagnosis. This figure has been adapted from the SIMPLE model and is composition of key nutrition care models applied internationally [27, 43, 46–48]. This is further detailed in Bell et al. [7].

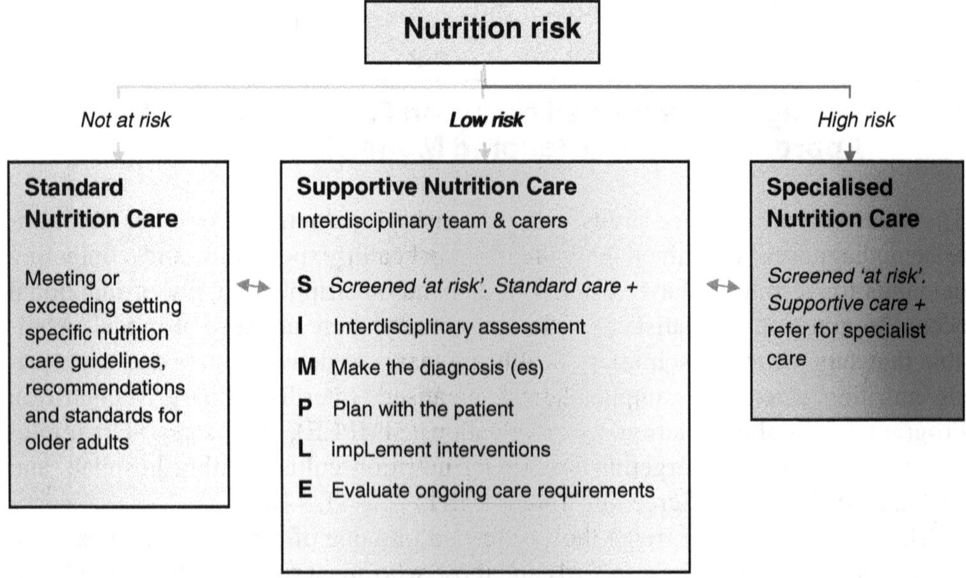

Fig. 1.2 A SIMPLE nutrition care approach. (Source: Adapted to fit from key nutrition care models [27, 43, 46–48])

1.5.2 A SIMPLE Case Example

An educational case example is now presented to illustrate how the SIMPLE model may be applied across practice settings.

Case Example

Mary is an 83-year-old female with hip fracture, admitted to a hospital with minimal dietetics services. She lost her husband 4 months ago, lives alone and has no children.

Anthropometry: *Height 162 cm, weight 82 kg and BMI 32; she has lost 10 kg in the last 6 months secondary to complications after cardiac surgery and sepsis on multiple recent admissions.*

Medical history: *Type 2 diabetes, high blood pressure, hyperlipidaemia, depressed and excessive alcohol intake.*

Pharmacy: *Cardiovascular drugs (cholesterol and blood pressure lowering), psychotropic drugs (antidepressant, anti-anxiety and sleeping aid) and oral hypoglycaemic agents for type 2 diabetes.*

Day 2 post-op rapport: *She has fever and chest infection. She has had hypoactive delirium since admission, and now the medical team is questioning whether she has underlying cognitive impairment and whether she might be drowsy due to overmedication for post-operative pains. She has had poor oral intake since admission. She gets standard hospital diet but without dessert and sweet bread because of her T2DM and obesity. A nurse has noticed that she coughed a couple of times while she was drinking her tea. There is a stage 2 pressure injury on her right heel.*

Cases like Mary's are encountered every day by staff working in geriatric care settings. It highlights the complexity of nutritional issues that need to be considered by the interdisciplinary team but also provides an example for SIMPLE supportive care.

1.5.2.1 S—Screen for Malnutrition

Mary will be identified as 'at risk' of malnutrition when she is screened using most internationally applied, validated malnutrition screening tools.

1.5.2.2 I—Interdisciplinary Assessment

Unfortunately, in many settings Mary would not have been screened for malnutrition risk and, even if positively screened, may not have met the clinical prioritisation criteria for specialist nutrition care. In many settings globally, access to timely dietitian or medical nutrition specialist care is simply not going to be available for Mary. Whether Mary would meet requirements for 'supportive' versus 'specialised' care will consequently be dependent on setting, but in this case, we suggest supportive, rather than standard care, should be considered as a minimum.

1.5.2.3 M—Make the Diagnosis (es)

Multiple nutrition-related diagnoses are evident, and the evidence-based recommendations for nutrition care are, at best, difficult to align but are more likely to be conflicting. For example, Mary has diabetes and is overweight, and she reports a long-standing low-cholesterol, 'low-sugar' diet; so she is happy about her weight loss. Unfortunately, Mary is also malnourished, in part reflecting restrictive dieting, excessive alcohol intake and poor intake associated with depression and social disconnection. In most settings, this will be the recognised priority in addressing Mary's nutritional diagnosis.

1.5.2.4 P—Plan with the Older Adult

Identifying the priority diagnosis and balancing nutrition co-diagnoses cannot generally be guided by evidence-based algorithms. Instead, clinical judgement and engagement with the older adult, their family, carers and treating teams are necessary in understanding and definition of shared treatment goals. In such cases, some components of nutrition care may be appropriately delivered by the interdisciplinary team, but only if they ask the right questions and work together with the older adult. What are their requirements and priorities? What does the evidence suggest? What is the treatment intent? What does the older adult want? If nutrition care is genuinely complex and likely to benefit from specialist attention, this should be prioritised wherever resources permit.

1.5.2.5 L—Implement Interventions

An evidence-based, multi-modal, interdisciplinary approach that promotes 'nutrition as a medicine', interdisciplinary nutrition care, food-service enhancements, improved nutrition knowledge and awareness and coordination of pre- and post-discharge nutrition care is likely to improve outcomes for older adults like Mary [31].

1.5.2.6 E—Evaluate Ongoing Care Requirements

Ensuring that individual and systems processes for the evaluation of ongoing care requirements are in place is a key component of integrated care. Where possible, engaging the older adult in self-monitoring should be a key priority and supported by post-discharge follow-up of nutrition by a general practitioner.

1.6 Bringing It All Together: Integrated Nutrition Care Across the Four Pillars of (Ortho) Geriatric Care

The following chapters of this book are written with older adults like Mary, and all those who care for her, firmly in mind. Chapters are centred around the key pillars of the call to action for orthogeriatric care [49]. These invoke the need to consider

(1) the core business of primary and secondary prevention strategies, (2) the interdisciplinary management of the acute period and (3) the rehabilitation phase, recognised as continuing for the rest of the older adult's life.

To support these three clinical pillars, a fourth is highlighted—the political pillar of creating national interdisciplinary alliances between relevant mainstream professional associations, to push for the policy change and multi-professional education that is needed if the first three are to gain impetus.

In considering these fundamental pillars of care, each chapter presents an evaluation of the current evidence for best practice, balanced with 'in field' applied understanding regarding how to balance 'best practice' with the realities of routinely confounding, and often conflicting, recommendations, conditions, resources perceptions, biases and team and older adult expectations.

The mantra of this book is that we should avoid applying prescriptive 'must do' algorithms or formulae, but readers will be challenged to consider their own local context and to decide how to prioritise efficient and effective nutrition care that matters to older adults, in the right place, at the right time, by the right healthcare providers. This approach will also support care across settings, whether medical nutrition specialist access, experiences and resources are readily accessible, limited or simply not available.

The purpose of Chap. 2 is to describe the nutritional recommendations for older adults and introduce the need to consider changes in requirements with age and disease. Chapter 3 shares knowledge about terminology and best practice for the nutrition care for older adult. Chapter 4 is about malnutrition prevention in older adults where many factors influence the nutritional intake, wellbeing and quality of life. This will introduce the need to consider acute or chronic diseases, and a reduced dietary intake plays a crucial role in developing malnutrition. A key aim of this chapter is to increase the nutritional-based knowledge of nurses and other healthcare providers to prevent malnutrition. Chapter 5 describes the practical aspects of nutrition support, including nutritional dense food, nutritional supplements and/or when enteral and parenteral nutrition may be used. The ethical aspects of nutrition support are also considered. This chapter also makes the case that perhaps the most critical tool in a dietitian or medical nutrition specialists toolkit is a clinically focussed food-service system.

Chapter 6 describes opportunities for nursing to demonstrate leadership in nutrition care, whether to supporting healthy eating to sustain healthy ageing and prevent and manage malnutrition; endocrine, immune system and organ dysfunction; muscle strength and function; bone health in older adults; or a combination of these. Considerations regarding assessment of hydration status, recommendations and guidelines for hydration, fluid intake and intravenous fluid therapy are provided in Chap. 7. Chapter 8 aims to untangling ageing, malnutrition, frailty, sarcopenia and function; these are different conditions with overlapping characteristics, consequences and interventional opportunities in older adults. These can often be hidden conditions; hence interdisciplinary awareness is needed for optimal identification and management. Chapter 9 aims to introducing bone health in older adult, what happens with ageing and how we diagnose osteoporosis. What we can do from a nutritional and non-nutritional perspective in preventing osteoporosis and supporting those with osteoporosis?

Many factors influence eating behaviour and nutritional status in older adults. Chapter 10 introduces the need to consider how to increase older adult motivation, factors that support or confound adherence to nutrition care, and reminds readers that eating habits are inseparably linked with people's physical and psychological health and wellbeing. An overarching aim of this chapter is to assist healthcare providers to consider psychological barriers that may lead older adults away from engaging with nutrition care and the importance of motivational interventions to support adherence to nutrition care. This chapter also provides useful insights and direction for further research.

Malnutrition prevention, detection and treatment in older adults benefit from an interdisciplinary approach, regardless of the care setting. The focus of Chap. 11 challenges the reader regarding how to engage older adults and teams in developing and sustaining models of nutrition care with an emphasis on interdisciplinary approaches. Implementation programmes are showcased that demonstrate the rationale and evidence for why and how to engage treating teams to spread and sustain nutrition care improvements across healthcare systems. Education improves interprofessional engagement with nutrition care across pillars. Chapter 12 details underpinnings and pragmatic approaches to education of healthcare providers. This will provide the reader with knowledge and skills to support interprofessional education that embeds evidence-based collaborative nutrition care and improves delivery for older adults. Key models supporting an interdisciplinary approach to nutrition care are covered in Chap. 13. Internationally applicable care pathways are presented that support interdisciplinary care for hospitals and to support integrated care beyond the hospital setting. The challenge of whether acute hospitals are the best environments to resolve malnutrition versus the need for interdisciplinary leadership, champions and resources to support scale and spread of nutrition care across the continuum is a common theme embedded across Chaps. 10–12.

Chapter 14 summarises the current evidence about the role of physical activity, exercise and physical rehabilitation with an emphasis on nutritional aspects. The focus of Chap. 15 is on the link between malnutrition and interventions in preventing and managing pressure injuries. Chapter 16 provides an overview of obesity, and body composition, and importantly targets an increased awareness of the limitations of commonly applied measure of muscle and body fatness such as the BMI. Chapter 17 provides an extension learning chapter to highlight that even detailed assessments that delineate muscle versus fat disregard the different types of fat and how these body fat mass should be considered not as simple energy storage but a complex human organ. The mouth is the first stage of digestion, and understanding oral health and oropharyngeal dysphagia as important factor in malnutrition are described in Chap. 18. Delirium is a common and serious complication in hospitalised older people. Poor nutrition and hydration are both risk factors for, and consequences of, delirium. Chapter 19 discusses the phenomenology of delirium and the role of nurses and other healthcare professionals in recognising, preventing and managing this serious complication. Interaction between food and drugs is a complex subject as prescribed drugs can affect the nutritional uptake of older adults and diet and timing of eating can change the efficacy of drugs. Consequently, Chapter 20 provides some detail on common supplementation and drug-food and food-drug interactions.

End-of-life care constitutes an important situation of extreme nutritional vulnerability for older adults. Feeding decisions often provoke wrenching moral and ethical questions for family members regarding whether to continue hand feeding or opt for tube feeding placement. Supporting older adults, and those who care for them, to make informed decision-making at the end of life is the focus on Chap. 21. This chapter provides practical examples that illustrate the unique complexities that should be considered when planning which, if any, medical nutrition therapies (by oral and artificial means) should be considered at the end of life.

1.7 Summary: Finishing Off with a List of New Questions

We have made the case that malnutrition is a wicked problem and noted that nutrition care is often provided across highly complex healthcare settings. Consequently, it would be naïve to conclude that malnutrition care in older adults is simple. We have suggested that reliance on specialists may delay or prevent timely, supportive nutrition care. However, we have also observed that timely, appropriate nutritional assessments and interventions are often overlooked or disregarded by 'in situ' interdisciplinary healthcare professionals, despite the high prevalence of nutrition-related diagnoses across geriatric populations and the potential cost benefits of early identification and treatment [5, 6, 27].

Successful and sustained nutrition care requires the engagement of older adults, carers and interdisciplinary teams using a knowledge translation approach. This, ideally, should foster tailoring of nutrition care using co-designed approaches. Interventions planned at the individual level should consider a shared decision-making approach, including informed consent and goal setting, and establishing monitoring and reassessment processes to identify whether interventions are effective and consistent with older adult goals and healthcare system deliverables [7, 50]. 'Cut and paste' approaches to nutrition care model reforms are less likely to be successful, either initially or sustained and spread [40, 51, 52].

We conclude that multi-modal, co-designed interventions, delivered by diverse healthcare workers, are pivotal to nutrition care of the older adult; these need to be integrated across acute care, rehabilitation and primary/secondary prevention in the community [45, 53–59]. Consequently, to finish this introductory chapter on a pragmatic note, we propose some nutrition-focussed questions that may be asked by nurses or other healthcare workers, regardless of setting (Table 1.2). This is not an exhaustive list but provides a useful place to start. A cross-reference to the relevant chapters in this book is provided, to provide insights into why these questions should be asked and what could be actioned in response to support integrated care for older adults like Mary who are at risk of malnutrition or already malnourished.

Table 1.2 Some useful nutrition-focussed questions to ask yourself when working with an older adult

Question	Key sources for further information
What are Mary's nutrition requirements, needs and preferences?	Chapter 2: Geriatrics and Nutritional Recommendations
Are Mary's requirements being met? Is Mary at risk of or already has a nutrition-related diagnosis or condition?	Chapter 3: Nutrition Care Process: Terminology and Best Practice Approaches
Could we have prevented Mary from becoming malnourished?	Chapter 4: Interdisciplinary Prevention of Malnutrition Chapter 5: Treatment of Malnutrition: Common Nutrition Support Prescriptions
Is it an essential nursing role to support nutrition care for Mary?	Chapter 6: Best Practice Nursing in Geriatrics: Role of Nutrition Care
Is Mary appropriately hydrated?	Chapter 7: Geriatrics and Orthogeriatrics: Hydration and Dehydration
Is Mary malnourished or frail, or is it something else?	Chapter 8: Health Impacts of Sarcopenia, Physical Dysfunction, Malnutrition and Cachexia
Why did Mary fracture her hip? And could we have prevented it?	Chapter 9: Skeletal Health in Older Adults Chapter 14: Role of Physical Activity for Older Adults: Nutritional Aspects
How do I engage Mary in her nutrition care?	Chapter 10: Psychological Barriers and Nutritional Care
How do I engage other team members in nutrition care?	Chapter 11: Nutritional Improvements: Spread and Sustainability
How can I improve the nutrition knowledge of all those who might influence Mary's nutrition care	Chapter 12: Nutritional Care: Role of Interprofessional Education for Interdisciplinary Cooperation
Who else might help to support nutrition care for Mary?	Chapter 13: Geriatric Malnutrition: A Multidisciplinary Approach
Is it worth the effort of trying to get Mary out of bed?	Chapter 14: Role of Physical Activity for Older Adults: Nutritional Aspects
Could we have prevented Mary's pressure injury? Will nutrition help?	Chapter 15: Prevention and Management of Malnutrition and PIs
I still don't understand why Mary is malnourished even though she is obese. Isn't fat just fat?	Chapter 16: BMI and Obesity Chapter 17: A Comprehensive Study of the Nutritional System
Is Mary just coughing or is she aspirating?	Chapter 18: Dysphagia in Older Adults
What do I do about the delirium?	Chapter 19: Hospitalized Older People, Nutrition and Delirium
How are the medicines interacting with the food or vice versa? Can food be a medicine?	Chapter 20: Elderly People and Food-Drug Interaction
In the end, just how much does food matter?	Chapter 21: End-of-Life Care, Ethics and Nutrition

References

1. World Health Organisation (2020) Malnutrition. https://www.who.int/news-room/q-a-detail/malnutrition
2. Agarwal E, Miller M, Yaxley A, Isenring E (2013) Malnutrition in the elderly: a narrative review. Maturitas 76(4):296–302
3. Elia M, Stratton RJ (2011) Considerations for screening tool selection and role of predictive and concurrent validity. Curr Opin Clin Nutr Metab Care 14(5):425–433
4. Bell JJ, Bauer JD, Capra S, Pulle RC (2014) Concurrent and predictive evaluation of malnutrition diagnostic measures in hip fracture inpatients: a diagnostic accuracy study. Eur J Clin Nutr 68(3):358–362
5. Bell JJ, Bauer JD, Capra S, Pulle RC (2014) Quick and easy is not without cost: implications of poorly performing nutrition screening tools in hip fracture. J Am Geriatr Soc 62(2):237–243
6. Bell JJ, Bauer J, Capra S, Pulle CR (2013) Barriers to nutritional intake in patients with acute hip fracture: time to treat malnutrition as a disease and food as a medicine? Can J Physiol Pharmacol 91(6):489–495
7. Bell JJ, Geirsdóttir ÓG, Hertz K, Santy-Tomlinson J, Skúladóttir SS, Eleuteri S et al (2021) Nutritional care of the older patient with fragility fracture: opportunities for systematised, interdisciplinary approaches across acute care, rehabilitation and secondary prevention settings. In: Falaschi P, Marsh D (eds) Orthogeriatrics: the management of older patients with fragility fractures. Springer International, Cham, pp 311–329
8. Burton-Shepherd A (2013) Preventing malnutrition in home-dwelling elderly individuals. Br J Community Nurs (Suppl Nutrition):S25–S31
9. Legrain S, Tubach F, Bonnet-Zamponi D, Lemaire A, Aquino JP, Paillaud E et al (2011) A new multimodal geriatric discharge-planning intervention to prevent emergency visits and rehospitalizations of older adults: the optimization of medication in AGEd multicenter randomized controlled trial. J Am Geriatr Soc 59(11):2017–2028
10. Bell CL, Tamura BK, Masaki KH, Amella EJ (2013) Prevalence and measures of nutritional compromise among nursing home patients: weight loss, low body mass index, malnutrition, and feeding dependency, a systematic review of the literature. J Am Med Dir Assoc 14(2):94–100
11. Adebusoye LA, Ajayi IO, Dairo MD, Ogunniyi AO (2012) Nutritional status of older persons presenting in a primary care clinic in Nigeria. J Nutr Gerontol Geriatr 31(1):71–85
12. Aliabadi M, Kimiagar M, Ghayour-Mobarhan M, Shakeri MT, Nematy M, Ilaty AA et al (2008) Prevalence of malnutrition in free living elderly people in Iran: a cross-sectional study. Asia Pac J Clin Nutr 17(2):285–289
13. Kabir ZN, Ferdous T, Cederholm T, Khanam MA, Streatfied K, Wahlin A (2006) Mini nutritional assessment of rural elderly people in Bangladesh: the impact of demographic, socioeconomic and health factors. Public Health Nutr 9(8):968–974
14. Volkert D, Beck AM, Cederholm T, Cereda E, Cruz-Jentoft A, Goisser S et al (2019) Management of malnutrition in older patients—current approaches, evidence and open questions. J Clin Med 8(7)
15. Cereda E, Pedrolli C, Klersy C, Bonardi C, Quarleri L, Cappello S et al (2016) Nutritional status in older persons according to healthcare setting: a systematic review and meta-analysis of prevalence data using MNA(®). Clin Nutr 35(6):1282–1290

16. Lacau St Guily J, Bouvard É, Raynard B, Goldwasser F, Maget B, Prevost A et al (2018) NutriCancer: a French observational multicentre cross-sectional study of malnutrition in elderly patients with cancer. J Geriatr Oncol 9(1):74–80
17. Cereda E, Veronese N, Caccialanza R (2018) The final word on nutritional screening and assessment in older persons. Curr Opin Clin Nutr Metab Care 21(1):24–29
18. Bell JJ, Pulle RC, Lee HB, Ferrier R, Crouch A, Whitehouse SL (2021) Diagnosis of overweight or obese malnutrition spells DOOM for hip fracture patients; a prospective audit. Clin Nutr 40(4):1905–1910
19. Dent E, Visvanathan R, Piantadosi C, Chapman I (2012) Nutritional screening tools as predictors of mortality, functional decline, and move to higher level care in older people: a systematic review. J Nutr Gerontol Geriatr 31(2):97–145
20. Rasheed S, Woods RT (2013) Malnutrition and quality of life in older people: a systematic review and meta-analysis. Ageing Res Rev 12(2):561–566
21. Al Snih S, Raji MA, Markides KS, Ottenbacher KJ, Goodwin JS (2005) Weight change and lower body disability in older Mexican Americans. J Am Geriatr Soc 53(10):1730–1737
22. Arnold AM, Newman AB, Cushman M, Ding J, Kritchevsky S (2010) Body weight dynamics and their association with physical function and mortality in older adults: the cardiovascular health study. J Gerontol A Biol Sci Med Sci 65(1):63–70
23. Ritchie CS, Locher JL, Roth DL, McVie T, Sawyer P, Allman R (2008) Unintentional weight loss predicts decline in activities of daily living function and life-space mobility over 4 years among community-dwelling older adults. J Gerontol A Biol Sci Med Sci 63(1):67–75
24. Chang M, Geirsdottir OG, Launer LJ, Gudnasson V, Visser M, Gunnarsdottir I (2020) A poor appetite or ability to eat and its association with physical function amongst community-dwelling older adults: age, gene/environment susceptibility-Reykjavik study. Eur J Ageing
25. Lackoff AS, Hickling D, Collins PF, Stevenson KJ, Nowicki TA, Bell JJ (2020) The association of malnutrition with falls and harm from falls in hospital inpatients: findings from a 5-year observational study. J Clin Nurs 29(3–4):429–436
26. Morley JE (2011) Assessment of malnutrition in older persons: a focus on the mini nutritional assessment. J Nutr Health Aging 15(2):87–90
27. Bell JJ, Young A, Hill J, Banks M, Comans T, Barnes R et al (2018) Rationale and developmental methodology for the SIMPLE approach: a systematised, interdisciplinary malnutrition pathway for impLementation and evaluation in hospitals. Nutr Diet 75(2):226–234
28. OECD (2019) Pensions at a Glance 2019
29. Division DoEaSA-P (2019) World population prospects 2019—highlights. United Nations, Affairs DoEaS, New York
30. Lee RJ, Collins PF, Elmas K, Bell JJ (2019) Restrictive diets in older malnourished cardiac inpatients: a cross-sectional study. Nutr Diet 78(2):121–127
31. Bell JJ, Bauer JD, Capra S, Pulle RC (2014) Multidisciplinary, multi-modal nutritional care in acute hip fracture inpatients—results of a pragmatic intervention. Clin Nutr 33(6):1101–1107
32. Young AM (2015) Solving the wicked problem of hospital malnutrition. Nutr Diet 72(3):200–204
33. Rittel HWJ, Webber MM (1973) Dilemmas in a general theory of planning. Pol Sci 4(2):155–169
34. Jeejeebhoy KN, Keller H, Gramlich L, Allard JP, Laporte M, Duerksen DR et al (2015) Nutritional assessment: comparison of clinical assessment and objective variables for the prediction of length of hospital stay and readmission. Am J Clin Nutr 101(5):956–965
35. Curtis LJ, Bernier P, Jeejeebhoy K, Allard J, Duerksen D, Gramlich L et al (2017) Costs of hospital malnutrition. Clin Nutr 36(5):1391–1396
36. Marques-Vidal P, Khalatbari-Soltani S, Sahli S, Coti Bertrand P, Pralong F, Waeber G (2018) Undernutrition is associated with increased financial losses in hospitals. Clin Nutr 37(2):681–686
37. Welsh TJ, Gordon AL, Gladman JR (2014) Comprehensive geriatric assessment—a guide for the non-specialist. Int J Clin Pract 68(3):290–293

38. Pioli G, Davoli M, Pellicciotti F, Pignedoli P, Ferrari A (2011) Comprehensive care. Eur J Phys Rehabil Med 47(2):265–279
39. Holmesland A-L, Seikkula J, Nilsen O, Hopfenbeck M, Erik AT (2010) Open dialogues in social networks: professional identity and transdisciplinary collaboration. Int J Integr Care 10:e53
40. Bell JJ, Rossi T, Bauer JD, Capra S (2014) Developing and evaluating interventions that are applicable and relevant to inpatients and those who care for them; a multiphase, pragmatic action research approach. BMC Med Res Methodol 14:98
41. Van Bewer V (2017) Transdisciplinarity in health care: a concept analysis. Nurs Forum 52(4):339–347
42. Rosenfield PL (1992) The potential of transdisciplinary research for sustaining and extending linkages between the health and social sciences. Soc Sci Med 35(11):1343–1357
43. Elia M (2003) In: Nutrition BAfPaE (ed) Screening for malnutrition: a multidisciplinary responsibility. Development and use of the malnutrition universal screening tool (MUST) for adults. BAPEN, Redditch
44. Keller H, Laur C, Atkins M, Bernier P, Butterworth D, Davidson B et al (2018) Update on the integrated nutrition pathway for acute care (INPAC): post implementation tailoring and toolkit to support practice improvements. Nutr J 17(1):2
45. Jensen GL, Compher C, Sullivan DH, Mullin GE (2013) Recognizing malnutrition in adults: definitions and characteristics, screening, assessment, and team approach. J Parenter Enteral Nutr 37(6):802–807
46. Keller H, Laur C, Valaitis R, Bell J, McNicholl T, Ray S et al (2017) More-2-eat: evaluation protocol of a multi-site implementation of the integrated nutrition pathway for acute care. BMC Nutr 3(1):13
47. Writing Group of the Nutrition Care Process/Standardized Language Committee (2008) Nutrition care process and model part I: the 2008 update. J Am Diet Assoc 108(7):1113–1117
48. Isenring EA, Bauer JD, Banks M, Gaskill D (2009) The malnutrition screening tool is a useful tool for identifying malnutrition risk in residential aged care. J Hum Nutr Diet 22(6):545–550
49. Dreinhöfer KE, Mitchell PJ, Bégué T, Cooper C, Costa ML, Falaschi P et al (2018) A global call to action to improve the care of people with fragility fractures. Injury 49(8):1393–1397
50. Jensen GL, Mirtallo J, Compher C, Dhaliwal R, Forbes A, Grijalba RF et al (2010) Adult starvation and disease-related malnutrition: a proposal for etiology-based diagnosis in the clinical practice setting from the international consensus guideline committee. J Parenter Enteral Nutr 34(2):156–159
51. Laur C, Bell J, Valaitis R, Ray S, Keller H (2018) The Sustain and Spread Framework: strategies for sustaining and spreading nutrition care improvements in acute care based on thematic analysis from the More-2-Eat study (Report). BMC Health Serv Res 18(1):930
52. Laur C, Valaitis R, Bell J, Keller H (2017) Changing nutrition care practices in hospital: a thematic analysis of hospital staff perspectives. BMC Health Serv Res 17(1):498
53. Keller H, Koechl JM, Laur C, Chen H, Curtis L, Dubin JA et al (2021) More-2-eat implementation demonstrates that screening, assessment and treatment of malnourished patients can be spread and sustained in acute care; a multi-site, pretest post-test time series study. Clin Nutr 40(4):2100–2108
54. Keller HH, Valaitis R, Laur CV, McNicholl T, Xu Y, Dubin JA et al (2019) Multi-site implementation of nutrition screening and diagnosis in medical care units: success of the More-2-eat project. Clin Nutr 38(2):897–905
55. Volkert D, Beck AM, Cederholm T, Cruz-Jentoft A, Goisser S, Hooper L et al (2019) ESPEN guideline on clinical nutrition and hydration in geriatrics. Clin Nutr 38(1):10–47
56. National Institute for Health and Clinical Excellence (NICE) (2006) Nutrition support in adults: oral nutrition support, enteral tube feeding and parenteral nutrition (clinical guideline 32)
57. Watterson C, Fraser A, Banks M (2009) Evidence based practise guidelines for the nutritional management of malnutrition in adult patients across the continuum of care. Nutr Diet 66:S1–S34

58. NICE (2012) NICE quality standard 24: quality standard for nutrition support in adults. NICE, London
59. Tappenden KA, Quatrara B, Parkhurst ML, Malone AM, Fanjiang G, Ziegler TR (2013) Critical role of nutrition in improving quality of care: an interdisciplinary call to action to address adult hospital malnutrition. J Parenter Enteral Nutr 37(4):482–497

2

Geriatrics and Nutritional Recommendations

Anne Marie Beck and Mette Holst

Abstract

The purpose of this chapter is to describe the nutritional recommendations for older adults and change in requirements with age and disease. Key factors influencing nutritional requirements, dietary intake, and nutritional status in old adults will be described, including specific nuances for geriatric and orthogeriatric patients.

Keywords

Nutritional recommendations · Nutritional status · Nutritional risk factors

---

This chapter is a component of Section 1: Nutritional Care in Old Age.
For an explanatiocn of the grouping of chapters in this book, please see Chap. 1: "Geriatrics and Orthogeriatrics: Providing Nutrition Care."

A. M. Beck (✉)
University College Copenhagen, Institute of Nursing and Nutrition, Copenhagen, Denmark

Dietetic and Nutritional Research Unit, Herlev-Gentofte University Hospital, Herlev, Denmark
e-mail: ambe@kp.dk

M. Holst
Department of Clinical Medicine, Centre for Nutrition and Bowel Disease, Aalborg University Hospital, Aalborg University, Aalborg, Denmark
e-mail: mette.holst@rn.dk

Learning Outcomes
By the end of this chapter, you will be able to:

- Report common nutritional risk factors among different groups of older adults.
- List examples of nutritional recommendations for old adults in relation to energy, protein, and vitamin D.
- Justify changes in requirements with age and diseases.
- Identify potentially modifiable risk factors for malnutrition in older adults.
- Describe aging-related characteristics that may impede accurate dietary assessment.

2.1 Nutritional Recommendations for Older Adults, Geriatric and Orthogeriatric Patients

This chapter will describe the nutritional recommendations for older adults focusing on where the recommendations differ from the requirement for younger people [1–5]. Many geriatric guidelines about food and nutrition are primarily valid for groups of healthy individuals with various levels of physical activity [2–4]. For individuals with diseases and other groups with special needs, dietary recommendations and the consequent dietary composition and energy content might have to be adjusted accordingly [1]. This section will also describe how nutritional requirements change in relation to aging and disease processes, with a specific focus on energy and protein and vitamin D.

2.2 Nutritional Recommendations for Older Adults

Dietary reference values (DRVs) for essential nutrients include the average requirement (AR), recommended intake (RI), upper intake level (UL), lower intake level (LI), and reference values for energy [2]. It is important to distinguish between the average requirement for a nutrient and the recommended intake of a nutrient. The recommended intake represents more than the requirement for the average person and covers the individual variations in the requirement for the vast majority of the population group (Fig. 2.1). Depending on the criteria used for setting the average requirement, the safety margin between the average requirement and recommended intake can vary [2]. In general, aging does not change the DRVs except for energy, protein, and vitamin D. However, it should be noted that low energy intake is recognized as a risk factor for macro- and micronutrient deficiency [2].

2.2.1 Energy Requirement and Recommended Intake

Daily energy expenditure tends to decline with age in the absence of disease mainly due to decreased fat-free mass (FFM) and decreased physical activity levels [2]. There are two main approaches able to be applied by interdisciplinary healthcare

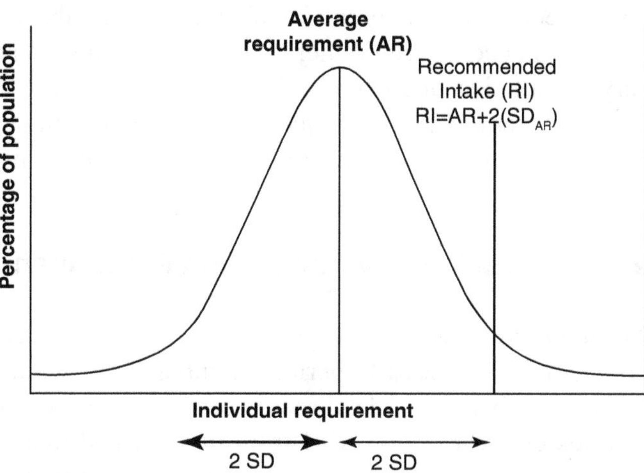

Fig. 2.1 Frequency distribution of an individual nutrient requirement. *SD* standard deviation. (With permission from [2]. https://www.norden.org/en/publication/nordic-nutrition-recommendations-2012)

providers in the clinical setting to estimate energy requirements. The factorial method calculates total energy expenditure from the resting (or basal) energy expenditure multiplied by a factor indicating physical activity level (PAL) [6]. An alternate method is the ratio method, which is an even more pragmatic approach whereby the subject's weight is multiplied by a specified caloric or kilojoule amount [6]. In the latter approach, the use of an adjusted body weight might be considered for older people who are obese. For older people with, e.g., a low body mass index, where weight gain might be relevant, the energy cost of weight gain may also be included. In these cases, one should be aware of the risk of refeeding (Chap. 3). While the factorial and ratio methods are broadly applied international in clinical settings, which method should be applied and what values to use are perhaps equally related to local practices and evidence-based values [2, 7–9]. Because estimates of requirements vary across different populations and clinical guidelines [1, 8, 9], we would recommend looking to country- or disease-specific recommendations. A useful good starting point is the E.S.P.E.N. guidelines for geriatrics which can be found here: https://www.espen.org/guidelines-home/espen-guidelines.

In this guideline about 30 kcal/kg BW is suggested as a rough estimate and general orientation for energy requirements in older persons. This guiding value needs individual adjustment regarding all relevant factors, i.e., gender, nutritional status, physical activity, and clinical condition. In addition, the aim of nutritional support (e.g., weight maintenance or increase) and acceptance and tolerance of the nutritional intervention need to be considered [1]. Because of great heterogeneity and large individual variation of energy requirements, even in healthy older persons, adequacy of energy intake needs to be controlled by close monitoring of body weight (taking water retention or losses into account), and intake adapted accordingly. "Injury factors" are applied in various settings for either the factorial method or the ratio method. These are generally not strongly evidenced, although consensus documents exist to support consideration of the increased requirements of acute or chronic disease [10]. Again, it should be noted that these are only a starting point and should include ranges rather than exact figures. Close monitoring should be prioritized above reliance on initial estimates, particularly in individuals considered likely to have particularly high requirements. It should be kept in mind that spontaneous oral energy intake of acutely hospitalized older patients is usually low and does not cover requirements [1]. Where accurate individual measures are necessary, alternative approaches, for example, indirect calorimetry or even doubly labeled water (DLW) technique in which stable isotopes (2H and 18O) are administered orally, could be considered, although these are primarily used for research.

2.2.2 Protein Requirement and Recommended Intake

Multimorbidity and chronic diseases are more frequent in older adults, and such conditions might lead to periodic temporary losses of body protein through catabolic exacerbations of the disease, temporary periods of bed rest, or loss of appetite. The losses must be replaced from the diet and thus represent an added need for dietary protein compared to the traditional recommendation defined as the lowest intake of protein to maintain nitrogen balance. In some cases positive nitrogen balance may not be achieved regardless of the amount of protein provided [2]. In addition, older individuals exhibit a gradual loss of muscle mass and strength with age (sarcopenia, Chap. 8). Sarcopenia may also occur in a variety of other nonnutritive factors, for example, in a sedated intensive care patients with induced paralysis, who will also lose muscle despite adequate protein and energy intakes [2].

A suggested minimum protein intake for many older adults across settings is 1.0–1.2 g protein/kg body weight (BW)/day. However, a systematic review suggested that a safe intake of up to at least 1.2–1.5 g protein/kg BW/day or approximately 15–20 E% represents an optimal intake level for older adults [2]. With decreasing energy intake (below 8 MJ/d), the protein E% should be increased accordingly [1, 2]. These recommendations are intended for the general population and not for groups or individuals with diseases or other conditions that affect their nutrient requirements. They are meant to be used for prevention purposes and are not specifically meant for treatment of diseases or significant weight reduction. Recommendations generally cover temporarily increased requirements, for example, during short-term mild infections or certain medical treatments. The recommended amounts are usually not suited for long-term infections, malabsorption, or various metabolic disturbances or for the treatment of persons with a nonoptimal nutritional status [1, 2].

In case of illness, protein requirements may even be further increased, e.g., due to inflammation, infections, and wounds. Very little is known about the protein needs of frail and multimorbid older persons, and scientific evidence, e.g., from intervention trials, is presently insufficient to derive concrete figures. Consequently, until more evidence is available, an intake of at least 1.0 g/kg BW/day should be ensured in all older persons, particularly in those at risk of malnutrition, e.g., frail and multimorbid persons, whose intake is often far below this amount [1]. Increased requirements, e.g., for muscle growth with strength training, for tissue regeneration in malnutrition or wound healing, or for increased metabolic demands in case of critical illness, should be met by appropriately increased intake [1]. Daily amounts of 1.2–1.5 g/kg BW/day have been suggested for older persons with acute or chronic illness and up to 2.0 g/kg BW/day in case of severe illness, injury, or malnutrition [1]. It is important to bear in mind that an insufficient intake of energy increases protein requirement. Thus, regarding protein status it is important to ensure not only adequate intake of protein but also appropriate intake of energy [1].

It is also worth noting that protein status is hard to estimate in daily clinical practice or community settings. Nitrogen balance remains the method of choice for determining the protein requirement in adults in the absence of validated or accepted alternatives and in the absence of a reliable biological marker of protein status [2]. However, N-balance is primarily measured for research purpose. Serum biomarkers as serum albumin and serum prealbumin or other biomarkers have not been shown to be valid method to estimate protein status [1].

2.2.3 Micronutrients and Dietary Fibers

With low energy intakes, it is difficult to meet the needs for all nutrients. In such cases supplementation with a multivitamin/mineral tablet and, where fiber intake appears inadequate or symptoms are suggestive of inadequacy, dietary fiber should be considered. For groups with a very low energy intake (<6.5 MJ or 1550 kcal), supplementation with a multivitamin/mineral tablet is recommended [1, 2].

Micronutrient recommendations vary according to populations, comorbidities, and national recommendations and clinical guidelines [5]. We recommend referral to national recommendations in the absence of disease (see some suggestions for further reading at the end of the chapter). Where multiple comorbidities exist and there is expected deficiency or deficiencies, a dietitian or medical nutrition specialist referral should be considered.

While a broad array of micronutrient deficiencies will be encountered by clinicians working with older adults, one that is most likely to be routinely identified is vitamin D. Vitamin D requirement is higher in older adults than in younger people. Apart from low dietary intake and limited time spent outdoors, the reason is that the amount of 7-dehydrocholesterol in the skin epidermis diminishes with age and the efficiency of conversion of this precursor into vitamin D is less effective than in younger individuals [2]. There is also some evidence that the PTH concentration tends to be higher among the older adults compared to younger adults at similar serum 25OHD concentrations.[1] This might indicate less efficient bioconversion due to diminished kidney function resulting in secondary hyperparathyroidism [2]. Further, the more rapid bone loss and higher fracture rate in older women than in men is related to diminished estrogen production in postmenopausal women [2]. More details about vitamin D recommendations, bone health, and osteoporosis can be found in Chap. 9.

[1] The circulating serum 25OHD concentration is regarded as a good marker of vitamin D status (2).

2.3 Nutritional Risk Factors in Older Adults

As shown in Fig. 2.2, multiple factors have been correlated with malnutrition in older adults. Nutritional risk factors include reduced appetite, female sex, social resources, poor physical function, poor self-related health, sensory function, chewing and swallowing problems, physical and cognitive impairment, and many other factors affecting the social, mental, and physical health of the old adult [11]. Chewing and swallowing problems due to dysphagia will be discussed in detail in Chap. 18.

Less emphasis has focused on nutritional risk factors that could be considered potentially modifiable. This was therefore the focus in a recent systematic review performed as part of the MaNuEL program [12]. Prospective cohort studies with

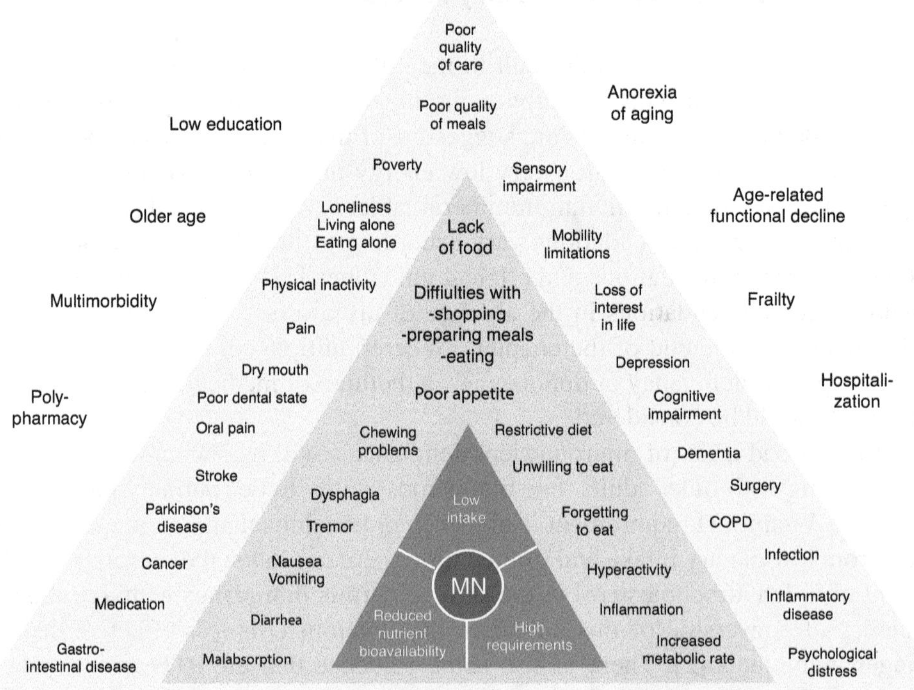

Fig. 2.2 DoMAP model. All factors—independent of the level—are regarded as (potential) "determinants" of MN meaning that they may contribute to the development of MN in a causative manner. The levels illustrate different modes of action: Level I (dark green): Central etiologic mechanisms; Level 2 (light green): Factors in this level directly lead to one of the three mechanisms in Level I (e.g., swallowing problems may directly cause low intake): Level 3 (yellow): Factors in this level may indirectly lead to one (or more) of the three central mechanisms through one (or more) of the direct factors in the light green triangle (e.g., stroke may cause low intake via dysphagia or difficulties with eating); surrounding factors in red are age-related changes and general aspects which also contribute to the development of MN, but act even more indirectly or subtle. *DoMAP* Determinants of Malnutrition in Aged Persons, *MN* malnutrition

participants of a mean age of 65 years or over in all settings were included. Malnutrition was defined as, e.g., low BMI or weight loss or as assessed by a screening tool [11]. The results are summarized in Table 2.1.

One, if not the most important, determinant of dietary intake in older persons is appetite which declines with age, referred to as anorexia of aging. The reported prevalence of anorexia of aging ranges from up to 25% in home dwellers to 62% in hospital populations and 85% in nursing home populations [13]. The consequences of anorexia of aging include the development of subsequent malnutrition, immunosuppression, sarcopenia, and frailty, which can reciprocally worsen appetite further [14]. This ultimately leads to adverse outcomes with higher rates of morbidity and mortality. The causes of anorexia of aging include changes in peripheral hormone signaling, gut motility, and sensory perception due to aging as well as social and environmental factors [13]. Regrettably, until now a uniform, unambiguous definition of anorexia of aging is lacking [15]. Screening tools for appetite assessment exist, for example, AHSPQ (Appetite, Hunger and Sensory Perception Questionnaire) or SNAQ (Simplified Nutritional Appetite Questionnaire); they are however not well established [15]. Further, in a recent systematic review, the authors concluded that there was a lack of clarity about whether anorexia of aging or malnutrition was the intervention target and that there was a need for standardized assessment so that effectiveness of a range of interventions could be fully explored [13].

Older adults have an increased risk at an insufficient protein intake because preferential consumption of protein-rich foods may decrease with aging [16]. Knowledge about the prevalence of low protein intake across different settings is limited. However, a meta-analysis applying data from four cohorts and four national surveys showed that the overall pooled prevalence of protein intake below recommended was up to 70% [16].

Table 2.1 Potentially modifiable nutritional risk factors for malnutrition in older adults (based on results from O'Keeffe et al. 2019 [11])

Risk factors	Determinants of malnutrition	Level of evidence
Hospitalization, eating dependency, poor self-perceived health, poor physical function, and poor appetite	Yes	Moderate
Loss of interest in life, access to meals and wheels, and modified texture diets	Yes	Low
Chewing difficulties, mouth pain, gum issues comorbidity, visual and hearing impairments, smoking status, alcohol consumption and physical activity levels, complaints about taste of food and specific nutrient intake	No	Moderate
Psychological distress, anxiety, loneliness, access to transport and well-being, hunger, and thirst	No	Low
Dental status, swallowing, cognitive function, depression, residential status, medication intake and/or polypharmacy, constipation, periodontal disease	Conflicting results	–

2.4 Estimating Intake in Older Adults

Assessment of dietary intake of older people requires particular care (Table 2.2). Diminished functions, disabilities, and health disorders may impair the ability to recall or record dietary intake correctly. In large epidemiological studies with older persons, generally the same dietary assessment methods as for younger age groups are applied—mainly food frequency questionnaires, diet histories, and multiple 24-h recalls—which all have their strengths and limitations regardless of age. It seems like these usual methods for dietary assessment are valid for older persons if they are physically and mentally healthy [15]. In clinical settings, food and hydration recording are most used method and can give good insight of food intake if healthcare providers, and if possible patient or family/friends, are involved in the process of food recording [15]. With increasing impairments, frailty, and disabilities, more time and effort should be invested in assessment of dietary intake needs among old adults.

These age-related issues are especially prevalent among old adults in short- or long-term institutional care, for example, hospitals and residential aged care homes. In these settings, direct observation, and direct measurement of dietary intake, is possible and should be used instead of or to assist self-reporting methods. Assistance from caregivers may be available, and information on food preparation, recipes, and usual portion sizes can be obtained from the kitchen personnel [15]. The gold standard in this setting is to weigh all meal components on the plate before and after meals, which may be a challenging task when snacks, in-between meals, and beverages also must be included. This method is extremely time-consuming and laborious and is generally reserved for research restricted to small patient groups [15]. Estimation methods are much more suitable regarding time and effort, and in clinical practice in geriatric institutions, plate diagrams with estimation of intake in quarters of the offered meal are widely used (Fig. 2.3) [15, 17, 18].

Table 2.2 Age-related characteristics that may impede accurate dietary assessment (based on Volkert and Schrader 2013 [14])

- Reduced capacity to deal with stress
- Physical limitations
  - Visual impairment
  - Hearing problems
  - Difficulties writing
- Mental impairment
  - Reduced short-term memory
  - Cognitive decline, dementia
  - Reduced communication skills: Limited attention, divagation
- Persons may not or only little be involved in food preparation

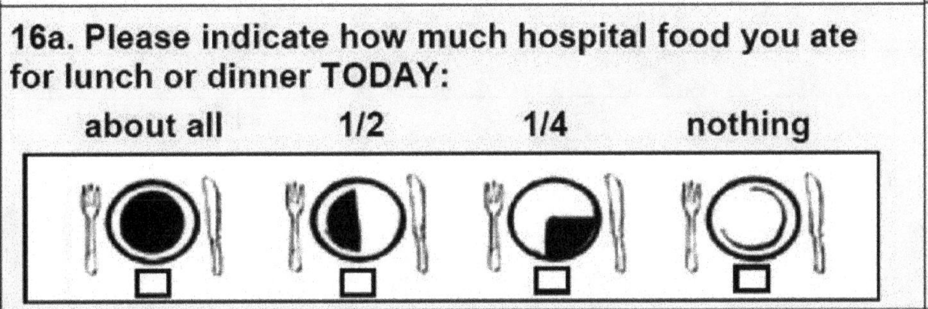

Fig. 2.3 Example of a simple estimation method to assess dietary intake, which can be used by the patients (from the Nutrition Day survey in hospitals [18] [https://www.nutritionday.org/])

2.5 Nutritional Status of Older Adults, Geriatric and Orthogeriatric Patients

Malnutrition, according to WHO definition, includes undernutrition (wasting, stunting, underweight), inadequate vitamins or minerals, overweight, obesity, and resulting diet-related noncommunicable diseases [19]. Overweight and obesity in old adults is described in Chap. 15. Malnutrition can be defined as "a state resulting from lack of intake or uptake of nutrition that leads to altered body composition (decreased fat free mass) and body cell mass leading to diminished physical and mental function and impaired clinical outcome from disease" [20]. Malnutrition can result from starvation, disease, or advanced aging (e.g., >80 years), alone or in combination [20]. Although there is no gold standard diagnosis for malnutrition, global consensus around core diagnostic criteria for malnutrition in adults in clinical settings is emerging [19]. With two-step approach for the malnutrition diagnosis, i.e., first screening to identify "at-risk" status using any validated screening tool and, second, assessment for diagnosis and grading the severity of malnutrition [21]. Other sections of this book detail nutritional assessment, nutritional diagnosis, and treatment (Chap. 3); malnutritional prevention (Chap. 4); nutritional support (Chap. 5); the overlap between co-diagnoses of malnutrition, sarcopenia, cachexia, and frailty (Chap. 8); and why systematized, interdisciplinary nutritional care is key to high-value, patient-centered outcomes (Chaps. 1 and 13).

As can be seen from Fig. 2.4, reported malnutrition prevalence rates vary considerably between and even within the settings. This might be explained by differences in age, morbidity, and functional status of included participants in the studies. Still, the results confirm that malnutrition prevalence markedly increases from community dwellers to geriatric and orthogeriatric patients and even further to residents in

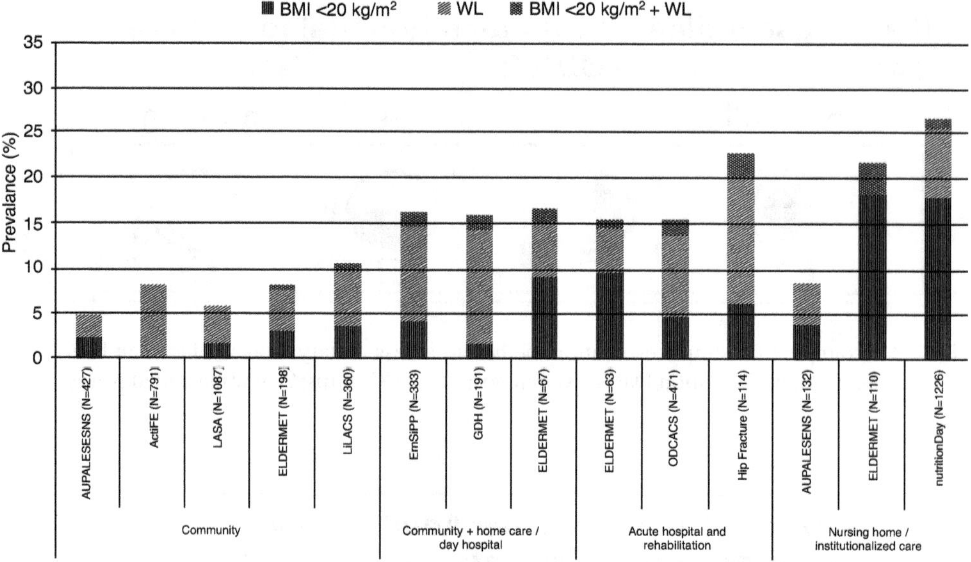

Fig. 2.4 Prevalences of malnutrition criteria based on low BMI, weight loss (WL) or both in older adults in different study samples by setting. (With permission from: Wolters M, Volkert D, Streicher M, Kiesswetter E, Torbahn G, O'Connor EM, et al. Prevalence of malnutrition using harmonized definitions in older adults from different settings – A MaNuEL Study. Clin Nutr. 2019;38(5):2389–98 [22])

nursing homes [22]. These findings are supported by the findings of reduced intake of energy during disease, due to among a high prevalence of nutritional risk factors. The complexity of malnutrition and nutritional risk factors in multimorbid old adults highlight the importance of interdisciplinary and multimodal interventions as also recommended by the E.S.P.E.N. guideline for geriatric patients [1]. These findings also highlight the need to proactively prioritize screening and interventional processes in the community settings (Chaps. 4 and 13).

2.6 Summary

Deterioration of nutritional status in older adults is commonly observed and is associated with impairment of recovery and rehabilitation. In older adults this can occur rapidly during acute illness or insidiously across time in response to diverse age or chronic disease-related factors. Insufficient energy and protein intake is a common cause of poor nutritional status in old age and specially during hospitalization. Older persons are generally at risk of malnutrition due to anorexia of aging but also several nutritional risk factors of which several might be modifiable. We conclude that malnutrition in older adults is a complex condition; interdisciplinary teamwork is needed to support and sustain a healthy nutritional status throughout the aging years.

Take-Home Points

- Impaired nutritional status is frequent among geriatric and orthogeriatric patients.
- Insufficient intake of energy, protein, and vitamin D is a significant problem among older adults, geriatric and orthogeriatric patients.
- Potentially modifiable nutritional risk factors should be taken into consideration when planning nutritional interventions.
- Ongoing monitoring should confirm whether the estimates of requirements (and intake) maintain or improve nutritional status over time.

References

1. Volkert D et al (2019) ESPEN guideline on clinical nutrition and hydration in geriatrics. Clin Nutr 38(1):10–47
2. Ministers, NCo (2014) Nordic Nutrition. Recommendations 2012. Integrating nutrition and physical activity
3. Brownie S, Muggleston H, Oliver C (2015) The 2013 Australian dietary guidelines and recommendations for older Australians. Aust Fam Physician 44(5):311–315
4. Age Scotland. Eat Well Age Well Project. (2020) Eat Well: A Guide for Older People in Scotland. https://www.eatwellagewell.org.uk/images/EatWellGuide2020.pdf
5. Shlisky J et al (2017) Nutritional considerations for healthy aging and reduction in age-related chronic disease. Adv Nutr 8(1):17–26
6. Gomes F et al (2018) ESPEN guidelines on nutritional support for polymorbid internal medicine patients. Clin Nutr 37(1):336–353
7. EFSA Panel on Dietetic Products, NaAENP (2016) Scientific opinion on dietary reference values for vitamin D. EFSA NDA Panel. EFSA J:145
8. Queensland Goverment. Estimating energy, protein & fluid requirementsfor adult clinical conditions. (2015) Consensus document from Dietitian/Nutritioists from the Nutrition Education Matreal Online "NEMO". Revised May 2015. https://www.scribd.com/document/295124816/Estimating-Energy-Protein-and-Fluid-Requirements-for-Adult-Clinical-Conditions
9. EatRight Academy of Nutrition and Dietetics. What are the caloric needs of healthy older adults (over age 65)? (2009) Adapted by the Academy of Nutrition and Dietetics from the American Academy of Pediatrics, Classifying Recommendations for Clinical Practice Guidelines, Pediatrics. 2004;114;874–877s. UWL:Energy needs 2009. https://www.andeal.org/recommendation-ratings
10. Dietitian/Nutritionists from the Nutrition Education Materials Online, N., team, Estimating energy, protein & fluid requirements for adult clinical conditions, p.f.r.f.a.c.c. Estimating energy, Editor. Queensland Government: Queensland Government.
11. O'Keeffe M et al (2019) Potentially modifiable determinants of malnutrition in older adults: a systematic review. Clin Nutr 38(6):2477–2498
12. Volkert D et al (2019) Development of a model on determinants of malnutrition in aged persons: a MaNuEL project. Gerontol Geriatr Med 5:2333721419858438
13. Cox NJ et al (2019) Assessment and treatment of the anorexia of aging: a systematic review. Nutrients 11(1):144
14. Chang M et al (2020) A poor appetite or ability to eat and its association with physical function amongst community-dwelling older adults: age, gene/environment susceptibility-Reykjavik study. Eur J Ageing
15. Volkert D, Schrader E (2013) Dietary assessment methods for older persons: what is the best approach? Curr Opin Clin Nutr Metab Care 16(5):534–540

16. Hengeveld LM et al (2020) Prevalence of protein intake below recommended in community-dwelling older adults: a meta-analysis across cohorts from the PROMISS consortium. J Cachexia Sarcopenia Muscle 11(5):1212–1222
17. Bjornsdottir R et al (2013) Validation of a plate diagram sheet for estimation of energy and protein intake in hospitalized patients. Clin Nutr 32(5):746–751
18. Worldwide N (2021) NutritionDay worldwide—benchmark & monitor your nutrition care. [cited 2021, 31]. https://www.nutritionday.org/
19. Organization WH (2020) Malnutrition-key facts, i. comprehensive implementation plan on maternal, and young child nutrition, adopted by member states through a world health assembly resolution in 2012. WHO, Geneva. https://www.who.int/news-room/fact-sheets/detail/malnutrition
20. Cederholm T et al (2017) ESPEN guidelines on definitions and terminology of clinical nutrition. Clin Nutr 36(1):49–64
21. Cederholm T et al (2019) GLIM criteria for the diagnosis of malnutrition—a consensus report from the global clinical nutrition community. J Cachexia Sarcopenia Muscle 10(1):207–217
22. Wolters M et al (2019) Prevalence of malnutrition using harmonized definitions in older adults from different settings—a MaNuEL study. Clin Nutr 38(5):2389–2398

3

Nutrition Care Process: Terminology and Best Practice Approaches

Mette Holst and Anne Marie Beck

Abstract

The purpose of this chapter is to share knowledge about terminology and best practice approaches for the nutrition care process, including nutritional screening, assessment, diagnosis, intervention, and monitoring. This will focus on nutrition care for older adults with or at risk of malnutrition, in their own home, hospital, or caring facilities.

Keywords

Screening · Malnutrition · Nutritional assessment · Nutritional status · Nutritional requirements · Nutritional therapy · Nutritional support

---

This chapter is a component of Section 1: Nutritional Care in Old Age.
For an explanation of the grouping of chapters in this book, please see Chap. 1: "Geriatrics and Orthogeriatrics: Providing Nutrition Care."

M. Holst (✉)
Centre for Nutrition and Intestinal Failure, Aalborg University Hospital and Department of Clinical Medicine, Aalborg University, Aalborg, Denmark
e-mail: mette.holst@rn.dk

A. M. Beck
University College Copenhagen, Copenhagen, Denmark

Dietetic and Nutritional Research Unit, Herlev-Gentofte University Hospital, Herlev, Denmark
e-mail: ambe@kp.dk

Learning Objectives

By the end of this chapter, you will be able to:

- Explain the nutrition care process for older adults.
- Explain incentives for nutritional screening and the key principles of successful screening.
- Describe the key elements of nutritional assessment and diagnosis.
- Describe how an intervention plan is made based on nutritional assessment, nutritional requirements, and nutrition impact factors.
- Describe the basic concepts of monitoring the efficacy of nutritional intervention.
- Describe the ethical aspects of when to introduce nutritional therapy and when to end.

Karen is 92 years old. For the past 5 years, she has lived in a residential aged care home. When she moved into her new home, she really came alive. There were people around her and staff to talk to. In addition to a little help in structuring daily life, remembering medicine, and small physical care tasks, Karen has largely managed on her own. In particular, she has enjoyed eating in the living room with the others for all meals. But for the past 3 weeks, Karen has been having problems with urinary tract infections. The antibiotics have given her stomach problems and she no longer like to get out of her own living room.

After 3 weeks, Karen's nurse Mary comes to visit to check up on the urinary tract infection. Karen is in bed, and it dawns on Mary that Karen has lost a lot of weight. On closer inspection, it becomes clear that Karen can barely stand on her feet. Although Karen is usually a little overweight (height 152 cm, weight 69 kg, BMI 30 kg/m^2), she has lost 4.5 kilos, including an obvious lot of muscle mass, which is seen on her arms, legs, and thorax. Asked how she eats, Karen says she has not felt like eating. She has nausea, the food does not taste like usual – in fact it tastes ugly – and she is also afraid of needing to go to the toilet when she has eaten. She no longer feels safe walking to the toilet on her own and is afraid that help will not make it in time. Upon closer inspection, Karen still has a fever, and she has fungus in her mouth.

In a kind and caring way, Mary advises Karen that the nutritional screening tool results show that Karen is at risk of malnutrition and might already be malnourished. In an easy-to-understand, simple way, Karen and Mary then discuss the implications of ongoing poor intake and consider whether it is time for food for comfort, food as a medicine, or a bit of both. Karen was very keen to improve her intake to prevent further nutrition deterioration to support her to get back to her usual function and lifestyle and was keen to regain her lost weight over the next 3 months. Together, they initiate a nutrition plan including cold soft meals and two oral nutritional supplements daily to start with. Mary then arranges for a dietitian to conduct a thorough assessment of Karen's nutritional status and to help with goal setting and a more specific nutrition care plan. A doctor is also called in to review antibiotics and look at Karen's mouth, and a physiotherapist is called in to make a physical rehabilitation plan for Karen. Last, but not least, the nurse makes an appointment with Karen and Karen's relatives. Together they agree that more help is needed in everyday life at the moment, more focus on small nutritious meals and a record of what Karen eats and drinks, increasing her regular weights to fortnightly, as well as a plan for mobilization. The nurse communicates the plan to the care team and documents appointments in Karen's care record, so that everyone can follow it and continuously document and revise over time.

3.1 The Nutrition Care Process

The nutrition care process (NCP) is a systematic sequence of distinct, but interrelated, steps to support to nutrition care for older adults like Karen [1, 2]. The NCP supports health professionals to detect the risk of protein-energy malnutrition, hereafter malnutrition, so that those who will benefit from nutrition care will be given the most appropriate individual nutritional therapy in due time. Malnutrition is a clinical disorder recognized under the International Classification of Diseases (ICD11) that encompasses starvation-related malnutrition and acute or chronic disease-related undernutrition [2–4]. Sarcopenia and frailty are nutrition-related conditions commonly associated with malnutrition and the geriatric syndrome [2, 5] (Fig. 3.1). The NCP aims to embrace all these areas of malnutrition.

How the NCP "looks" across settings and populations is in principle the same, but the work tools may be designed differently; Fig. 3.2 depicts the nutrition care process as presented by the Academy of Nutrition and Dietetics [1, 6, 7]. We draw your attention to the outer circles of the NCP model. While not the focus of this chapter, these constructs will be addressed by ensuing chapters to ensure the systems, resources, and infrastructure are in place to support the right nutrition care processes, delivered to the right older person, at the right time, and in the right place.

The NCP is traditionally applied by dietitians and medical and nursing nutrition specialists worldwide to deliver or coordinate malnutrition care, by applying a common framework for nutrition care, focused nutrition care documentation, and application of evidence-based guidelines. Nutrition care models for patients with or at risk of malnutrition are also available which support directing nutrition care to low, moderate, or high nutritional risk. Such approaches support timely and efficient malnutrition care processes to moderate-risk patients where specialist nutrition care is unlikely to be available or add value beyond the care able to be provided by nurses, other interdisciplinary healthcare providers, volunteers, family, and friend. This approach also not only engages diverse healthcare providers in nutrition care processes but also directs nutrition specialist resources to where there are most needed [8–11] (Chaps. 1 and 13).

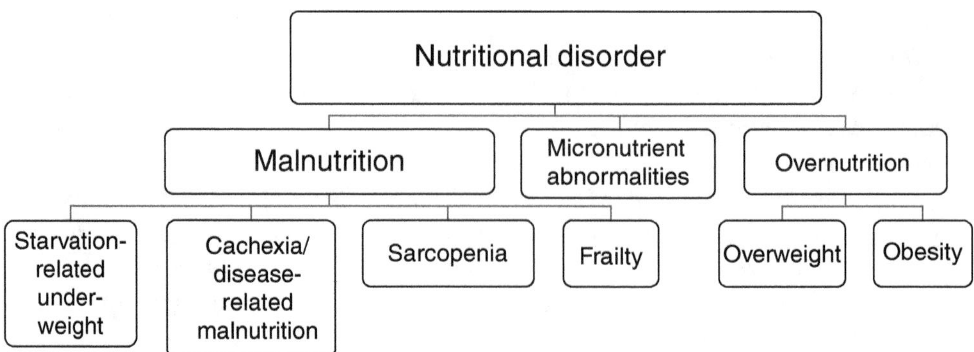

Fig. 3.1 The conceptual tree of nutritional disorders [1, 2]. (Reprinted from Clin Nutr, 34(3), T Cederholm, I Bosaeus, R Barazzoni, et al. A conceptual tree of nutritional disorders., p. 335–341., with permission from Elsevier)

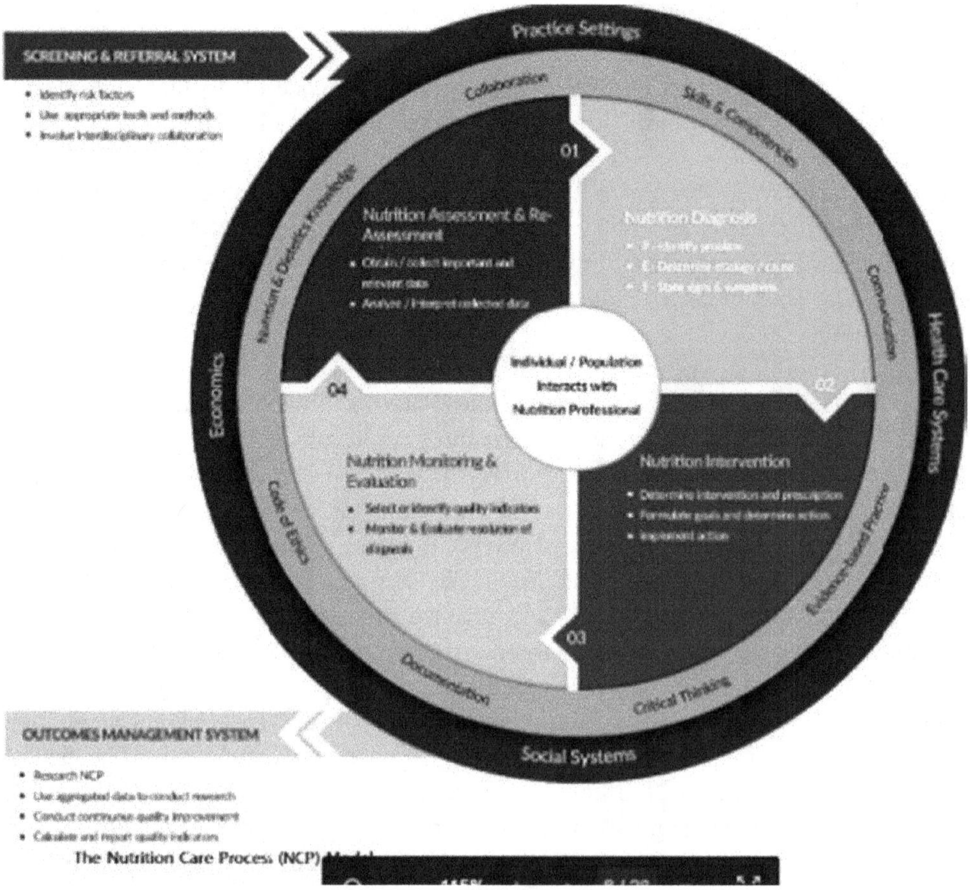

Fig. 3.2 Nutrition care process and model [1, 7]. (Reprint from Journal of the Academy of Nutrition and Dietetics, 117(12) William I. Swan,Angela Vivanti, Nancy A. Hakel-Smith, Brenda Hotson, Ylva Orrevall, Naomi Trostler, Kay Beck Howarter, Constantina Papoutsakis. Nutrition Care Process and Model Update: Toward Realizing People-Centered Care and Outcomes Management p. 2003–2014. with permission from Elsevier)

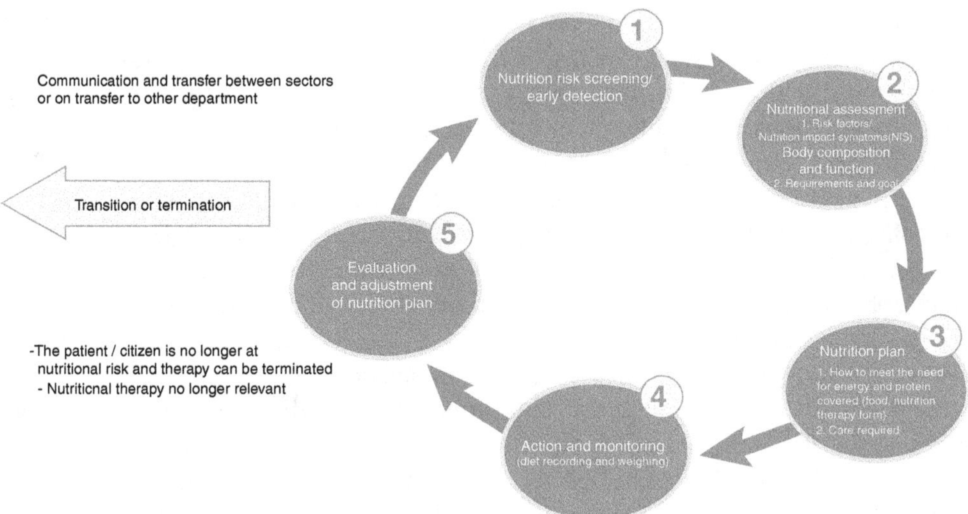

Fig. 3.3 The Multiprofessional Nutrition Care Process model. (Model by author Mette Holst)

Our case study above highlights the importance of nonspecialized nutrition care actions that can be performed by diverse healthcare providers and carers, wherever older adults are cared for in practice. Therefore, a multiprofessional approach which is based on the NCP, but to a greater extent clarifies the elements of the NCP model into action elements, is presented in the Multiprofessional Nutrition Care Process model (Fig. 3.3). The remainder of this chapter is based on the Multiprofessional Nutrition Care Process model, to highlight opportunities for nurses and the multiprofessional teams working with and around nurses to deliver nutrition care processes to older adults with or at risk of malnutrition.

3.2 Nutritional Screening/Risk Detection

Systematic nutritional risk detection, or malnutrition risk screening, has multiple aims, including identifying nutritional status, the need for nutritional intervention, and those who are at risk of negative outcomes such as infections, prolonged healing, or death, due to their nutritional status [12–15]. For our case study, a screening tool was applied that detected nutritional risk, informed the need for nutritional intervention, and also alerted the nurse and older adult to the relationship between poor nutrition intake and outcomes.

Malnutrition risk screening should be performed in all subjects interfacing with healthcare services, whether in hospital, community, or aged care home settings. Depending on the care setting, screening should be performed within the first 24 to 48 h after first contact and thereafter at regular intervals. The screening process allows healthcare providers to target prevention and treatment of undernutrition to relevant individuals in a timely manner. One of the most important things we can do to prevent the negative consequences of malnutrition is to commence nutritional therapy as early as possible, because we know that the greater the weight loss, the greater the risk of negative outcomes; and in older, multimorbid adults, regaining lost muscle is at best difficult and in many cases unachievable.

ESPEN (the European Society for Clinical Nutrition and Metabolism) and ASPEN (American Society for Parenteral and Enteral Nutrition) recommend using validated screening tools [5, 16–18]. Malnutrition screening tools mostly combine weight loss, reduced food intake, and disease activity. When targeting community-dwelling older adults, physical and functional status, nutrition intake, and chronic conditions may be prioritized in addition to current nutritional status, whereas in the hospitalized patient, acute disease should also be considered in combination with the above. The various screening tools are validated in different settings and weigh the different parameters differently [19]. Unintentional weight loss is routinely included as a measure in screening tools regardless of setting and is used by itself also in primary early detection of malnutrition. Unplanned weight loss is the most readily available and best validated parameter for early detection of nutritional risk. When looking for weight loss in a course of treatment, it is important to look not only at the latest weight but at the entire course of treatment. If older adults, or those caring for them, are unable to answer if they have lost weight within a specified time period, many tools ascribe an "at risk" score, in order not to miss the opportunity for nutritional intervention in a person who might benefit [20]. In nursing homes and in frail community-dwelling older adults, monthly weighing is consequently recommended.

Although our case study was a clear-cut positive screen, no nutritional screening tool is perfect. For example, a patient with cardiac cachexia may not have lost weight due to fluid overload, or may still report a reasonable appetite, and still be at risk of malnutrition. Screening healthcare providers must apply critical thinking and clinical judgment. Treating teams may also choose to consider groups of older adults with specific conditions or treatment requirements "at risk," for example, those admitted to intensive care or acute hip fracture units.

The result of the nutritional screen should trigger predefined actions. For those not at nutritional risk, standard nutrition care processes, for example, a general diet hospital, feeding assistance where required, and adequate time to eat, should be offered. Regardless of setting, older adults initially screened "not at risk" should be rescreened at specified time points to detect any change in risk status. Subjects who are found to be at risk need to undergo nutritional assessment [13].

3.3 Nutritional Assessment and Diagnosis

3.3.1 Nutrition Impact Symptoms

A nutritional assessment will acquire sufficient information about nutrition impact symptoms (NIS), body composition and function, stress metabolism, psychological and psychosocial parameters, as well as nutritional requirements to inform nutritional diagnosis(es), goal setting, and care planning (Fig. 3.3).

Some assessment data is provided as person-centered outcome measures; biases such as recall, interpretation, and wanting to please should be taken into consideration. Nutritional assessment in many older adults is further complicated by multimorbidity, cases of acute illness and hospitalizations, and disabilities in combination with nutrition-related problems such as dysphagia, decreased appetite, fatigue, and muscle weakness. The crossover between malnutrition, physical dysfunction, sarcopenia, frailty, and cachexia in aging further contributes to diagnostic difficulties (Chap. 8).

The purpose of the NIS assessment is to detect, reduce, or remove barriers to eating and ensure that the nutrition plan can take into account physiological, psychosocial, and environmental changes related to eating (Table 3.1). Chapters 2 and 4 highlight additional determinants of malnutrition.

Further investigation and relevant treatment should be initiated in relation to modifiable NIS factors detected. Our case study highlights how nurse Mary identified reversible nutrition impact symptoms and, together with Karen and other healthcare team members, actioned interventions that aligned with shared goals. Our case also highlights the need for dieticians, nurses, medical professionals, and other healthcare providers to work together. The multiprofessional team contributes a broader perspective than nutrition alone and may help to identify changeable barriers to nutrition intake. A systematic approach to both the NCP and assessing NIS is recommended, in order to understand the greater picture of the individual nutrition intake disturbances; there are many determinants of malnutrition and different tools for NIS assessment (Chaps. 2 and 4). As an example, the Nutrition Impact Symptoms Score for symptoms impacting on food intake [21] is built on PG-SGA, which is one of the best validated NIS instruments for cancer patients [22].

Table 3.1 Commonly reported nutrition impact symptoms

Medical/physiological	*Psychosocial*
Altered tastes and smells	Carer burden
Anorexia of aging, lack of appetite, or early satiety	Social isolation
Cognitive impairment, delirium, or dementia	Food or financial insecurity
Depression	Poor emotional well-being
Dry mouth	Self-administered dietary restrictions and preferences
Dysphagia (swallowing difficulty)	*Environmental*
Fatigue	Older adult, clinician, and community beliefs, biases, and perceptions
Gastrointestinal upset, e.g., nausea, vomiting, diarrhea, constipation	Misinformation and misdirection and treatment biases
Lack of teeth or ill-fitting dentures	
Malabsorption or endocrine issues	
Medical comorbidities	
Mouth sores	
Pain	
Polypharmacy or medication side effects	
Prescribed dietary restrictions	

3.3.2 Nutritional Diagnosis

The Global Leadership Initiative on Malnutrition (GLIM) criteria is a recent global initiative and consensus initiative convened by several of the major global clinical nutrition societies and experts [16]. The purpose is to be able to make a "nutritional diagnosis" for malnutrition, which clarifies which factors contribute to nutritional risk (Table 3.2). This should make the intervention effort more action oriented.

The procedure is first an "early detection" of nutritional risk applying a validated screening tool as described above. This informs a thorough assessment which

Table 3.2 GLIM criteria: phenotypic and etiologic criteria for the diagnosis of malnutrition

Phenotypic criteria*			Etiologic criteria*	
Weight loss (%)	Low body mass index (kg/m^2)	Reduced muscle mass[a]	Reduced food intake or assimilation	Inflammation
>5% within the past 6 months or >10% beyond 6 months	<20 if <70 years or <22 if >70 years	Reduced by validated body composition measuring techniques[a]	≤50% of ER >1 week, or any reduction for >2 weeks, or any chronic GI condition that adversely impacts food assimilation or absorption	Acute disease/ injury or chronic disease-related
	Asia: <18.5 if <70 years or <20 if >70 years			

Thresholds for severity grading of malnutrition into stage 1 (moderate) and stage 2 (severe) malnutrition			
	Phenotypic criteria[a]		
	Weight loss (%)	Low body mass index (kg/m^2)[b]	Reduced muscle mass[c]
Stage 1/moderate malnutrition (requires one phenotypic criterion that meets this grade)	5–10% within the past 6 months or 10–20% beyond 6 months	<20 if <70 years, <22 if ≥70 years	Mild to moderate deficit (per validated assessment methods—see below)
Stage 2/severe malnutrition (requires one phenotypic criterion that meets this grade)	>10% within the past 6 months or >20% beyond 6 months	<18.5 if <70 years, <20 if ≥70 years	Severe deficit (per validated assessment methods—see below)

[a]Severity grading is based upon the noted phenotypic criteria, while the etiologic criteria described in the text and Fig. 3.4 are used to provide the context to guide intervention and anticipated outcomes

[b]Further research is needed to secure consensus reference BMI data for Asian populations in clinical settings

[c]For example, appendicular lean mass index (ALMI, kg/m^2) by dual-energy absorptiometry or corresponding standards using other body composition methods like bioelectrical impedance analysis (BIA), CT, or MRI. When not available or by regional preference, physical examination or standard anthropometric measures like mid-arm muscle or calf circumferences may be used. Functional assessments like handgrip strength may be used as a supportive measure [16, 23]

consists of the criteria: phenotypic (unplanned weight loss, BMI, or muscle mass) and etiologic, which considers reduced dietary intake and disease state (Table 3.2 and Fig. 3.4).

Of the phenotypic criteria, muscle mass is the most important indicator of survival or complications. During active disease, we know that weight loss mainly takes place in the muscle mass. The bottom line is that muscle mass is the fastest "food" for those who have not received enough energy and protein for combustion. In addition, muscle mass is an indicator of maintaining physical activity. Therefore, it is also primarily muscle mass we look at when we make a more thorough assessment of body composition. Sarcopenia is a syndrome that is defined predominantly by the simultaneous occurrence of lower skeletal muscle mass, strength, and function in older adults. Sarcopenia significantly impacts self-reported quality of life and physical activity level as well as function and is associated with inadequate protein intake and/or reduced physical activity [24].

Muscle mass is monitored in different ways. Commonly reported trusted methods for application in research include dual-energy X-ray absorptiometry (DXA), magnetic resonance index (MRI), and computerized tomography (CT). Access to these is limited in most clinical settings, costs can be prohibitive, and radiation exposure also needs consideration for the latter (Fig. 3.5).

Until ready access to trusted methods is available in the clinic, we have various tools to use.

Commonly applied measures of muscle mass in clinical settings globally are the calf circumference and upper arm circumference measures. These are of low cost, are easy to perform, and generally correlate with trusted methods. However, their precision is reduced in obese subjects [25]. Although broad uptake is yet to be realized, ultrasound has demonstrated potential for application as a measure of muscle

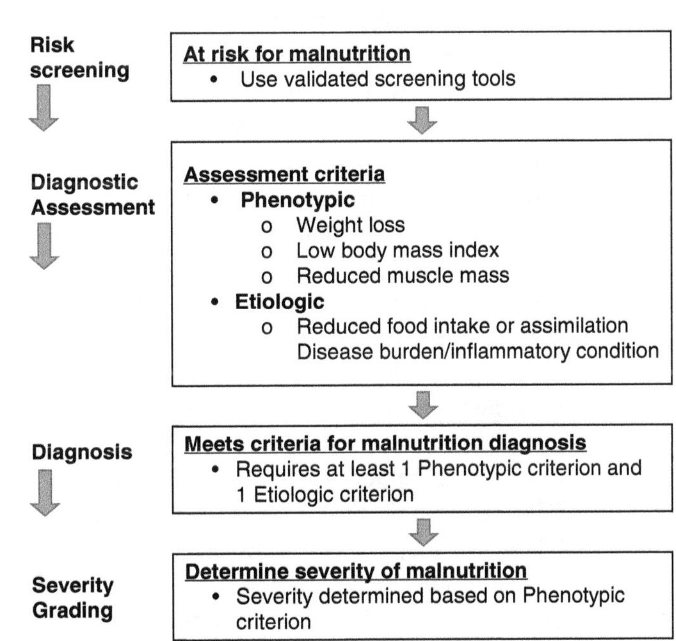

Fig. 3.4 GLIM criteria [16]. (Copyright © 2018 Elsevier Ltd., the European Society for Clinical Nutrition and Metabolism and American Society for Parenteral and Enteral Nutrition. All rights reserved. https://www.ncbi.nlm.nih.gov/pmc/articles/PMC6438340/figure/jcsm12383-fig-0001/)

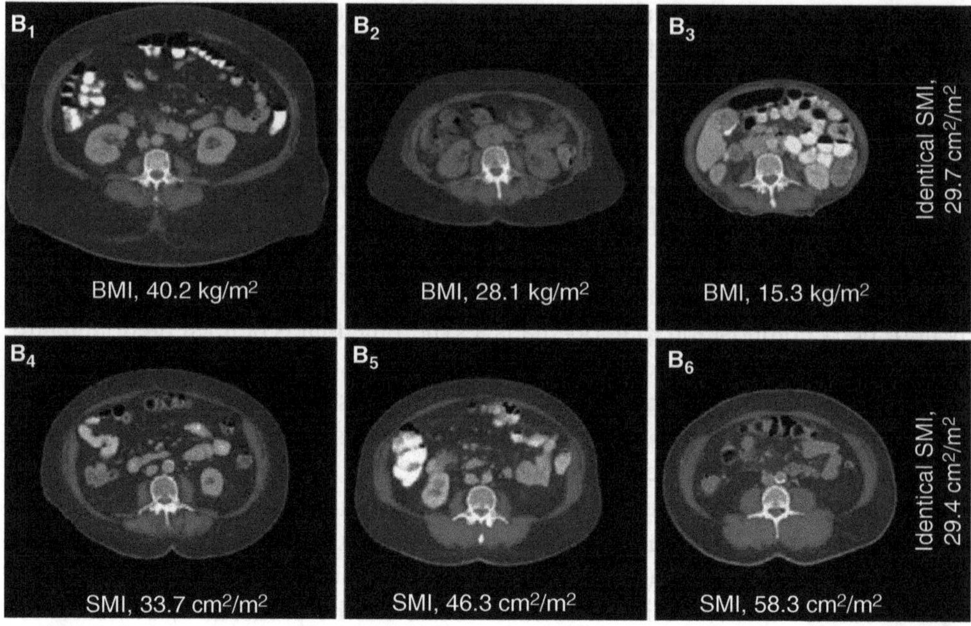

Fig. 3.5 Skeletal muscle mass and different BMI vs same body size with different skeletal muscle mass (Martin L. et al. [23]) B_1, B_2, and B_3 show the same skeletal muscle mass index (SMI) but different body mass index (BMI), that is, the same amount of muscle mass for different body size. B_4, B_5, and B_6, shown in Fig. 3.5 show the same BMI with different SMI, that is, the same body size with different amount of muscle mass (Martin L. et al. [22]). (With permission from Martin, L., et al., Cancer cachexia in the age of obesity: skeletal muscle depletion is a powerful prognostic factor, independent of body mass index. J Clin Oncol, 2013. 31(12): p. 1539–47. https://doi.org/10.1200/JCO.2012.45.2722)

mass. Bioimpedance (BIA) is relatively easily accessible and quick to read and translate into results. It is increasingly applied across a variety of patients and settings by trained healthcare providers. BIA measures the amount and ratio of fat, muscle tissue, and fluid. This is done by the device sending a weak current through the tissue and measuring the different resistances for each tissue type. A reliable bioimpedance measurement requires a little rigor in the method, for example, bladder emptying shortly prior to measurement and fasting and avoidance of moderate or intense physical activity. The latter, however, should probably be passable in many clinical settings. BIA is not appropriate for those with pacemakers and is unlikely to be accurate in those with fluid overload or electrolyte imbalance. As a doubly indirect method, BIA has limited precision and is poorly correlated with sarcopenia in at least some older adult populations [25, 26]. However, we would suggest that at present, BIA provides a valuable source of clinical setting muscle mass information, if the right validated device and methodological process is applied.

The GLIM criteria allow for functional assessments to be used as a supportive measure. There are many ways of measuring muscle strength and function, noting these have traditionally been applied to assess status before an intervention or the effect of an intervention. Handgrip strength, gait speed (4- or 6-min walk at a usual

Table 3.3 EWGSOP2 sarcopenia cut-off points for physical strength [27]

Test	Cut-off points for men	Cut-off points for women
EWGSOP2 sarcopenia cut-off points for low strength by chair stand and grip strength		
Grip strength	<27 kg	<16 kg
Chair stand	>15 s for five rises	
ASM	<20 kg	<15 kg
ASM/height^2	<7.0 kg/m^2	<5.5 kg/m^2
EWGSOP2 sarcopenia cut-off points for low performance		
Gait speed	≤0.8 m/s	
SPPB	≤8 point score	
TUG	≥20 s	
400-m walk test	Non-completion or ≥ 6 min for completion	

From: EWGSOP2. Sarcopenia: revised European consensus on definition and diagnosis [27]

pace, and measure the distance in meters), chair-stand test which measures time taken to rise five consecutive times from a chair as quickly as possible without arm rests, or 30-s chair-stand test, where the number of times raised in 30 s is counted, are among the single parameters measured and recommended (Table 3.3 EWGSOP2 [27]). Combined estimates including patient-reported outcomes are often used as well [28].

For our case study above, although Karen had a relatively high BMI, she had lost more than 5% of body weight. As such she meets the phenotypic criteria for malnutrition diagnosis, without the need for further scanning, clinical, or functional assessment. Regarding BMI, this case draws attention to the fact that both sarcopenia and malnutrition can occur in all weight classes, i.e., in older adults who are already thin but also in those who are in "healthy," overweight, or obese categories (Chaps. 8 and 16).

3.3.3 Etiologic Criteria

When we look at the etiologic criteria of GLIM, the question "Have you eaten less than you usually do in the past week" is well validated, included in many screening tools, and directly associated with unplanned weight loss. Many healthcare providers work with quartiles and thus do not go for a specific figure, but a rough estimate. Nurse Mary probably asked something like "Have you eaten as you usually do in the past week or less than usual?" And in response to Karen's answer, she would probably have questioned further to ask if she had eaten 50, 75, or maybe only 25% of usual. Further questions may consider if poor intake has continued for a longer time period. Where time allows and where appropriate, a detailed dietary history may be undertaken. Although this may take some time and level of skill to assess, a detailed history will provide a good impression of food and fluid intake adequacy and potentially reversible barriers and enablers to this (Fig. 3.4) [29].

For assessment of comorbid disease activity, it would be helpful to have a biomarker which could inform a malnutrition diagnosis or whether an older adult needs nutritional treatment or not. Unfortunately, despite its popular application in clinical and research settings, albumin levels are more likely to reflect overall disease rather than nutritional status or requirements. A systematic review assessed the role of albumin in otherwise healthy subjects who had a very small dietary intake, mainly due to anorexia nervosa. The study showed that serum albumin and prealbumin levels were maintained even at a marked weight loss, and they were only lowered during extreme hunger – that is, at a BMI below 11 [30, 31]. Many other blood markers have been tested, but none have been shown to be adequately sensitive to nutritional status to be used as stand-alone malnutrition markers [32, 33]. We would not recommend testing albumin or other blood markers for our case study, as these are likely to be influenced by the acute phase response due to her active infections. That is not to say that laboratory measures should not be considered; electrolytes; vitamin and mineral; endocrine, renal, and liver function tests; protein; and immune measures may be appropriate to be considered when undertaking a thorough nutritional assessment. For example, Karen has been indoors for some time, and a vitamin D test may be appropriate, if she is not receiving supplements (Chap. 9). As an older adult, if not already supplemented, B12 may also be worth considering in case she has poor absorption. Although our case is not at risk of refeeding syndrome, for the prevention and management of refeeding syndrome, it is recommended to initially test and monitor patients with blood tests at the start of nutritional treatment, especially if they have had a greater weight loss or a greatly reduced dietary intake for longer than a week [34].

3.3.4 Estimating Requirements

The next logical step in the nutrition care process is to estimate an individual's requirements for energy, protein, fluid, and other macro- and micronutrients. This is described in Chap. 2. However, in our case it was simply a ballpark clinical judgment call by nurse Mary that Karen's intake of protein and energy was greatly reduced for >2 weeks and clearly inadequate to meet her requirements.

3.3.5 Nutritional Diagnosis

The nurse must always make an individual assessment of the older adult's current situation, which will form the basis for the clinical decisions chosen in consultation with the patient. Best practice in nutritional nursing care can be found in Chap. 6.

A thorough nutritional assessment will inform a nutritional diagnosis; a well-crafted nutritional diagnosis will not only highlight a modifiable nutritional problem but also document underlying etiologies, signs, and symptoms [1, 7]. It is clear from above that Karen should have a documented diagnosis of malnutrition; and this should also be discussed with the older adult. While we have focused on malnutrition, it is important to note the diversity of nutritional diagnoses commonly observed in older adults across the continuum of care [6]. For our case, a key second diagnosis might be "inadequate protein, energy, and micronutrient intake, related to medication-related GIT upset, mouth ulcers, and fear of incontinence, evidenced by intake <50% of requirements and weight loss >5% over the past 3 weeks".

3.4 The Nutrition Plan and Care Required

The nutrition plan targets individualized nutritional therapy approaches most likely to meet the older adult's nutritional requirements and address the nutritional diagnosis(es) and shared treatment goals (Chaps. 1, 5, 10, 11, 13, and 21). For those with active nutrition care goals, the care required generally follows a three-step process as briefly outlined below and detailed in Chap. 5.

Step 1: Energy- and protein-dense food/fortified foods including snack meals and Oral Nutritional Supplements (ONS) [11].

Older persons with malnutrition or at risk of malnutrition should be offered energy- and protein-dense foods. Fortified food, additional snacks, and/or finger food may be used in order to facilitate dietary intake [5]. Many studies have shown that it is especially difficult to achieve an adequate protein intake without the use of nutritional supplements for people at nutritional risk [35]. Consequently, hospitalized older persons with malnutrition or at risk of malnutrition should also be offered ONS, in order to improve dietary intake and body weight and to lower the risk of complications and readmission [5].

Restrictive diet deprescription should be considered by treating teams for older adults with or at risk of malnutrition. Those at nutritional risk who would normally follow a special diet such as patients with heart disease, kidney disease, diabetes, and obesity often require a more energy- and protein-rich diet during illness. In the case of heart and kidney disease, the nutrition plan may require planning in consultation with a dietitian or, alternatively, may be deprescribed by the treating medical team where intake is likely to be inadequate. Similarly, an acutely unwell inpatient with diabetes may be better off receiving extra insulin and more frequent blood sugar monitoring rather than a sugar-free or low-fat diet that may lead to further nutritional status decline. Weight loss diets are not recommended during periods of illness and should only be resumed when the older adult is healthy or in a stable phase of the disease course, only if, after careful consideration, they remain appropriate [5] (Chap. 16). The need for careful across team communication is especially crucial where multimorbid patients are vulnerable to mixed advice from multiple specialities regarding what is "healthy" (Chaps. 1 and 13). Although not mentioned in the case study above, Karen was not taking her supplements as she thought they were bad for her diabetes. This was observed by her doctor who assured her that the supplements were a very important medicine to support her recovery.

Our case highlights the need for nurses and multiprofessional healthcare providers to advocate for individualized, nutrition care planning and decision-making. Team members should also ensure relevant information is provided and equally understood and clarify goals and expectations as core factors for patient-focused nutrition care (Chaps. 10–12). A practical and considerate approach will provide the individual and/or relatives with information of when to get help if it gets difficult to follow the plan and where to get help specifically, including name of the professional, phone number/e-mail, and office hours. Both are preferably individualized and written down for the individual to take home. It is also important that nutrition care is coordinated to be applied by healthcare providers across contexts. It also must be clear to all who is the primary responsible clinician for these coordination tasks [36].

There is a lot of care associated with food, meals, and nutritional nursing, and it can be a difficult balancing act to meet the individual person's wishes, preferences, and needs, while meeting the needs for energy and protein. Healthcare providers are recommended to be aware of the possibilities for creating social communities in a hospital ward, in a nursing home, or in the citizen's immediate environment, to enable those people who want to eat with others. The importance of clinically focused foodservice systems is further discussed in Chap. 5.

The nurse and other healthcare providers who serve the day's meals must take on a "hosting role" in connection with the meal before, during, and after the meal, with thoughts on how the best meal is created in the current context. It is a well-known fact that the duration of the meal, eating with others, the surroundings, and the meal influence how much and what one eats [37, 38]. An appetite-stimulating environment supports the person's desire to eat, for example, by removing unpleasant odors and ventilating the living room and cleaning up. In addition, our case highlights the importance of nurse's tasks to make sure that the older adult has received the necessary help for oral and hand hygiene and toileting before the meal is served.

Step 2: Enteral tube feeding.

For older adults who are unable to consume adequate nutrition orally, tube feeding may be an option. ESPEN recommends tube feeding for those patients, including older persons with reasonable prognosis, for whom oral intake is expected to be impossible for more than 3 days or expected to be below half of energy requirements for more than 1 week, despite interventions to ensure adequate oral intake, in order to meet nutritional requirements and maintain or improve nutritional status [5, 39]. The older person should of course be sufficiently informed and give consent, where the option of tube feeding is considered in their best interest [5, 40].

Patients with dysphagia, intensive care patients, cancer patients, as well as patients who have lost the urge to eat due to discomfort from illness or treatment will often be able to be helped with a tube for a period of time. Enteral tube feeding, also called "enteral nutrition," can be given as complete and partial nutrition to patients. Details regarding enteral tube feeding are provided in Chap. 5. Our example older adult (Karen) had previously documented in her advanced care plan that should she be acutely unwell with a chance for recovery and unable to eat, she was willing to receive short-term tube feeding, although she did not want any long-term feeding tube devices placed if she did not have capacity to make that decision.

Step 3: Parenteral nutrition.

Parenteral nutrition (PN) should be reserved for those who are unable to ingest or absorb adequate nutrition through their gastrointestinal tract. Parenteral nutrition can be administered through an intravenous (iv) approach. Central iv accesses are often used, but with a duration of a few days, parenteral nutrition can also be provided using peripheral iv access. Older persons with reasonable prognosis and active treatment goals (expected benefit) are recommended to be offered PN if oral and enteral intake are expected to be impossible for more than 3 days or expected to be below half of energy requirements for more than 1 week, in order to meet nutritional requirements and maintain or improve nutritional status [5]. Details regarding administration and monitoring of patients on parenteral nutrition are provided in Chap. 5.

3.4.1 Nursing Care Required for Nutritional Therapy

Each of the above three steps will fail in the absence of supportive nursing care. In many countries, the hospital, home-care, or aged care home nurse plans and performs the daily care of the patient and assesses the patient's need for help in connection with eating and coordinates with the involved healthcare professionals. This can of course differ between countries. Studies have shown that patients with poor intake find it difficult to ask the nursing staff for help with eating, which means that the nurse must pay special attention to assessing these patients' care needs. Assistance with eating can in practice be shared with other healthcare staff, volunteers, family, and friends around the patient. Chapters 6 and 10 describe the nursing care efforts in detail.

3.5 Action and Monitoring

In this phase, the practical enactment of the nutritional support plan is performed, monitored, and documented (Chap. 6). Ongoing evaluation is planned for and made, depending on setting and severity of nutritional risk. Local or national standards for community and hospital may provide actual standards for action and monitoring [8, 9]. When initiating nutritional therapy or a special diet for an older adult at nutritional risk, it is crucial that the effort is documented, evaluated, and adapted during the process. Karen was going along well in life. Perhaps not unexpectedly, she became ill suddenly, probably due to her chronic diseases. She then self-isolates and lost her desire to eat not only due to multiple acute nutrition impact symptoms but also because the community and socializing around the meal were lost. It is crucial that nurses and other staff who serve or prepare the food for the older adult consider that the day's meals also have a social significance for the older adult and relatives. Nurses and other healthcare providers are ideally placed to identify factors in the environment that may affect the appetite.

The best and most widely used monitoring method is diet recording of the patient's dietary intake. Where possible, self-monitoring, or involvement in monitoring, should be considered. This allows active engagement, and feedback can be used in the guiding conversations with the patient, including relatives when possible and relevant. Based on a diet registration, the healthcare provider or dietitian and the patient can discuss problems around meals and meal frequency and can clarify the individual patient's issues, wishes, and need for help. Documentation of the individual agreement is necessary, as it will ensure that the patient, for example, will be offered the right help in all eating situations. Increasingly across settings, diet registration forms are being implemented that integrate with electronic work tools on computers or apps on phones and tablets. The individual abilities, as well as tools, infrastructure, and resources available, will determine the choice of registration method. However, the 24-h recall method, while a relatively good tool for intake adequacy assessment, does not help neither the nursing staff nor the patient to improve the patient's intake across the course of the day. Conversely, a "real-time" time registration method is recommended for actual motivation [41–43]. The nurse and other nursing staff handle the diet registration and are responsible for documenting the result of the patient's intake in the medical record.

Weight and especially serial weights are routinely applied as a monitoring parameter, but weight alone is an uncertain parameter in older adults with, for example, dehydration or overhydration. Regardless of the setting for weighing, it is advised to weigh the subject in the same kind of clothes and shoes, every time. While many weigh without shoes, weighing in light shoes and indoor clothing is recommended in the older, as shoes may help prevent them from slipping on the floor. Weighing circumstances, for example, clothes and type of weighing scale, should be documented. Height may be measured standing back to a wall without shoes to the nearest centimeter (cm). If height is unable to be accurately measured standing, for example, due to kyphosis, one approach is to measure the patient in bed with the patient lying flat and stretched, measuring from top head to heel. Other proxy height measurement measures, for example, ulna measurement, are recommended across settings and populations [44].

There are a broad variety of other monitoring opportunities that should be considered including biochemical, clinical, physiological, and functional measures, psychosocial changes, and older adult knowledge, understanding, and adherence to shared treatment plans (Chaps. 4 and 5). Clear documentation of monitoring measures and results can form the basis for an interdisciplinary discussion of the older adult's nutrition plan, and as per our case above, this may include, for instance, dietitians, pharmacists, physicians, physiotherapists, occupational therapists, social workers, or speech pathologists (Chaps. 13 and 18).

3.6 Evaluation and Adjustment of Nutrition Plan

The above monitoring measures can be used to evaluate and adjust the nutrition plan. For example, the dietitian or nurse uses the total daily intake and the monitored weight to determine if the client has achieved, or is making progress toward, the planned goals. Otherwise, the plan must be adjusted. Furthermore, NIS should be reconsidered, to evaluate whether changes should be made and whether interdisciplinary healthcare providers should be referred. When the individual demonstrates adequate intake and weight stabilization, the monitoring frequency can decrease.

3.7 Discharge from Hospital or Handover to Another Caretaker

With consent of the older adult, it may be appropriate to provide information to the next care-person, for them to be able to support high-quality nutrition care. Information about actual weight, nutrition plan including consistency modifications, nutritional requirements and goals, allergies, or other food restrictions or preferences (e.g., cultural or religious requirements) should be followed by recommendations for monitoring and motivation, as well as how the individual and other carers are engaged. If the individual has cognitive impairment, information should also include likes and dislikes for foods and feeding preferences.

3.8 End of Nutritional Therapy

Nutritional therapy is ended when goals are met. Even where the goals are not quite met, where the acute condition is stabilized, and if individual is able to self-monitor and has sufficient capability, opportunity, and motivation, it may be appropriate to discharge the patient from nutrition specialist care. However, encouraging mealtimes, supporting adequate food and fluid intake, and monitoring nutrition intake, impact symptoms, and related outcome measurements remains a core role for nurses like Mary. For older and particularly multimorbid or institutionalized older adults, we know that diseases and life events may rapidly again put the individual back at risk. Therefore, regular nutritional screening in line with local recommendations is required unless other events suggest screening should be more frequent.

3.9 Ethical Considerations

The main aim of geriatric medicine including geriatric nutritional therapy is to optimize functional status of the older person and, thus, to ensure greatest possible autonomy and best possible quality of life. There is sufficient consensus that oral nutrition, apart from providing nutrients, has significant psychological and social functions, enables sensation of taste and flavor, and is a mediator of pleasure and well-being. Therefore, oral options of nutrition are routinely the first choice and should include encouragement and time to eat, high-quality food choices, and consideration of the need for dedicated assisted feeding, even if these may prove difficult, time-consuming, resource intensive, and demanding. Sufficient training of caregivers should be provided [5, 43].

According to the ESPEN guideline on ethical aspects of artificial nutrition and hydration [40], the ethical principles "autonomy, beneficence, non-maleficence and justice" have to be applied in the act of medical decision-making. In life-threatening situations where a well-founded decision cannot be made, across many cultures and settings, the principle *in dubio pro vita* (when in doubt, favor life) should be considered. Autonomy does however not mean that an older adult has the right to obtain every treatment they wish or request, if this particular treatment is not medically indicated. Furthermore, the guideline states that a competent patient has the right to refuse a treatment after adequate information even when this refusal would lead to his or her death, although again we note differences across cultures and settings in this regard [40].

For nutrition and hydration in dementia, the guideline claims that the decision to discontinue artificial feeding might be misunderstood as an order "do not feed" as nutrition is associated with life and its absence with starvation. For patients with eating difficulties requiring support, an individual care plan has to be established. Especially the guideline states that in regard to medical decisions at the end of life, appropriate terminology has to be carefully chosen. In palliative care, artificial nutrition has become an integral part, allowing increased survival in terminal cases where the individual would otherwise have died from starvation and not primarily from their malignant disease. In the terminal state, it may be considered difficult to end or decrease nutrition or fluid therapy, even if this might benefit the patient. It is thus recommended that from the very beginning of nutritional therapy, the treatment is evaluated every time the patient is seen in the clinic, just as with all other medication and treatment. This is of course especially required in progressive or terminal diseases such as cancer, lung fibrosis, Parkinson's, or motor neurone disease. Ethical issues are covered in further detail in Chap. 21.

3.10 Summary

Karen lives in a nursing home. However, Karen could just the same live in her own home and may in that case even for a short while need hospitalization or a relief stay in a care home. Regardless of setting, requirements for good nutritional practice and care remain the same. While these nutrition care processes may be at times directed by a nutrition care specialist, they are reliant on all members of the healthcare team to work together.

Take-Home Points

- Nurses are ideally placed to lead nutrition care process actions.
- The nutrition care process must engage the older adult, family and friends as appropriate, and diverse healthcare providers.
- Nutrition impact symptom assessment is vital to detect, remove, or reduce barriers to eating.
- The older adult is center of the nutrition plan and needs to agree on short- and long-term goals.
- Nutrition care for the old person with, or at risk of, malnutrition should not be limited to the acute care setting or short-term follow-up.

References

1. Swan WI et al (2017) Nutrition care process and model update: toward realizing people-centered care and outcomes management. J Acad Nutr Diet 117(12):2003–2014
2. Cederholm T et al (2015) Diagnostic criteria for malnutrition—an ESPEN consensus statement. Clin Nutr 34(3):335–340
3. The L (2019) ICD-11. Lancet 393(10188):2275
4. White JV et al (2012) Consensus statement: academy of nutrition and dietetics and American Society for Parenteral and Enteral Nutrition. J Parenter Enteral Nutr 36(3):275–283
5. Volkert D et al (2019) ESPEN guideline on clinical nutrition and hydration in geriatrics. Clin Nutr 38(1):10–47
6. Swan WI et al (2019) Nutrition care process (NCP) update part 2: developing and using the NCP terminology to demonstrate efficacy of nutrition care and related outcomes. J Acad Nutr Diet 119(5):840–855

7. Lacey K, Pritchett E (2003) Nutrition care process and model: ADA adopts road map to quality care and outcomes management. J Am Diet Assoc 103(8):1061–1072
8. Bell JJ et al (2018) Rationale and developmental methodology for the SIMPLE approach: a systematised, interdisciplinary malnutrition pathway for impLementation and evaluation in hospitals. Nutr Diet 75(2):226–234
9. Keller H et al (2018) Update on the integrated nutrition pathway for acute care (INPAC): post implementation tailoring and toolkit to support practice improvements. Nutr J 17(1):2
10. Falaschi P Orthogeriatrics. Springer International, Cham
11. Bell JJ et al (2021) Nutritional care of the older patient with fragility fracture: opportunities for systematised, interdisciplinary approaches across acute care, rehabilitation and secondary prevention settings. In: Falaschi P, Marsh D (eds) Orthogeriatrics: the management of older patients with fragility fractures. Springer, Berlin, pp 311–329
12. Kondrup J et al (2003) ESPEN guidelines for nutrition screening 2002. Clin Nutr 22(4):415–421
13. Cederholm T et al (2017) ESPEN guidelines on definitions and terminology of clinical nutrition. Clin Nutr 36(1):49–64
14. Reber E et al (2019) Nutritional risk screening and assessment. J Clin Med 8(7):1065
15. Elia M, Stratton RJ (2011) Considerations for screening tool selection and role of predictive and concurrent validity. Curr Opin Clin Nutr Metab Care 14(5):425–433
16. Cederholm T et al (2019) GLIM criteria for the diagnosis of malnutrition—a consensus report from the global clinical nutrition community. Clin Nutr 38(1):1–9
17. Keller H et al (2020) Global leadership initiative on malnutrition (GLIM): guidance on validation of the operational criteria for the diagnosis of protein-energy malnutrition in adults. JPEN J Parenter Enteral Nutr 44(6):992–1003
18. Mueller C et al (2011) A.S.P.E.N. clinical guidelines. J Parenter Enteral Nutr 35(1):16–24
19. Skipper A et al (2020) Adult malnutrition (undernutrition) screening: an evidence analysis center systematic review. J Acad Nutr Diet 120(4):669–708
20. Volkert D et al (2019) Management of malnutrition in older patients—current approaches, evidence and open questions. J Clin Med 8(7):974
21. MacLaughlin HL et al (2018) The nutrition impact symptoms (NIS) score detects malnutrition risk in patients admitted to nephrology wards. J Hum Nutr Diet 31(5):683–688
22. Jager-Wittenaar H, Ottery FD (2017) Assessing nutritional status in cancer: role of the patient-generated subjective global assessment. Curr Opin Clin Nutr Metab Care 20(5):322–329
23. Martin L et al (2013) Cancer cachexia in the age of obesity: skeletal muscle depletion is a powerful prognostic factor, independent of body mass index. J Clin Oncol 31(12):1539–1547
24. Verlaan S et al (2017) Nutritional status, body composition, and quality of life in community-dwelling sarcopenic and non-sarcopenic older adults: a case-control study. Clin Nutr 36(1):267–274
25. Bauer JM, Morley JE (2020) Editorial: body composition measurements in older adults. Curr Opin Clin Nutr Metab Care 23(1):1–3
26. Zambone MA, Liberman S, Garcia MLB (2020) Anthropometry, bioimpedance and densitometry: comparative methods for lean mass body analysis in elderly outpatients from a tertiary hospital. Exp Gerontol 138:111020
27. Cruz-Jentoft AJ et al (2019) Sarcopenia: revised European consensus on definition and diagnosis. Age Ageing 48(1):16–31
28. Ferrucci L et al (2007) Disability, functional status, and activities of daily living. In: Birren JE (ed) Encyclopedia of gerontology, 2nd edn. Elsevier, New York, pp 427–436
29. Bell JJ et al (2021) Nutritional care of the older patient with fragility fracture: opportunities for systematised, interdisciplinary approaches across acute care, rehabilitation and secondary prevention settings. In: Falaschi P, Marsh D (eds) Orthogeriatrics: the management of older patients with fragility fractures. Springer International, Cham, pp 311–329
30. Lee RJ et al (2019) Restrictive diets in older malnourished cardiac inpatients: a cross-sectional study. Nutr Diet 78:121–127
31. Keller U (2019) Nutritional laboratory markers in malnutrition. J Clin Med 8(6):775
32. Fruchtenicht AVG et al (2018) Inflammatory and nutritional statuses of patients submitted to resection of gastrointestinal tumors. Rev Col Bras Cir 45(2):e1614

33. Merker M et al (2020) Association of baseline inflammation with effectiveness of nutritional support among patients with disease-related malnutrition: a secondary analysis of a randomized clinical trial. JAMA Netw Open 3(3):e200663
34. Friedli N et al (2020) Refeeding syndrome is associated with increased mortality in malnourished medical inpatients: secondary analysis of a randomized trial. Medicine (Baltimore) 99(1):e18506
35. Stratton RJ, Elia M (2007) Who benefits from nutritional support: what is the evidence? Eur J Gastroenterol Hepatol 19(5):353–358
36. Holst M, Rasmussen HH, Unosson M (2009) Well-established nutritional structure in Scandinavian hospitals is accompanied by increased quality of nutritional care. e-SPEN, Eur e-Journal Clin Nutr Metab 4(1):e22–e29
37. Wikby K, Fägerskiöld A (2004) The willingness to eat. Scand J Caring Sci 18(2):120–127
38. Nieuwenhuizen WF et al (2010) Older adults and patients in need of nutritional support: review of current treatment options and factors influencing nutritional intake. Clin Nutr 29(2):160–169
39. Weimann A et al (2006) ESPEN guidelines on enteral nutrition: surgery including organ transplantation. Clin Nutr 25(2):224–244
40. Druml C et al (2016) ESPEN guideline on ethical aspects of artificial nutrition and hydration. Clin Nutr 35(3):545–556
41. Holst M, Ofei KT, Skadhauge LB, Rasmussen HH, Beermann T (2017) Monitoring of nutrition intake in hospitalized patients: can we rely on the feasible monitoring systems? J Clin Nutr Metab 1:1
42. Holst M, Zacher N, Østergaard T, Mikkelsen S (2019) Disease related malnutrition in hospital outpatients—time for action. Int J Food Sci Nutr Res 1(1):e000349
43. Holst M, Rasmussen HH, Laursen BS (2011) Can the patient perspective contribute to quality of nutritional care? Scand J Caring Sci 25(1):176–184
44. Marinos Elia CR, Stratton R, Todorovic V, Evans L, Farrer K (2008) THE 'MUST' EXPLANATORY BOOKLET a guide to THE 'malnutrition universal Screening tool' ('MUST') for adults. BABEN

4

Interdisciplinary Prevention of Malnutrition

Patrick Roigk and Fabian Graeb

Abstract

A healthy nutritional intake is required to prevent malnutrition. Furthermore, nutrition is associated with improved quality of life in older adults. Simultaneously, many factors influence nutritional intake in later life. Onset and progression of acute or chronic diseases and a reduced dietary intake play a crucial role in developing malnutrition. Malnutrition is associated with poor outcomes such as pressure injury, increased length of hospital stays and increased mortality. The aim of the chapter is to increase the nutritional-based knowledge of the interdisciplinary team to prevent malnutrition in all its forms. Therefore, this chapter offers evidence-based information to support interdisciplinary prevention of malnutrition in older adults across diverse healthcare settings.

Keywords

Malnutrition prevention · Risk factors · Nutritional care · Prevention · Public health · Malnutrition

---

This chapter is a component of Section 1: Nutritional Care in Old Age.
For an explanation of the grouping of chapters in this book, please see Chap. 1: 'Geriatrics and Orthogeriatrics: Providing Nutrition Care'.

P. Roigk (✉)
Department of Clinical Gerontology and Geriatric Rehabilitation, Robert-Bosch-Hospital, Stuttgart, Germany
e-mail: Patrick.roigk@rbk.de; https://www.rbk.de

F. Graeb
Faculty Social Work, Education and Nursing Science, Hochschule Esslingen - University of Applied Sciences, Esslingen, Germany
e-mail: fabian.graeb@hs-esslingen.de; https://www.hs-esslingen.de

Learning Outcomes
By the end of this chapter, you will be able to:

- Know your role within the process of preventing malnutrition.
- Demonstrate awareness of the nutritional needs of older adults.
- Identify older adults at risk of malnutrition.
- Understand and apply opportunities to prevent malnutrition.

4.1 Malnutrition and Its Risk Factors

Enjoying a wide variety of nutritious foods supports older adults to stay healthy and feel well. Insufficient nutrition leads to a loss of health-related resources, particularly in older age. Although definitions vary globally, according to the recent ESPEN consensus and terminology of clinical nutrition [1, 2], malnutrition is defined as:

- A serious reduced body mass (i.e. BMI <18.5 kg/m^2) **or**
- An unintended weight loss ($>5\%$ in 6 months or $>10\%$ beyond 6 months) **and either**
- A BMI <20 kg/m^2 (<70 years)/a BMI 22 $<$kg/m^2 (≥ 70 years) **or** serious reduced muscle mass (i.e. FFMI <15 kg/m^2 in women, <17 kg/m^2 in men).

The risk of malnutrition increases when the older adult does not reach a minimum of 50% of requirements for more than 3 days or when factors are influencing the dietary intake [3]. Based on research findings, up to 50% of the older persons in hospital settings are malnourished [4–6]. A recent meta-analysis from Cereda et al. (2016) demonstrates differing amounts of malnutrition across settings: community (3.1%), outpatients (6.0%), home-care services (8.7%), hospital (22.0%), nursing homes (17.5%), long-term care (28.7%) and rehabilitation/sub-acute care (29.4%), based on the Mini Nutritional Assessment® [4].

The reasons why persons develop malnutrition are multifactorial (Chaps. 2, 3, and 10); consequently, a multifactorial approach is needed (Chap. 13). Malnourished persons may be grouped into those with inadequate intake, reduced uptake or bioavailability of nutrients or increased requirements caused by acute or chronic disease [7]. For example, an older adult may become malnourished because they continue adhering to a restrictive, 'healthy lifestyle' diet into their later life, despite evidence of reduced intake or absorption and increased requirements associated with co-morbid disease. We note that healthcare organisations, expert recommendations and/or individual clinicians often fail to advocate for 'stop dieting' or to evaluate restrictive diets [8].

The model Determinants of Malnutrition in Aged Persons (DoMAP) highlights these and many other major direct or indirect influencing factors of malnutrition in older adults (Fig. 4.1). The main etiologic mechanisms are placed in the middle of the model (level 1 = dark green). The factors in the light green triangle (level

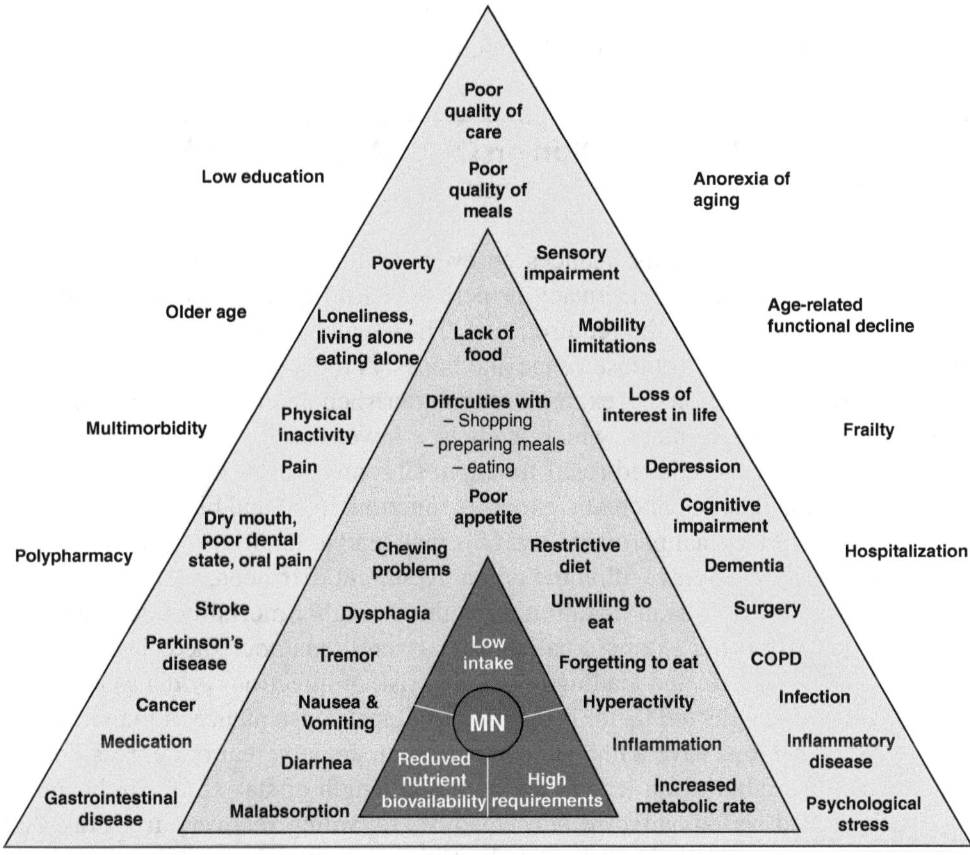

Fig. 4.1 DoMAP model: Determinants of Malnutrition in Aged Persons [9]

2 = lighter green) are the determinants, which directly lead to one of the main factors, for example, hyperactivity leading directly to high requirements. The third level (yellow) contains determinants, which indirectly lead to one or more central mechanisms through factors in level 2. For example, the side effect of medication may lead to poor appetite and to a lower intake. Around the pyramid are typical age-related factors which are additionally influencing the process of malnutrition [9].

Some factors like hospitalisation or polypharmacy might be starting points of developing malnutrition. Other factors like frailty or multimorbidity may progressively worsen the nutritional status of the older adult. If the treatment of older adults with or at risk of malnutrition is individualised to identified determinants of malnutrition, outcomes are improved whether measured by functional status, quality of life or mortality [10]. A recent systematic review analysed socioeconomic factors which contribute the development of malnutrition in older adults. The authors analysed a higher risk not only for persons with a low educational level (odds ratio (OR), 1.48; 95% (CI), 1.33–1.64; $p < 0.001$) but also for those who live alone (OR, 1.92; 95% CI, 1.73–2.14; $p < 0.001$) and are single, widowed or divorced (OR, 1.73; 95% CI, 1.57–1.90; $p < 0.001$) and for persons with a low income level (OR, 2.69; 95% CI, 2.35–3.08; $p < 0.001$). Therefore, nutritional care should be treated in a multifactorial way and must also be aware for socioeconomic aspects in the daily work regarding different types of older adults [11].

4.2 Impact of Malnutrition on Older Adults, Healthcare Systems and the Community

Malnutrition has major consequences on every organ system in the human body [12]. In case of a dietary inadequacy or period of fasting, the body mobilises the functional reserve to meet the requirements. This occurs across diverse parts of the body including muscles, adipose tissue and bones. A reduced muscle mass leads to a reduced muscle function, for example, a malnourished older adult with associated reduced cardiac muscle mass, which leads to a lower cardiac output. This down-regulation results in a reduced renal function. Chronic malnutrition may also correspond with changes in pancreatic exocrine function, intestinal blood flow, villous architecture and intestinal permeability. This may lead to the loss of ability to reabsorb water and electrolytes within the colon. Resultant diarrhoea, with all its negative consequences, from skin irritation through to a higher mortality rate, may then occur, particularly if our example patient was severely malnourished. The immune system may also be affected leading to a higher risk of infections or delayed wound healing. An often neglected factor is the psychological consequence of malnutrition. Malnourished persons have a higher risk to develop anxiety, fear or depression. All these effects of malnutrition lead to an increased length of stay (LOS) in hospitalised patients and serious adverse consequences regarding recovery from disease, trauma and surgery [13]. However, malnutrition is not only associated with an increased risk of mortality in hospitalised older patients but also in community-dwelling older adults. All these facts have major consequences not only for individuals but also for the society [14]: in the European Union, about 20 million patients are diagnosed with diseases which are related to malnutrition. This leads to costs up to € 170 billion in Europe annually [15, 16].

4.3 General Nutritional Care and Prevention of Malnutrition

Every setting and specific patient group needs an individualised and multifactorial approach to prevent malnutrition. On the European level, the European Society for Clinical Nutrition and Metabolism (ESPEN) publishes Guidelines and Consensus Papers on specific topics for specific settings that will be updated from time to time. The latest guideline, which addresses the needs of older people, was published in 2019 [4]. It is common that these guidelines have to be adapted or updated to the country-specific needs and the recommendations of the certain professional societies. For example, in Germany, the German Society for Nutritional Medicine (DGEM) and the German Network for Quality Development in Nursing have developed and published guidelines and standards for different settings, different health professionals and target groups [17–19].

The goal of a clinical nutrition intervention in older adults is to maintain or improve the quality of life and to ensure the intake of an appropriate amount of energy, nutrients, micronutrients and fluids [18]. In order to know how much energy is needed in older adults, knowledge about the calculation of energy intake can be helpful. The basal metabolic rate (BMR) describes the rate which a person needs to maintain the basic function of the body. In older adults, the BMR may be crudely estimated as 20 kcal/kg body weight (BW) per day. However, the daily energy expenditure depends highly on the level of physical activity (PAL), but also on age and weight of the person, and any additional requirements of acute or chronic disease, or malabsorption. The more active a person is, the more energy will be needed (Table 4.1). The PAL in older adults is usually estimated 1.2 to 1.4 [3]. Additional details on nutritional requirements are provided in Chap. 2.

Healthy nutrition should be well balanced, but specific recommendations vary widely [21]. A rudimentary approach to intake and distribution of macronutrients (carbohydrates, fat and proteins) may consider a practical guide: '50% – 30% – 20%'. However, these values have to be understood as approximate 'ballparks' that should vary depending on individual and population-based requirements, recommendations and norms. **Carbohydrates** are the most important nutrient for humans in terms of quantity and providing energy for the body. In addition to supplying the body with energy and essential fatty acids, **fats** also serve as a component of body structures such as cell membranes or as a starting substance for other biologically active substances. **Proteins** play an important role in muscle growth and life itself. Proteins are made of about 20 amino acids. A lack of proteins leads to a loss of muscle strength and a higher risk of falls [22]. However, the amount varies by the nutritional status, PAL, disease and tolerance of the person [23]. The Harvard School of Public Health offers information on their website about rich, environmental-friendly and healthy sources of proteins [24]. Many studies, reviews and recommendations suggest prioritising minimally processed plant-based protein sources (Table 4.2), eggs and lower-fat dairy and white meats (e.g. fish, poultry) over red meat and suggest limiting or avoiding processed meats.

Table 4.1 Energy consumption for various activities as measured by basal metabolic rate [20]

PAL	Examples
1.2–1.3	Exclusively sedentary or lying way of life (frail, dependent, bedbound people)
1.4–1.5	Exclusively sedentary activity with little or no strenuous leisure activity (office workers, precision mechanics)
1.6–1.7	Sitting activity, temporary additional energy expenditure for walking and standing activities, little or no strenuous leisure activity (laboratory technicians, students, assembly line workers)
1.8–1.9	Mostly moving and standing work (housewives, nursing staff, waiters, mechanics, craftsmen)
2.0–2.4	Physically demanding professional work or very active leisure activities (construction workers, farmers, forest workers, miners, competitive athletes)

Table 4.2 Categorised examples for plants rich in proteins [24]

Legumes	Lentils, beans (adzuki, black, fava, chickpeas/garbanzo, kidney, lima, mung, pinto, etc.), peas (green, snow, snap, split, etc.), edamame/soybeans (and products made from soy: tofu, tempeh, etc.), peanuts
Nuts and seeds	Almonds, pistachios, cashews, walnuts, hazelnuts, pecans, hemp seeds, squash and pumpkin seeds, sunflower seeds, flax seeds, sesame seeds, chia seeds
Whole grains	Kamut, teff, wheat, quinoa, rice, wild rice, millet, oats, buckwheat

In case that most of the proteins comes from plants, a mix of different sources should be ensured. For healthy older adults, a diet should include at least 1.0–1.2 g protein/kg body weight/day. For certain older adults who have acute or chronic illnesses, 1.2–1.5 g protein/kg body weight/day may be indicated, with even higher intake for individuals with severe illness or injury [23].

In case of a renal insufficiency, the protein intake must be adapted to the stage of the disease.

Micronutrients (vitamins and minerals) cannot be produced in the body and consequently must be derived from the diet. Vitamins are involved in various important processes, such as the structure and protection of cells. For example, some vitamins play a crucial role in the formation of bones or in blood. In addition, vitamins contribute significantly to the regulation of metabolism and can also be part of enzymes. Unlike fats, carbohydrates and proteins, vitamins are not used as building blocks or as an energy source. Vitamins can be distinguished in fat-soluble (A, D, E, K) and water-soluble (C, B1, B2, B6, B12, niacin, pantothenic acid, biotin, folic acid). They can be stored differently in the body. Additional to that, there are many other minerals—such as the trace elements nickel, cobalt, copper, manganese, chromium and molybdenum and ultra-trace elements such as arsenic, lead, boron and silicon. Reference values can be found in recommendations of expert societies such as specialist societies of Germany, Austria and Switzerland (D-A-CH).

Critical nutrients and micronutrients in older age include **calcium** and **vitamin D**. Calcium and vitamin D are the most important nutrients in bone health and muscle function (Chap. 8). Vitamin D promotes protein synthesis and calcium and phosphate transport in muscles [25]. The Food and Agriculture Organization (FAO) recommended 800–1000 mg calcium per day in men and women over 50 years [26]. The main resource of calcium is dairy but also mineral water or green vegetables, e.g. broccoli and curly kale [27]. The vitamin D intake by food is limited. The production of vitamin D takes place in the skin by exposing to ultraviolet B rays. Differences of skin colour, age, how much the skin has been exposed to the sun or the latitude in which the persons live are factors to be considered when making recommendations regarding sun exposure times [28]. In Germany, it is recommended for adults to expose their hands, face and arms to the sun for at least 5 to 15 min between 12:00 and 15:00 per day in the summertime. In winter, the time of exposure should triple. Information about the time which should be spent in the sun to produce an appropriate amount of vitamin D can be found on webpages of the country-specific professional societies. However, the production of vitamin D within the skin and exposure to ultraviolet B rays is limited in older adults. Therefore, vitamin D should routinely be supplemented. The recommended daily amount of vitamin D intake varies between the countries and populations. The International Osteoporosis Foundation (IOF) and many national recommendations recommend for seniors aged 60 years and over a supplement at a dose of 800 to 1000 IU/day.

4.4 The Role of Physical Activity and Training in Malnutrition Prevention

Ageing has multiple consequences on every cell of the human body. The loss of muscle mass in older age is caused by a reduced protein synthesis [23]. Furthermore, inactivity with anabolic resistance is a contributor to develop sarcopenia [29]. Good nutrition, especially protein intake, can help slow down age-related functional decline. In combination with exercise, it is possible to maintain muscle functioning [30]. A meta-analysis of effects of progressive resistance strength training showed positive effects to improve physical functioning and improving strength and the performance of easy and complex activities on older people [31]. The ESPEN expert group recommends practical guidance for maintaining muscle health and physical function for older adults above 65 years. This includes daily physical activity for all older adults, as long as activity is possible; additionally, resistance training should be offered, when possible, as part of an overall fitness programme [23]. Additional information on physical activity, exercise and physical rehabilitation is provided in Chap. 14.

4.5 Opportunities for Nurses and Other Healthcare Providers to Prevent Malnutrition

The prevention and treatment of malnutrition needs a comprehensive approach by healthcare providers across the continuum of care (Chaps. 1, 6, and 13). The quality indicators in Table 4.3 highlight examples of nutritional care opportunities to prevent malnutrition in older adults. They are divided in three topics: general aspects, organisational aspects and educational aspects.

4.6 Additionally, Good to Know

We have included the following points of interest observed across years of providing care for older adults with malnutrition:

- Older adults with normal weight or obesity could also have undetected malnutrition [1]!
- The sarcopenia phenotype is associated with malnutrition (Chap. 8) [37].
- A potential life-threatening metabolic condition in malnourished persons after starting (mainly) parenteral feeding is the refeeding syndrome. Therefore, the

Table 4.3 Opportunities for interdisciplinary healthcare providers to prevent malnutrition in older adults

General aspects	
Nutrition screening and assessment	• The screening and assessment of malnutrition should be embedded in admission, clinic and general practice processes • Older adults screened at risk of malnutrition should receive a thorough nutrition assessment within 24–48 h (Chap. 3) [10] • Older persons should be monitored and considered at high risk for dehydration [32]
High-quality, nutrient-dense food choices	• A varied diet, rich in macronutrients and micronutrients (e.g. protein, calcium), should be offered regularly • Food sources should provide additional energy and protein when the older adult is acutely unwell, recovering from illness, or malnourished [3] • Older adults in hospitals, aged care settings and other facilities should have the opportunity to select different diets from a high-quality menu • Offered food should include local produce prepared in line with what older persons usually consume in everyday life [19, 33] • Nutrient-dense snacks and fluids should be available 24 h/day, particularly in case of caring for patients with dementia • In case of swallowing or chewing problems, texture-modified products with an appetizing structure (i.e. moulded foods) are preferred [34]
Limit unnecessary or restrictive diets	• Highly restrictive diets (e.g. extreme ketogenic diets, gluten-free diet without medical reasons or fruitarian) should be avoided [3] • Consider deprescription of weight loss or lifestyle disease diets (e.g. lipid-modifying diets) in those with or at risk of malnutrition • Fasting periods and restrictive surgical/procedural diets should be minimised, especially before/after surgery or procedures [19]
Consider nutritional supplements	• Oral nutritional supplements rich in energy and nutrients should be offered where indicated and aligning with treatment goals [3, 10] • Micronutrients (e.g. vitamin D, calcium, multivitamins) should be supplemented in line with local guidelines
Organisational-related aspects	
Assistance	• Mealtime assistance should be offered when necessary, ensuring adequate time to eat, with the goal to support self-independency [3, 19] • Pre-meal toileting and mobilisation assistance, for example, to a dining room or out of bed
Environment	• The eating environment should be pleasant. An additional dining room on the ward supports the social aspects of dining [3, 19] • De-cluttering of meal trays and serving tables
Mealtime interruptions	• Diagnostic procedures or medical professional visits should be planned in the time between the mealtimes [19] • Encourage families and friends to support food and fluid intake at mealtimes

(continued)

Table 4.3 (continued)

Team care processes	• Dietician, nurses and medical professionals should have scheduled meetings to support nutritional care of malnourished patients (Chap. 11) [35] • Clinical governance processes should be in place to support nutritional care
Educational aspects	
Older adults and carers	• Older adults and their relatives should get information and education to prevent and treat malnutrition [19] • Consumers should be included in co-designing nutrition education materials
Interdisciplinary healthcare providers	• Staff should be well prepared to support nutritional care with consideration to qualifications, skills and responsibilities [19, 36] • Staff should understand who to refer for ongoing supportive or specialist nutritional care and how to do this • Nursing specialists in nutritional care should be a part of the team in order to spread knowledge and to address the topic on the ward [35]
Influencers and advocates	• Healthcare administrators, policymakers, professional bodies and politicians should all be engaged to prevent malnutrition • Robust data and reports should be prepared and presented to support prevention of malnutrition across the lifecycle and continuum of care

start of the nutrition should be slowly 'step by step', in persons who are extremely underweight, with massive weight loss in a short time period or after prolonged starvation [2].

- Oral nutrition should be preferred wherever possible, with dedicated feeding assistance and encouragement; combination of oral and enteral or parenteral feeding is also possible [9].
- Participate on the nutrition day. It's a worldwide annual systematic collection and analysis of data in hospital wards, intensive care units and nursing homes. It can be used to demonstrate the benefits of nutritional care in a systematic, periodic way [38].

4.7 Limits of Preventing Malnutrition

The change of the nutritional status like losing appetite or weight can be a part of the physiological process and thus a part of ageing. On the other hand, a worsening nutritional status can influence the health status in a negative way or can also be the result of chronic or acute diseases, e.g. cancer, dementia or renal failure. In some cases, malnutrition can be an expression of a personal decision of the older adult, particularly in end-of-life situations [39]. Besides the goal to maintain or improve the weight and nutritional status of the older adult, good nutritional care should always consider the aspects of quality of life and what matters to the older adult. Therefore, clinical nutrition should keep in mind the ethical aspects of nutrition. Especially in end-of-life situations (Chap. 21), the following points should be considered:

- Reversible symptoms, which disturb appetite and enjoyment, like nausea, emesis, pain and chewing and swallowing problems, should be detected and treated.
- Older adults should eat the food they want to eat.
- Needs and wishes of the older adult should be followed.
- In end-stage disease, voluntary refusal to eat and drink should be discussed in the multidisciplinary team and accepted, when reversible symptoms are unable to be identified.
- To identify the older adult's will, advanced care planning could be helpful with all involved formal (and informal) caregivers.

4.8 Implementation of Malnutrition Interventions

The efficacy of implemented malnutrition interventions depends on different factors. A systematic review from Murimi et al. (2017) found four major factors which support the efficacy of interventions: interventions that lasted ≥5 months, having ≤3 focused objectives, appropriate design and use of theories [40]. To address these factors or adapt the findings in the individual organisation, an implementation plan is necessary. Implementation frameworks and theories which aim to change both patient and healthcare provider behaviour exist [41–43]; Chap. 10 is devoted to implementation approaches that support sustaining and spreading nutritional care improvements. Implementation planning should consider influencing individuals, structures and processes both within and external to the organisation [44]. An additional priority is to have sustainable financial support for the new structures and processes to support ongoing treatment provided by supportive interdisciplinary healthcare providers and nutritional care specialists. In terms of the counselling of patients, a theoretical underpinning and ongoing education of the interdisciplinary team members and specialists is required. All mentioned elements should be integrated as a part of a quality improvement system which is supported by data that is evaluated and reported regularly; this will enable continuous improvement of the nutritional care provided to older adults across healthcare settings.

Take-Home Points

Many hospitals and nursing homes globally are already working with guidelines or expert standards. However, this does not mean that a good nutritional care is implemented in the daily practice [45, 46]. To self-assess application of learning to practice, the following practical questions should be answered:

- Is the offered food made in a way you (or your grandparents) would enjoy?
- Is the whole care process focused on the needs and wishes of the older adults/residents?

- Do you know the macronutrients and micronutrients?
- Do you screen and assess all older adults/residents for malnutrition risk regularly?
- Do you know who is responsible in the nutritional process of your organisation?
- Is the nutritional process standardised and implemented in a quality improvement system of your organisation?

References

1. Cederholm T, Bosaeus I, Barazzoni R, Bauer J, van Gossum A, Klek S et al (2015) Diagnostic criteria for malnutrition—an ESPEN consensus statement. Clin Nutr 34:335–340. https://doi.org/10.1016/j.clnu.2015.03.001
2. Cederholm T, Barazzoni R, Austin P, Ballmer P, Biolo G, Bischoff SC et al (2017) ESPEN guidelines on definitions and terminology of clinical nutrition. Clin Nutr 36:49–64. https://doi.org/10.1016/j.clnu.2016.09.004
3. Volkert D, Beck AM, Cederholm T, Cruz-Jentoft A, Goisser S, Hooper L et al (2019) ESPEN guideline on clinical nutrition and hydration in geriatrics. Clin Nutr 38:10–47. https://doi.org/10.1016/j.clnu.2018.05.024
4. Cereda E, Pedrolli C, Klersy C, Bonardi C, Quarleri L, Cappello S et al (2016) Nutritional status in older persons according to healthcare setting: a systematic review and meta-analysis of prevalence data using MNA®. Clin Nutr 35:1282–1290. https://doi.org/10.1016/j.clnu.2016.03.008
5. Cereda E, Veronese N, Caccialanza R (2018) The final word on nutritional screening and assessment in older persons. Curr Opin Clin Nutr Metab Care 21:24–29. https://doi.org/10.1097/MCO.0000000000000431
6. Lacau St Guily J, Bouvard É, Raynard B, Goldwasser F, Maget B, Prevost A et al (2018) NutriCancer: a French observational multicentre cross-sectional study of malnutrition in elderly patients with cancer. J Geriatr Oncol 9:74–80. https://doi.org/10.1016/j.jgo.2017.08.003
7. Agarwal E, Miller M, Yaxley A, Isenring E (2013) Malnutrition in the elderly: a narrative review. Maturitas 76:296–302. https://doi.org/10.1016/j.maturitas.2013.07.013
8. Lee RJ, Collins PF, Elmas K, Bell JJ (2021) Restrictive diets in older malnourished cardiac inpatients: a cross-sectional study. Nutr Diet 78:121–127. https://doi.org/10.1111/1747-0080.12590
9. Volkert D, Kiesswetter E, Cederholm T, Donini LM, Eglseer D, Norman K et al (2019) Development of a model on determinants of malnutrition in aged persons: a MaNuEL project. GGM 5:1–8. https://doi.org/10.1177/2333721419858438
10. Schuetz P, Fehr R, Baechli V, Geiser M, Deiss M, Gomes F et al (2019) Individualised nutritional support in medical inpatients at nutritional risk: a randomised clinical trial. Lancet 393:2312–2321. https://doi.org/10.1016/S0140-6736(18)32776-4
11. Besora-Moreno M, Llauradó E, Tarro L, Solà R (2020) Social and economic factors and malnutrition or the risk of malnutrition in the elderly: a systematic review and meta-analysis of observational studies. Nutrients 12:737. https://doi.org/10.3390/nu12030737
12. Saunders J, Smith T (2010) Malnutrition: causes and consequences. Clin Med (Lond) 10:624–627. https://doi.org/10.7861/clinmedicine.10-6-624
13. Norman K, Pichard C, Lochs H, Pirlich M (2008) Prognostic impact of disease-related malnutrition. Clin Nutr 27:5–15. https://doi.org/10.1016/j.clnu.2007.10.007
14. Sanchez-Rodriguez D, Locquet M, Reginster J-Y, Cavalier E, Bruyère O, Beaudart C (2020) Mortality in malnourished older adults diagnosed by ESPEN and GLIM criteria in the SarcoPhAge study. J Cachexia Sarcopenia Muscle 11(5):1200–1211. https://doi.org/10.1002/jcsm.12574
15. Freijer K, Tan SS, Koopmanschap MA, Meijers JMM, Halfens RJG, Nuijten MJC (2013) The economic costs of disease related malnutrition. Clin Nutr 32:136–141. https://doi.org/10.1016/j.clnu.2012.06.009

16. Arribalzaga EB (2009) Valoración de la circunferencia de la pantorrilla Como indicador de riesgo de desnutrición en personas mayores [valuation of the circumference of the calf like indicator of risk of malnutrition in senior persons]. Nutr Hosp 24:368–369
17. Valentini L, Volkert D, Schütz T, Ockenga J, Pirlich M, Druml W et al (2013) Leitlinie der Deutschen Gesellschaft für Ernährungsmedizin (DGEM): DGEM-Terminologie in der Klinischen Ernährung. Aktuel Ernahrungsmed 38:97–111. https://doi.org/10.1055/s-0032-1332980
18. Volkert D, Bauer M, Frühwald T, Gehrke I, Lechleitner M, Lenzen-Großimlinghaus R et al (2013) Klinische Ernährung in der Geriatrie: Leitlinie der Deutschen Gesellschaft für Ernährungsmedizin (DGEM) in Zusammenarbeit mit der GESKES, der AKE und der DGG. Akt Ernähr Med 38:e1–e48. https://doi.org/10.1055/s-0033-1343169
19. DNQP (2017) Expertenstandard Ernährungsmanagement zur Sicherung und Förderung der oralen Ernährung in der Pflege, 1st edn. Hochschule Osnabrück, Osnabrück
20. Mathias D (2018) Physical activity level. In: Mathias D (ed) Fit und gesund von 1 bis Hundert. Springer, Berlin, p 15. https://doi.org/10.1007/978-3-662-56307-6_11
21. Venn BJ (2020) Macronutrients and human health for the 21st century. Nutrients 12:2363. https://doi.org/10.3390/nu12082363
22. Rizzoli R, Bonjour J-P (2004) Dietary protein and bone health. J Bone Miner Res 19:527–531. https://doi.org/10.1359/JBMR.040204
23. Deutz NEP, Bauer JM, Barazzoni R, Biolo G, Boirie Y, Bosy-Westphal A et al (2014) Protein intake and exercise for optimal muscle function with aging: recommendations from the ESPEN expert group. Clin Nutr 33:929–936. https://doi.org/10.1016/j.clnu.2014.04.007
24. Harvard School of Public Health (2021) The nutrition source. Protein. http://www.hsph.harvard.edu/nutritionsource/what-should-you-eat/protein/. Accessed 2 Apr 2021
25. Morelli S, de Boland AR, Boland RL (1993) Generation of inositol phosphates, diacylglycerol and calcium fluxes in myoblasts treated with 1,25-dihydroxyvitamin D3. Biochem J 289(Pt 3):675–679. https://doi.org/10.1042/bj2890675
26. FAO (2001) Human vitamin and mineral requirements: report of a joint FAO/WHO expert consultation Bangkok, Thailand. http://www.fao.org/3/a-y2809e.pdf. Accessed 3 Nov 2020
27. IOF (2020) Calcium content of common foods. https://www.osteoporosis.foundation/patients/prevention/calcium-content-of-common-foods. Accessed 3 Nov 2020
28. Wacker M, Holick MF (2013) Sunlight and vitamin D: a global perspective for health. Dermatoendocrinology 5:51–108. https://doi.org/10.4161/derm.24494
29. Dickinson JM, Volpi E, Rasmussen BB (2013) Exercise and nutrition to target protein synthesis impairments in aging skeletal muscle. Exerc Sport Sci Rev 41:216–223. https://doi.org/10.1097/JES.0b013e3182a4e699
30. Boirie Y (2009) Physiopathological mechanism of sarcopenia. J Nutr Health Aging 13:717–723. https://doi.org/10.1007/s12603-009-0203-x
31. Liu C-J, Latham NK (2009) Progressive resistance strength training for improving physical function in older adults. Cochrane Database Syst Rev 2009:CD002759. https://doi.org/10.1002/14651858.CD002759.pub2
32. Hooper L, Bunn D, Jimoh FO, Fairweather-Tait SJ (2014) Water-loss dehydration and aging. Mech Ageing Dev 136–137:50–58. https://doi.org/10.1016/j.mad.2013.11.009
33. Hauner H, Beyer-Reiners E, Bischoff G, Breidenassel C, Ferschke M, Gebhardt A et al (2019) Leitfaden Ernährungstherapie in Klinik und Praxis (LEKuP). Aktuel Ernahrungsmed 44:384–419. https://doi.org/10.1055/a-1030-5207
34. Farrer O, Olsen C, Mousley K, Teo E (2016) Does presentation of smooth pureed meals improve patients consumption in an acute care setting: a pilot study. Nutr Diet 73:405–409. https://doi.org/10.1111/1747-0080.12198
35. Reber E, Strahm R, Bally L, Schuetz P, Stanga Z (2019) Efficacy and efficiency of nutritional support teams. J Clin Med 8(9):1281. https://doi.org/10.3390/jcm8091281
36. Volkert D, Chourdakis M, Faxen-Irving G, Frühwald T, Landi F, Suominen MH et al (2015) ESPEN guidelines on nutrition in dementia. Clin Nutr 34:1052–1073. https://doi.org/10.1016/j.clnu.2015.09.004

37. Cruz-Jentoft AJ, Bahat G, Bauer J, Boirie Y, Bruyère O, Cederholm T et al (2019) Sarcopenia: revised European consensus on definition and diagnosis. Age Ageing 48:16–31. https://doi.org/10.1093/ageing/afy169
38. Schindler K, Pichard C, Sulz I, Volkert D, Streicher M, Singer P et al (2017) nutritionDay: 10 years of growth. Clin Nutr 36:1207–1214. https://doi.org/10.1016/j.clnu.2016.11.004
39. Felder S, Lechtenboehmer C, Bally M, Fehr R, Deiss M, Faessler L et al (2015) Association of nutritional risk and adverse medical outcomes across different medical inpatient populations. Nutrition 31:1385–1393. https://doi.org/10.1016/j.nut.2015.06.007
40. Murimi MW, Kanyi M, Mupfudze T, Amin MR, Mbogori T, Aldubayan K (2017) Factors influencing efficacy of nutrition education interventions: a systematic review. J Nutr Educ Behav 49:142–165.e1. https://doi.org/10.1016/j.jneb.2016.09.003
41. Nilsen P (2015) Making sense of implementation theories, models and frameworks. Implement Sci 10:53. https://doi.org/10.1186/s13012-015-0242-0
42. Kwasnicka D, Dombrowski SU, White M, Sniehotta F (2016) Theoretical explanations for maintenance of behaviour change: a systematic review of behaviour theories. Health Psychol Rev 10:277–296. https://doi.org/10.1080/17437199.2016.1151372
43. Bluethmann SM, Bartholomew LK, Murphy CC, Vernon SW (2017) Use of theory in behavior change interventions. Health Educ Behav 44:245–253. https://doi.org/10.1177/1090198116647712
44. Laur C, Valaitis R, Bell J, Keller H (2017) Changing nutrition care practices in hospital: a thematic analysis of hospital staff perspectives. BMC Health Serv Res 17:498. https://doi.org/10.1186/s12913-017-2409-7
45. Fleischer N, Klewer J (2011) Untersuchung des Ernährungsmanagements vor und während der Implementierung des nationalen Expertenstandards Ernährungsmanagement zur Sicherstellung und Förderung der oralen Ernährung in der Pflege in einer stationären Altenpflegeeinrichtung. HBScience 2:143–149. https://doi.org/10.1007/s16024-011-0037-4
46. Volkert D, Weber J, Kiesswetter E, Sulz I, Hiesmayr M (2019) Nutritional situation in German hospitals—results of the nutritionDay project 2018. Ernährungs Umschau 66:204–211. https://doi.org/10.4455/eu.2019.045

5

Treatment of Malnutrition: Common Nutrition Support Prescriptions

Mette Holst, Ólöf G. Geirsdóttir and Jack J. Bell

Abstract

Malnutrition is observed in around one in three hospital inpatients; this harmful ICD10-AM-coded disease is a strong independent predictor of adverse older adult and healthcare outcomes, mortality, and treatment costs globally, particularly in multimorbid, older adults. Despite recognition of malnutrition as a disease, nutrition support prescriptions are often not valued as the medicine to treat it. This chapter is devoted to the common nutrition support prescriptions for treating malnutrition: (1) protein- and energy-dense and/or fortified foods, fluids, and menus (HPHE support); (2) oral nutrition supplements; (3) enteral tube feeding; and (4) parenteral nutrition.

M. Holst
Centre for Nutrition and Intestinal Failure, Aalborg University Hospital, Aalborg University, Aalborg, Denmark

Department of Clinical Medicine, Aalborg University, Aalborg, Denmark
e-mail: mette.holst@rn.dk

Ó. G. Geirsdóttir
Faculty of Food Science and Nutrition, School of Health Science, University of Iceland, Reykjavík, Iceland
e-mail: ogg@hi.is

J. J. Bell (✉)
Allied Health, The Prince Charles Hospital, Chermside, Queensland, Australia

School of Human Movement and Nutrition Sciences, The University of Queensland, St Lucia, QLD, Australia
e-mail: jack.bell@health.qld.gov.au

Keywords

Malnutrition · Nutrition support · Enteral nutrition · Parenteral nutrition · Nutrition assessment

Learning Objectives
By the end of this chapter, you will be able to:

- Describe the rationale for shared decision-making and informed consent.
- List key questions for older adults and teams to consider prior to commencing, changing, or ceasing nutrition support.
- Apply a systematic approach to nutrition support in older adults.
- Justify the rationale for prescribing HPHE support, oral nutrition supplements, enteral, and parenteral nutrition.
- Value nutrition support actions as medicines prescribed for malnutrition, a harmful, life-limiting disease in older adults.
- Value the need for the involvement of relatives and/or interdisciplinary teams to support nutrition prescriptions in older adults.

5.1 Nutrition Support in Older Adults: A Hard Edge Best Balanced by Shared Decision-Making, Informed Consent, and Ethical Insight

Nutrition support (or artificial nutrition) definitions consider care processes provided when unassisted oral intake of food and liquids fails to provide adequate nutrients to meet an individual's estimated requirements [1, 2]. Nutrition support considers prescription of protein- and energy-dense and/or fortified foods, drinks, and menus (HPHE support), oral nutrition supplements (ONS), enteral tube feeding (hereafter enteral nutrition), and parenteral nutrition (PN).

According to the European Society for Clinical Nutrition and Metabolism (ESPEN), artificial nutrition and hydration are a medical intervention; as such these require an indication, a therapeutic goal, the will of the older adult, and consent of the competent older adult or alternative decision-maker [1]. Whether to commence, continue, or withdraw artificial nutrition support in older adults is often a difficult decision. Such decisions should not be made in isolation by a single team member, neither should this be a burden placed on a single older adult or their carer, and may require advice from experts or guiding literature (Chap. 21) [1].

Many guidelines, recommendations, and algorithms for nutrition support exist [1–8]. These often require clinical judgment to apply in real-world individuals across treatment contexts that may be different from where recommendations were developed or considered to be applied. Nutrition support processes can improve outcomes for older adults, and their service providers and funders, and are recommended across many settings [4, 8, 9]. However, a balanced approach also should consider the inconsistency of evidence for nutrition support [10, 11]. There are risks associated with nutrition support, particularly where prescriptions are required to deliver all nutrient and fluid needs; these can be associated with under- or overprescription and/or complications associated with invasive delivery devices that require skilled insertion and careful management. Potential complications associated with the provision of nutrition support are often poorly reported, with a high degree of bias demonstrated across many studies [4, 10].

Not surprisingly, given these complexities, interdisciplinary team management of nutrition support is considered best practice. Teams are able to provide expert advice across nutrition care processes, for example, regarding the appropriateness of nutrition support modalities, and recommendations for when it may be appropriate to transition across one or more feeding modalities (Chaps. 6 and 11–13) [4, 12].

What is most important, however, is to include the older adult, or their decision-maker, in these processes [13]. Shared decision-making is the pinnacle of patient-centered care; Table 5.1 highlights key questions for older adults and teams to consider prior to commencing, changing, or ceasing nutrition support [1, 4, 9, 13–15].

Table 5.1 An example nutrition support checklist

• Is there an indication for nutrition support, a therapeutic goal, and informed consent?
• What clinical conditions/comorbidities will influence outcomes?
• Is the older adult actually at risk of refeeding syndrome? If so what do I need to do?
• Is the proposed goal(s) and treatment(s) feasible and realistic?
• Are treating team capabilities and professional and ethical boundaries secured?
• Does this represent ethically appropriate, transparently allocated resources?
• What are the alternative options?
• What is the expected duration and treatment intent of nutrition support?
• What are the risks, burdens, and benefits of the treatment versus no-treatment options?
• How will these influence quality of life or health-related quality of life?
• Is it worth a trial of treatment?
• What are the review timeframes, options, and processes for ongoing care, clinical handover, or discontinuation?
• What are the older adult's treatment preferences and refusal rights?
• What is the older adult's nutrition status and diagnosis(es)?
• Are there any cultural, religious, or legal considerations?
• Does the older adult have adequate health literacy to make an informed consent decision?
• Is it the will of the older adult to proceed?
• Does the older adult have close relatives or carers who are, with consent, informed and encouraged to support nutrition care?
• Are shared goals, decisions, and informed consent processes considered and documented?
• Are nutrition assessment and reassessments, diagnoses, goals, interventions, and monitoring processes appropriately undertaken and documented in line with locally endorsed recommendations, procedures, and/or guidelines?
• Is an interdisciplinary care team organized to support nutrition care across the continuum?

5.2 Applying a Systematic Approach to Nutrition Support in Older Adults

Systematic nutrition care processes should guide delivery of nutrition support. Building on previous chapters and international models, we propose a SIMPLER approach to nutrition support (Table 5.2) [3, 6, 7, 16]. We also strongly recommend nutrition support is administered and governed by locally endorsed recommendations, guidelines, and procedures, overseen by nutrition support teams and/or specialists.

5.3 Protein- and Energy-Dense and/or Fortified Foods, Fluids, and Menus

Regardless of setting, there is strong consensus that older persons with or at risk of malnutrition should be offered energy- and protein-dense foods and fluids and/or fortified foods; we refer to these as high-protein/high-energy (HPHE) support opportunities. What these look like across global settings are understatedly diverse. These should be texture-modified where oropharyngeal dysphagia and/or chewing problems are evident (Chap. 18) [4]. Additional finger foods or snacks should also be available and offered [4].

A crucial element for HPHE support is accessibility for both the individual and for the care staff that offer them. It is of essential importance that, for example, nutritional drinks and snacks are stored close to the patient and are able to be offered outside of set mealtimes and that these products are cooled or easily heated and completely ready for serving. For people with reduced appetite and dietary intake, it is also important that the portion size is minimized. This may limit the amount of vegetables and fiber consumed. Offering a multivitamin tablet is therefore often necessary for patients who receive "energy- and protein-dense foods," so that the vitamin and mineral needs are optimally covered (Chaps. 2–4). In some care settings, the size of a "small portion" is not implied, and therefore portion sizes may need to be described in detail.

Processes and system opportunities must be leveraged so that the consistency and composition of the diet can be tailored to deliver nutritional needs, both at

Table 5.2 SIMPLER nutrition support processes [3, 6, 7, 16]

Screen for relevant nutrition diagnoses
Investigate and assess using an ABCDEF approach: anthropometry, biochemistry, clinical, diet and drugs, environment and estimated requirements, function
Make the nutrition diagnosis(es)
Plan with the patient including shared goal setting, informed consent discussion regarding treatment versus no-treatment options, and risks versus benefits implement interventions including nutrition support, education, care integration, and clinical handover
Evaluate continuously; ongoing reassessment, monitoring and reviewing of individual patients
Review practice through nutrition care process and policy reforms, recommendations, and research

patient population and individual levels accounting for medical, psychosocial, cultural, and environmental factors. Standards and accreditation processes, quality assurance and risk management, policies, funding and resource allocation, industry and political lobbying, and educational, professional, technological, and research processes should all be engaged to ensure high-quality HPHE food choices are readily available to older adults at risk of malnutrition, across the continuum of care. We especially encourage facility administrators to consider the growing evidence base that demonstrates that high-quality menus and foodservice systems improve nutritional intake, the proportion of patients meeting nutritional requirements, and patient satisfaction, while simultaneously reducing food waste and cost [17].

Most importantly, we implore older adults and interdisciplinary teams to identify malnutrition as a harmful disease and value HPHE foods and fluids as the primary medicine to treat it [18].

5.4 Oral Nutrition Supplements

Despite dedicated efforts, achieving an adequate protein intake and energy intake through HPHE support alone is not possible, particularly in multimorbid older adults [11]. Where requirements are unlikely to be met, older adults with malnutrition, or those at risk of malnutrition and with chronic conditions, should also be offered ONS, in order to improve dietary intake and body weight and to lower the risk of complications and readmission [4].

ONS are available in different flavors and are energy and protein rich; most also provide additional micronutrients. These drinks routinely have a long shelf life and so can be consumed as a snack when off the ward or out of the house. Where ONS are offered, there is strong consensus that these provide at least 400 kcal/day, including 30 g or more of protein/day, and continue for 4 weeks or more [4]. When ONS are offered to an older person, recommendations support continuing for at least 1 month, with ongoing monthly assessment of efficacy and expected benefit [4].

At times older adults may be unable to meet their protein and energy requirements despite HPHE support and ONS prescription, due to the reduced desire or ability to consume or absorb nutrients and/or increased requirements of acute or chronic conditions. In such cases enteral or parenteral tube feeding may be indicated [1].

5.5 Artificial Tube Feeding

Nutrition support, in particular EN and PN, are considered as medical treatments rather than basic cares. Consequently, these should only be applied in situations where there is a realistic chance of improving or maintaining the older adult's condition and quality of life [1, 4]. In older adults with inadequate nutritional intake in the terminal or palliative phase of illness, comfort feeding should be offered [4]. Other circumstances, for example, where risks are considered to outweigh the expected benefits, will demand interdisciplinary assessment and clinical judgment, and determining older adult wishes and realistic treatment goals, noting that sometimes trials of tube feeding may be appropriate to consider [1, 4]. In the following sections, we provide an overview of EN and PN. However, we refer the reader to locally endorsed policies, procedures, and guidelines that must be enacted and audited to adequately govern artificial tube feeding in older adults.

5.5.1 Enteral Nutrition

In older persons with active treatment goals, enteral tube feeding (enteral nutrition (EN)) should be considered where oral intake is expected to be below half of energy requirements for more than 1 week, or absent for more than 3 days, despite attention to promote oral intake adequacy [4]. Where EN aligns with shared treatment goals, this should be initiated without delay [4]. The ongoing benefits and potential risks of EN require regular assessment, reassessment, and monitoring processes directed by locally endorsed procedures and guidelines. A review should also be undertaken whenever there is a change in condition or treatment planning [4]. Wherever possible and safe to do so, oral intake should still be encouraged throughout the duration of EN.

5.5.1.1 Feeding Tube Types

Depending on physiological, physical, environmental, and personal factors, feeding tubes can be via nasogastric, nasojejunal, orogastric, orojejunal, gastrostomy, or jejunal routes. The most common are the nasogastric tubes (NGT) and PEG (percutaneous endoscopic gastrostomy), both of which feed directly into the stomach. With lifelong tube feeding, a low-profile balloon gastrostomy, or PEG button, may be used, which is less obtrusive to the older adult. The button probe also empties into the stomach. In addition, there are also probes that empty further into the intestine, for example, PEGJ probes (PEG with jejunal tube extension). Alternatively, a tube may be entered directly through the abdomen at the jejunum (e.g., surgical jejunostomy). A typical course is to start with the insertion of a nasogastric feeding tube through the nose, and later, if the need for prolonged tube feeding is assessed, a longer-term feeding device is implanted.

5.5.1.2 Tube Placement

Installation of naso-enteral feeding tubes should be performed by those trained in the procedure; this is usually a nurse or medical professional. Preparation and involvement of the older adult, good time, and a calm environment are important. Complications to placement due at times occur, for example, malpositioning into the lungs or accidental removal. In many settings, X-ray control is prescribed, where the guide wire in the nasal probe clarifies the location of the probe. There may be local agreements regarding control of location, where X-ray control is deselected, for example, in very restless patients/cerebrally affected patients.

The PEJ catheter or the PEGJ probe can be inserted in connection with a surgical operation. PEG, PEGJ, and button probe insertions require a scopic procedure when tube feeding is needed over a longer period of time, i.e., more than 3 months. There is a small risk of intestinal perforation or other complications during construction; although rare, these may have life-threating or ending consequences [19]. These should be inserted by appropriate trained specialists.

It is necessary for the nurse to make sure that the written prescriptions are in place and that the location of the probe after construction has been seen and approved by the medical professional before starting the nutrition.

5.5.1.3 Tube Considerations and Care Requirements

There are many considerations regarding tube care and requirements; institutions must have local guidelines/procedures and access to experts who may assist or give advice regarding management and care requirements for tubes [20]. It is important that the nurse, dietitian, or other accountable healthcare provider is aware of these local procedures for identifying the type of probe, the site of insertion and the place of discharge, and management processes. For example, PEG versus PEGJ tubes may look similar. However, while bolus feeding via PEGs is generally acceptable, PEGJs should not be used for bolus administration of tube feeding as it empties into the middle of the small intestine and not into the ventricle. Similarly, when "exercising" probes as part of good practice management, some probes, for example, PEGs, may require rotating, while rotating PEGJs is routinely not recommended. Leaving nasogastric tubes in situ for extended periods without appropriate management practices may lead to a pressure injury. Similarly, gastrostomy insertion sites should be observed for signs of infection; older adults should be provided with management education where appropriate.

5.5.1.4 Checking Placement

Before each administration of nutrition, fluid or medicine, ensure the probe is positioned correctly in line with local standards or recommendations. Commonly recommended methods to check positioning include reading the markings on the probe at the insertion site and/or pH values of aspirates. In many settings it is suggested to start with slow administration, for example, with 20–30 mL of water, where no resistance may be experienced; the patient should be observed for signs of misplacement, such as cough, nausea, and respiratory effects.

5.5.1.5 Flushing Tubes

Tubes should be flushed regularly. Local guidelines and fluid and medication requirements will all need to be considered when determining individual flush volumes and frequencies, for example, four hourly flushes for continuous feeds with at least 30 mL, flushes of water before and after medication, before and after intermittent or bolus feedings, and when pump feeds are commenced or stopped. Flushing the tube promptly after gastric aspiration for pH testing, but not before, is often recommended. It may be appropriate to provide increased or additional water flushes or to meet fluid requirements. It is commonly recommended for continuous pump feeds to use the Y port on the feeding tube when flushing to maintain a closed system. Disconnecting the feeds to flush is not recommended. Where a tube is not actively being used for feeding purposes, for example, during trials of oral intake, or is being used for alternative purposes, local guidelines for flushing should be considered.

5.5.1.6 Feeding Regimens and Modality

Dependent on settings, dietitians or medical staff prepare an individual tube feeding plan, which is usually prescribed and documented in the medical record. Several sections of hospitals have also prepared guiding nutritional instructions, which contain a standard start-up of tube nutrition. In this way, the nurses can ensure the patient a faster start-up of tube feeding, which can later be adapted by a dietitian or medical nutrition specialist. For patients in need of enteral nutrition, several different types of feeding tubes can be constructed.

The choice feeding modality should consider the older adult's individual needs and preferences with the aim to provide safe enteral nutrition and hydration appropriate to the clinical status, in addition to functional and quality of life issues [15]. Optimal feeding times and modality remain inconclusive; we would recommend considering local, national, and/or disease-specific recommendations when choosing feeding modality. Options include, for example, pump versus gravity feeding or bolus, continuous, intermittent, or overnight feeding approaches. Which method chosen should consider the advantages and disadvantages of each mode of feeding, interdisciplinary team recommendations, clinical judgment, treatment goals, additional therapies and medications, and what matters to the older adult.

There are a broad variety of enteral tube feeding preparations available globally; product-specific recommendations are beyond the remit of this text. The final product prescribed is guided by individual requirements, evidence-based recommendations for macro- and micronutrients, costs, logistics, tube feeding hardware (e.g., pumps, giving sets), care provider contracts, and purchasing agreements.

5.5.1.7 Formula Handling and Management

When setting up and dismantling, local hygiene measures must always be observed, as tube feeding must be considered as a food that can be contaminated by improper handling. The manufacturer's product instructions should always be observed. All feeds should be cross-checked according to local prescribing practices and visually inspected, and the use by date noted prior to administration. Aseptic technique should always be applied when handling feeds. Medications, water, dye, or pancreatic/biliary fluids should not be added enteral nutrition formulas. Hang times should be governed by both the product description and local practice requirements. Local practices should also be in place for what is required when breaking ready-to-hang, "closed" systems.

5.5.2 Parenteral Nutrition (PN)

PN is a form of nutrition support administered through an intravenous (iv) approach. Where aligned with treatment goals and expected benefit, recommendations support offering older adults PN where combined oral and enteral tube intake is expected to be impossible for more than 3 days or below half of energy requirements for more than 1 week.

Parenteral nutrition is a prescription drug. The nutrition plan is often planned by the medical professional in consultation with the dietitian and nurse, with consideration to the individual's fluid, macronutrient (energy, protein, fat, carbohydrate), and micronutrient requirements. Addition of vitamins and minerals must be performed under aseptic conditions or provided separately.

Parenteral nutrition often has a slow administration time of 10–16 h. Setup time should ideally be planned accounting for the patient's daily rhythm and other treatment requirements. Administration of parenteral nutrition can be given briefly, as full or supplementary nutrition, or for some older adults for life, for example, for those with short bowel syndrome. While central iv accesses are predominantly applied in most settings, for short durations or where central access is not an option, parenteral nutrition can also be set up using peripheral access. There is generally a difference in the concentration of preparations for use via central and peripheral routes; these are routinely highlighted on the products for administration. In case of lifelong administration, the parenteral nutrition can be given at home under the guidance and control of nutrition support teams or services. Other patient groups with gastrointestinal obstruction may also be discharged with parenteral nutrition to the home for longer or shorter periods, but routinely with a requirement for hospital or specialist outpatient review. Knowledge of the work around parenteral nutrition has also become a relevant area for the nurse specialists in addition to dietitians and medical professionals.

While interdisciplinary management of PN is globally considered best practice, how this "looks," what will be prescribed, who will prescribe it, and how this will be monitored will vary according to health service resources and infrastructure, specialist staff availability, patient populations and treatment settings, clinical and professional governance, and sociocultural factors. We strongly recommend that PN is administered and audited in line with locally endorsed policies, procedures, and guidelines that must be in place to govern safe, effective parenteral nutrition.

5.6 Preventing and/or Managing Nutrition Support Complications

5.6.1 Medications

Medications, whether ONS, EN, PN, or other medications and pharmaceutical products, should always be administered according to local guidelines and medication-specific recommendations. These should account for food-drug and drug-nutrient interaction (Chap. 20). Many medicines, in addition to prescribed tube feeds, can be administered through EFT devices. However, the administering healthcare professional must always check what is appropriate to administer via EN or PN tubes, for example, whether current tablets are appropriate to be crushed and given via an NGT. We recommend discussion with local pharmacist and treating medical professional and setting specific recommendations.

5.6.2 Aspiration

Underlying illnesses, acute complications, procedures, medications, changing levels of consciousness, feeding tube (mis)placement, and feeding positions are all risk factors for aspiration. Interdisciplinary teams should screen for dysphagia and implement safe swallowing strategies and modified diets where indicated and appropriate (Chap. 18). Dedicated attention to oral hygiene and mouthcares may reduce the risk of aspiration pneumonia. For patients receiving enteral tube feeding, a check should be undertaken to confirm that the feeding tube is in the proper position before initiating feedings. Elevating the head of bed for individuals on bedrest should be considered, both during and for a period after feeding, ensuring positioning and supported to prevent sliding down in bed and creating shear forces [12]. Although evidence is limited, avoiding excessive feeding tube rates or bolus volumes and considering continuous pump feeding over bolus feeding where patients have demonstrated intolerance to gastric bolus feeding may be appropriate [12, 21–23]. Where high risk of aspiration, demonstrated intolerance to gastric feeding or in older adults with demonstrated reflux and aspiration of gastric contents, jejunal feeding should be considered [12]. Recent consensus guidelines also suggest avoiding supplementary overnight tube feeding in older adults with a hip fracture due to lack of beneficial effects, patient burden, and poor tolerance [4]. All efforts should be made to minimise use of sedation and prevent delirium [4, 12] the administration of gastric enteral feedings. The relative risks and benefits of promotility agents should also be considered [12].

5.6.3 Gastrointestinal Upset

Diverse factors influence gastrointestinal status. Patients receiving nutrition support are often observed to experience constipation, diarrhea, or gastrointestinal obstruction; in many cases these are independent of the nutrition support approach prescribed, for example, underlying illness or disease, infections (e.g., *Clostridium difficile*), antibiotics, and other medications. Medication review should consider both potential causes (e.g., antibiotics, magnesium, laxatives) and prescription of antiemetics (vomiting) or medications to manage diarrhea. For patients with ongoing vomiting, a reduced pump feeding rate or change to continuous feeding may be appropriate if the patient is receiving bolus feeding. For patients with bolus feeding, it should be confirmed that the feeding device is in the gastric ventricle. For all patients with severe or prolonged gastrointestinal upset, it is important to assess whether the patient is receiving adequate fluid to maintain fluid balance.

5.6.4 Delayed Gastric Emptying or Gastroparesis

Numerous medications impair gastric emptying, particularly opiates, some antidepressants, and dopamine. Again, the relative risks and advantages of gastric emptying agents/prokinetics should be considered. Post-pyloric feeding should also be considered where ongoing. Although recommendations and practices for monitoring gastric residual volumes vary widely, recommendations support avoiding withholding EN for gastric residual volumes (GRVs) <500 mL in the absence of other signs of intolerance and implementing measures to reduce risk of aspiration for volumes between 250 and 500 mL [12].

5.6.5 Hyperglycemia

Where hyperglycemia is observed, medical staff should be informed prior to changing nutrition support prescriptions. Hyperglycemia is commonly observed in acutely unwell, multimorbid older adults; opportunities for medical management, rather than restricting dietary or tube feeding intake, should be carefully considered by the treating team particularly in older adults with demonstrated inadequate intake or malnutrition. This approach is supported by recent guidelines strongly recommending that in older patients with diabetes mellitus, malnutrition and risk of malnutrition shall be managed according to recommendations for malnourished older persons without diabetes mellitus [4].

5.6.6 Refeeding Syndrome

There is limited consensus regarding the diagnosis and management strategies for refeeding syndrome [12, 24]. Recent consensus guidelines recommend starting early and gradually increasing EN or PN in malnourished older adults in 3 days, supplementing thiamine even in the case of suspected mild deficiency, while monitoring and correcting blood levels of phosphate, magnesium, and potassium and glucose [4, 12]. We recommend referring to locally endorsed guidelines for refeeding management.

5.7 Summary

Nutrition support in older adults is often complex and is best overseen by interdisciplinary nutrition support teams. However, the daily work of delivering nutrition support is routinely undertaken by the older adults themselves, family and friends, nurses, and other interdisciplinary healthcare providers. Shared goal setting and decision-making is the pinnacle of patient-centered care. We implore healthcare providers to work together with older adults to identify malnutrition as a harmful, life-limited disease that may be treated with nutrition support, wherever this aligns with what matters to the older adult.

Take-Home Points

- Artificial nutrition and hydration are a medical intervention; as such these require an indication, a therapeutic goal, the will of the patient, and consent of the competent patient or alternative decision-maker.
- Patients and interdisciplinary teams must identify malnutrition as a harmful disease and value HPHE foods and fluids as the primary medicine to treat it.

- Where requirements are unlikely to be met, older adults with malnutrition, or those at risk of malnutrition and with chronic conditions, should be offered ONS.
- In older persons with active treatment goals, enteral tube feeding should be considered where oral intake is expected to be below half of energy requirements for more than 1 week or absent for more than 3 days.
- Where aligned with treatment goals and expected benefit, older adults should be offered PN where combined oral and enteral tube intake is expected to be impossible for more than 3 days or below half of energy requirements for more than 1 week.

References

1. Druml C, Ballmer PE, Druml W, Oehmichen F, Shenkin A, Singer P et al (2016) ESPEN guideline on ethical aspects of artificial nutrition and hydration. Clin Nutr 35(3):545–556
2. National Institute for Health and Clinical Excellence (NICE) (2006) Nutrition support in adults: oral nutrition support, enteral tube feeding and parenteral nutrition (clinical guideline 32)
3. Bell JJ, Young A, Hill J, Banks M, Comans T, Barnes R et al (2018) Rationale and developmental methodology for the SIMPLE approach: a Systematised, Interdisciplinary Malnutrition Pathway for impLementation and Evaluation in hospitals. Nutr Diet 75(2):226–234
4. Volkert D, Beck AM, Cederholm T, Cruz-Jentoft A, Goisser S, Hooper L et al (2019) ESPEN guideline on clinical nutrition and hydration in geriatrics. Clin Nutr 38(1):10–47
5. Volkert D, Beck AM, Cederholm T, Cereda E, Cruz-Jentoft A, Goisser S et al (2019) Management of malnutrition in older patients-current approaches, evidence and open questions. J Clin Med 8(7):974
6. Swan WI, Vivanti A, Hakel-Smith NA, Hotson B, Orrevall Y, Trostler N et al (2017) Nutrition care process and model update: toward realizing people-centered care and outcomes management. J Acad Nutr Diet 117(12):2003–2014
7. Cederholm T, Barazzoni R, Austin P, Ballmer P, Biolo G, Bischoff SC et al (2017) ESPEN guidelines on definitions and terminology of clinical nutrition. Clin Nutr 36(1):49–64
8. Mueller C, Compher C, Ellen DM (2011) A.S.P.E.N. clinical guidelines: nutrition screening, assessment, and intervention in adults. J Parenter Enter Nutr 35(1):16–24
9. Tappenden KA, Quatrara B, Parkhurst ML, Malone AM, Fanjiang G, Ziegler TR (2013) Critical role of nutrition in improving quality of care: an interdisciplinary call to action to address adult hospital malnutrition. J Parenter Enter Nutr 37(4):482–497
10. Feinberg J, Nielsen EE, Korang SK, Halberg Engell K, Nielsen MS, Zhang K et al (2017) Nutrition support in hospitalised adults at nutritional risk. Cochrane Database Syst Rev 5:CD011598
11. Stratton RJ, Elia M (2007) A review of reviews: a new look at the evidence for oral nutritional supplements in clinical practice. Clin Nutr Suppl 2(1):5–23
12. Boullata JI, Carrera AL, Harvey L, Escuro AA, Hudson L, Mays A et al (2017) ASPEN safe practices for enteral nutrition therapy [Formula: see text]. JPEN J Parenter Enteral Nutr 41(1):15–103
13. King PC, Barrimore SE, Pulle RC, Bell JJ (2019) "I Wouldn't Ever Want It": a qualitative evaluation of patient and caregiver perceptions toward enteral tube feeding in hip fracture inpatients. J Parenter Enter Nutr 43(4):526–533
14. Barry MJ, Edgman-Levitan S (2012) Shared decision making — the pinnacle of patient-centered care. N Engl J Med 366(9):780–781
15. Mon AS, Pulle C, Bell J (2018) Development of an 'Enteral tube feeding decision support tool' for hip fracture patients: a modified Delphi approach. Aust J Ageing 37(3):217–223
16. Bell JJ, Geirsdóttir ÓG, Hertz K, Santy-Tomlinson J, Skúladóttir SS, Eleuteri S et al (2020) Nutritional care of the older patient with fragility fracture: opportunities for systematised, interdisciplinary approaches across acute care, rehabilitation and secondary prevention settings. In: Orthogeriatrics. Springer, Cham, pp 311–329

17. McCray S, Maunder K, Barsha L, Mackenzie-Shalders K (2018) Room service in a public hospital improves nutritional intake and increases patient satisfaction while decreasing food waste and cost. J Hum Nutr Dietet 31(6):734–741
18. Bell JJ, Bauer J, Capra S, Pulle CR (2013) Barriers to nutritional intake in patients with acute hip fracture: time to treat malnutrition as a disease and food as a medicine? Can J Physiol Pharmacol 91(6):489–495
19. Milanchi S, Wilson MT (2008) Malposition of percutaneous endoscopic-guided gastrostomy: guideline and management. J Minim Access Surg 4(1):1–4
20. ESPEN Webinar Enteral accesses for enteral nutrition in adults . Nutrition E. Enteral Nutrition, Adults and Adolescents (>15 yr) (2021). https://www.google.com/search?rlz=1C1GCEA_enIS778IS778&sxsrf=ALeKk03SJdw8ztTt7iOiQgPqyzRkci_3g:1625224667813&q=Nutrition+E.+Enteral+Nutrition,+Adults+and+Adolescents+(%3E15+yr).+2021;(November+2018).&spell=1&sa=X&ved=2ahUKEwiegIXYocTxAhUygv0HHcGsBDUQBSgAegQIARAz&biw=1280&bih=577. November 2018.
21. Bischoff SC, Austin P, Boeykens K, Chourdakis M, Cuerda C, Jonkers-Schuitema C et al (2020) ESPEN guideline on home enteral nutrition. Clin Nutr 39(1):5–22
22. Gkolfakis P, Arvanitakis M, Despott EJ, Ballarin A, Beyna T, Boeykens K et al (2021) Endoscopic management of enteral tubes in adult patients - Part 2: Peri- and post-procedural management. European Society of Gastrointestinal Endoscopy (ESGE) Guideline. Endoscopy 53(2):178–195
23. Torsy T, Saman R, Boeykens K, Duysburgh I, Van Damme N, Beeckman D (2018) Comparison of two methods for estimating the tip position of a nasogastric feeding tube: a randomized controlled trial. Nutr Clin Pract 33(6):843–850
24. Matthews-Rensch K, Capra S, Palmer M (2021) Systematic review of energy initiation rates and refeeding syndrome outcomes. Nutr Clin Pract 36(1):153–168

6

Best Practice Nursing in Geriatrics: Role of Nutrition Care

Lina Spirgienė, Gytė Damulevičienė, Gabriele Bales and Jack J. Bell

Abstract

Evidence-based guidelines, recommendations and standards are considered the cornerstone of 'best practice' in nursing care. However, what optimal nutrition care of older adults actually looks like in real-world settings is also dependent on age, disease and care contexts and, perhaps most importantly, what matters to the older adult.

This chapter is a component of Part I: Nutritional Care in Old Age.
For an explanation of the grouping of chapters in this book, please see Chap. 1: 'Geriatrics and Orthogeriatrics: Providing Nutrition Care'.

L. Spirgienė (✉)
Department of Nursing and Care, Faculty of Nursing, Medical Academy, Lithuanian University of Health Sciences, Kaunas, Lithuania
e-mail: lina.spirgiene@lsmuni.lt

G. Damulevičienė
Department of Geriatrics, Lithuanian University of Health Sciences, LT, Kaunas, Lithuania
e-mail: gyte.damuleviciene@lsmuni.lt

G. Bales
Advanced Practice Nurse, University Department of Geriatric Medicine Felix Platter, Basel, Switzerland
e-mail: gabriele.bales@felixplatter.ch

J. J. Bell (✉)
Allied Health, The Prince Charles Hospital, Chermside, Queensland, Australia

School of Human Movement and Nutrition Sciences, The University of Queensland, St Lucia, QLD, Australia
e-mail: jack.bell@health.qld.gov.au

Keywords

Nurses · Nursing staff · Malnutrition · Nutritional support · Older adults · Professional role

Learning Outcomes
At the end of the chapter, the reader will be able to:

- Describe why 'best practice' nursing care should consider individualised nutrition care actions across age, disease and care setting spectra.
- List key opportunities for nurses to coordinate, lead, deliver and evaluate supportive nutrition care processes.

Aunty Esther lived on a small island in the Torres Strait. Aunty was fit and healthy across her early adult years, living a traditional lifestyle including growing and harvesting local fruits and vegetables, fishing and collecting shellfish. However, over the years, as the island became progressively 'westernised', Aunty's diet changed, she reduced her exercise, and she consequently gained weight. By the time she had reached her early 50s, Aunty had developed obesity (class 3), type 2 diabetes, chronic kidney disease and heart disease. Aunty did not want to leave the island for any medical care and instead chose to entrust her healthcare to Mia, the community nurse. Over the next decade, Aunty and Mia worked together to manage her multiple conditions with a 'diet-only' approach, in line with Aunty's treatment preferences. In her mid-60s, Aunty essentially stopped eating for several months after her two sons were lost at sea. With support and care from nurse Mia, Aunty eventually recovered some of her lost muscle stores and enjoyed living with her granddaughter and extended family until her early 70s. Following a severe stroke, Aunty was cared for by her family and nurse Mia for a short time before she passed away, sitting outside on her woven coconut mat, surrounded by those she loved. Aunty Esther was proud to have never left her island home, and the only healthcare she ever consented to was provided by Mia, the community nurse.

6.1 What Is 'Best Practice' Nursing Nutrition Care?

Best practice is characterised as 'directive, evidence-based and quality-focused' care [1]; surrogate terms and related concepts include optimal care, evidence-based guidelines and practice, practice development and standards of care [1, 2]. To achieve best practice in nutrition care in older adults, evidence-based guidelines, recommendations and standards of care should underpin patient-focused care that is implemented into daily nursing practice [1]. Across global settings, evidence-based guidelines and care standards that are relevant and appropriate to direct care in multimorbid older adults may be absent, competing or even contradictory. What is 'optimal care' will also need to consider the value of healthcare, which is defined primarily by care that matters to the older adult, with consideration given to the resources required to provide that care, in addition to diverse other barriers and enablers to care [3, 4]. As highlighted in Chap. 1, best practice should also support transitioning towards transdisciplinary care approaches, where [1] traditional professional boundaries are transcended; [2] knowledge, skills and accountabilities are integrated and shared; and [3] the focus is on solving real-world, complex nutrition problems, in partnership with the older adult and those who care for them [5].

How does this apply to nursing best practice in nutrition care? In many settings, nutrition specialists, for example, dietitians, medical nutrition specialists and nutrition support nurse practitioners, have been considered best *qualified* to deliver nutrition care processes [6, 7]. A recent systematic review has demonstrated that nurses can safely provide oral nutritional supplements, food or fluid fortification or enrichment, give education and dietary counselling to geriatric patients and patients' carers and administer nutrition care across professions; as such nurses are well placed to support essential processes of nutrition care to older adults [8]. As highlighted in our case study above, nurses are often best *positioned* to lead, coordinate and/or deliver 'best practice' nutrition care processes (Chap. 1) [9]. However, we also suggest that nurses should not be required to do this in isolation; for our case study above, in all but the most under-resourced settings, it would be important for nurse Mia to be embedded in a broader interdisciplinary team including medical and nutrition specialists.

Our case example builds on previous chapters highlighting that the spectrum and progression of nutrition care is evolving and can range from dietary management of lifestyle diseases to preventing, screening, identifying and managing malnutrition or other nutrition-related conditions and, ultimately, caring for those in the last stages of life by supporting food and fluids for comfort. It highlights that what should be defined as 'best practice' changes over the course of life and disease processes and fundamentally should be measured by delivering care that matters to the patient [10]. This emphasises a key point; in older, multimorbid adults, the actual individual care provided will at times be different to nutrient or disease-specific treatment recommendations endorsed by individual professions, societies or nations particularly where these have not been co-designed with culturally diverse, multimorbid, older adults.

Globally, nurses support coordination of patient-centric care processes across aging, disease and care setting spectra that require tailoring of care to the individual patient [11]. Nurses are highly attuned to individual patient's care needs and preferences; have highly developed skills in working across disciplines, systems and healthcare settings; and routinely translate evidence-based guidelines and recommendations into best practice, patient-centred care. A pivotal role for nursing is also to manage care conflicts and unrealistic expectations, whether these are directed from older adults and carers or individuals and teams caring for them [12]. Nurses actively support shared decision-making and goal setting and are well placed to observe where previous goals or care recommendations require review and recognise and encourage specialist care [re]referral where this is appropriate [13]. Finally, in many settings globally, nurses are firmly established in clinical, policy, education and research leadership, governance and advocacy roles [14].

We consequently propose that nurses are well connected, brokering interdisciplinary team members, who are particularly well placed to coordinate, lead and deliver 'best practice' nutrition care processes and improvements.

6.2 Leading Supportive Nutrition Care for Older Adults with or at Risk of Malnutrition: An Example of Best Practice in Nursing Care

Nutrition care screening pathways exist that support triaging malnutrition care according to nutrition risk screening outcomes [15–17]. One example is the Systematised, Interdisciplinary Malnutrition Program for impLementation and Evaluation (SIMPLE) [15]. This approach triages screening three risk categories: standard, supportive or specialised nutrition care. What 'supportive' nutrition care processes look like should ultimately be determined by local teams with consideration to patient- and context-specific factors; this should consider different stages of nutrition care process models applied internationally (Fig. 6.1) [15–19]. Across settings, enabling systematised, interdisciplinary 'supportive' nutrition care processes

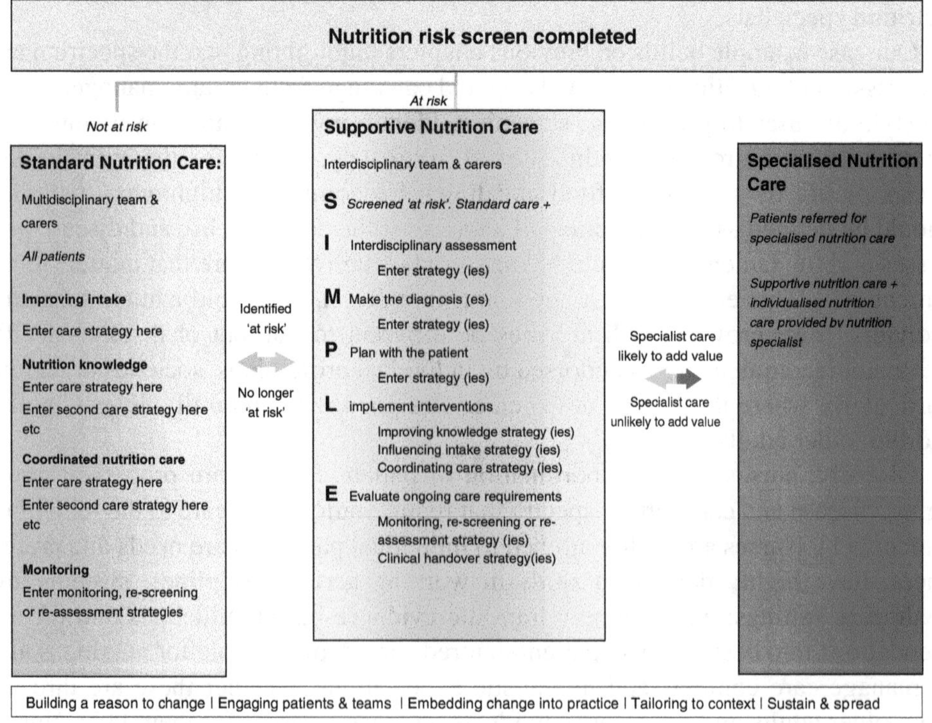

Fig. 6.1 A SIMPLE approach to supportive nutrition care [9]

where appropriate, rather than relying on specialist care delivery, has demonstrated improved and sustained patient-reported nutrition experience measures and healthcare outcomes, whilst simultaneously directing specialist resources to where they are most urgently required [20–22].

Take-Home Checklist

- Table 6.1 provides a supportive nutrition care checklist for older adults with or at risk of malnutrition [15, 18, 19, 23]. We note that each and every one of these will not necessarily provide a useful grounding point for nurses aspiring to lead, coordinate and model best practice supportive nutrition care in older adults.

Table 6.1 Supportive nutrition care checklist for older adults with or at risk of malnutrition [9, 15, 18, 19, 23]

Service and setting level
• Evidence-based guidelines, care standards, accreditation processes, policies and operating procedures guide interdisciplinary nutrition and hydration care for older adults
• Interdisciplinary nutrition care committees meet regularly with regularly reviewed terms of reference and supporting governance processes
• Nutrition support teams or specialists are accessible to refer for specialist nutrition care
• On presentation and repeat nutrition screening, processes are embedded applying validated instruments; these should be audited and reported at least annually
• Social care and facility foodservices systems support timely access to safe, high-quality, nutrient-dense food choices in line with older adult requirements, individual and sociocultural preferences and preferred eating times
• Fortified food and additional snacks or finger food are available to support adequate dietary intake
• In longer-stay healthcare and home care facility settings, food intake shall be supported by a home-like, pleasant dining environment to support adequate dietary intake and maintain quality of life
• High-quality, aesthetically pleasing texture-modified, enriched foods are available for those with chewing problems or signs of oropharyngeal dysphagia
• Processes are established and audited that avoid or minimise nil by mouth and restrictive diets associated with surgery, procedures or tests
• Patient-reported nutrition experience measures (nPREMS) and outcomes measures (PROMs) guide provision of care and care improvements
• Processes are enacted to identify, document and benchmark nutrition-related complications (e.g. hospital-acquired malnutrition, falls, pressure injuries, skin tears and wound dehiscence)
• Nutrition education and curriculum are embedded in interdisciplinary healthcare professional training, orientation and re-entry processes
Individual-level audits, documentation and/or patient-reported experience measures demonstrate:
• Interdisciplinary team members deliver multicomponent supportive nutrition care processes
• Older adults or carers of those screened at risk report awareness of risk status when audited
• Specific supportive nutrition care processes actioned at point of screening
• ABCDEF approach to nutrition assessment (anthropometric, biochemistry, clinical, dietary, environmental and psychosocial and functional variables)
• Key nutrition assessment metrics (e.g. height, weight, BMI) recorded within specified timeframes
• Nutrition diagnoses (e.g. malnutrition) recorded within specified timeframes

(continued)

Table 6.1 (continued)

• Malnutrition-related hospital-acquired complications identification and intervention (e.g. malnutrition, pressure injury, skin tear, fall, delirium) • All at-risk or malnourished older adults, or their caregivers where appropriate, report receiving individualised nutritional information and education • Shared nutrition goal setting and multimodal interventions • Medicine and supplement (prescribed or self-prescribed) review to support nutrition care and limit adverse drug-nutrient and food-drug interactions • Pre-meal toileting, mealtime positioning and eating environment support enjoyment of meals • Adequate time to eat, encouragement and assistance with meals where required • Mealtime assistance, encouragement and support provided by interdisciplinary healthcare providers, volunteers, family, friends and carers • High levels of older adult satisfaction with meals and mealtimes • Low levels of food waste • Oral nutritional supplements (ONS) or enteral or parenteral nutrition is offered where food fortification and dietary counselling are not sufficient to meet nutrition requirements, and these align with shared goals and treatment intent • Prescribed diets and nutritional supplements reviewed and deprescribed where appropriate • Clinical handover and integration of nutrition care across care settings

References

1. Nelson AM (2014) Best practice in nursing: a concept analysis. Int J Nurs Stud 51(11): 1507–1516
2. DiMaria-Ghalili RA, Gilbert K, Lord L, Neal T, Richardson D, Tyler R et al (2016) Standards of nutrition care practice and professional performance for nutrition support and generalist nurses. Nutr Clin Pract 31(4):527–547
3. Teisberg E, Wallace S, O'Hara S (2020) Defining and implementing value-based health care: a strategic framework. Acad Med 95(5):682–685
4. Grol R, Grimshaw J (2003) From best evidence to best practice: effective implementation of change in patients' care. Lancet (Lond, Engl) 362(9391):1225–1230
5. Van Bewer V (2017) Transdisciplinarity in health care: a concept analysis. Nurs Forum 52(4):339–347
6. DiMaria-Ghalili RA, Gilbert K, Lord L, Neal T, Richardson D, Tyler R et al (2016) Standards of nutrition care practice and professional performance for nutrition support and generalist nurses. Nutr Clin Pract 31(4):527–547
7. Writing Group of the Nutrition Care Process/Standardized Language Committee (2008) Nutrition care process and model part I: the 2008 update. J Am Diet Assoc 108(7):1113–1117
8. ten Cate D, Ettema RGA, Huisman-de Waal G, Bell JJ, Verbrugge R, Schoonhoven L et al (2020) Interventions to prevent and treat malnutrition in older adults to be carried out by nurses: a systematic review. J Clin Nurs 29(11–12):1883–1902
9. Bell JJ, Geirsdóttir ÓG, Hertz K, Santy-Tomlinson J, Skúladóttir SS, Eleuteri S et al (2020) Nutritional care of the older patient with fragility fracture: opportunities for systematised, interdisciplinary approaches across acute care, rehabilitation and secondary prevention settings. In: Orthogeriatrics. Springer, Cham, pp 311–329
10. Kingsley C, Patel S (2017) Patient-reported outcome measures and patient-reported experience measures. BJA Educ 17(4):137–144
11. Kitson A, Marshall A, Bassett K, Zeitz K (2013) What are the core elements of patient-centred care? A narrative review and synthesis of the literature from health policy, medicine and nursing. J Adv Nurs 69(1):4–15
12. Johansen ML (2012) Keeping the peace: conflict management strategies for nurse managers. Nurs Manag 43(2):50
13. Truglio-Londrigan M, Slyer JT (2018) Shared decision-making for nursing practice: an integrative review. Open Nurs J 12:1–14

14. Heinen M, van Oostveen C, Peters J, Vermeulen H, Huis A (2019) An integrative review of leadership competencies and attributes in advanced nursing practice. J Adv Nurs 75(11):2378–2392
15. Bell JJ, Young A, Hill J, Banks M, Comans T, Barnes R et al (2018) Rationale and developmental methodology for the SIMPLE approach: a Systematised, Interdisciplinary Malnutrition Pathway for impLementation and Evaluation in hospitals. Nutr Dietet 75(2):226–234
16. Keller H, Laur C, Atkins M, Bernier P, Butterworth D, Davidson B et al (2018) Update on the Integrated Nutrition Pathway for Acute Care (INPAC): post implementation tailoring and toolkit to support practice improvements. Nutr J 17(1):1–6
17. Elia M (2003) Screening for malnutrition: a multidisciplinary responsibility. In: Nutrition BAfPaE (ed) Development and use of the Malnutrition Universal Screening Tool (MUST) for adults. BAPEN, Redditch
18. Swan WI, Vivanti A, Hakel-Smith NA, Hotson B, Orrevall Y, Trostler N et al (2017) Nutrition care process and model update: toward realizing people-centered care and outcomes management. J Acad Nutr Diet 117(12):2003–2014
19. Cederholm T, Barazzoni R, Austin P, Ballmer P, Biolo G, Bischoff SC et al (2017) ESPEN guidelines on definitions and terminology of clinical nutrition. Clin Nutr 36(1):49–64
20. Bell JJ, Bauer JD, Capra S, Pulle RC (2014) Multidisciplinary, multi-modal nutritional care in acute hip fracture inpatients - results of a pragmatic intervention. Clin Nutr 33(6):1101–1107
21. Bell Jack J, Young Adrienne M, Hill J, Banks MD, Comans T, Barnes R (2021) Systematised, Interdisciplinary Malnutrition Program for impLementation and Evaluation (SIMPLE) delivers improved hospital nutrition care processes and patient reported experiences – an implementation study. Nutr Diet. Early view: https://doi.org/10.1111/1747-0080.12663
22. Keller H, Koechl JM, Laur C, Chen H, Curtis L, Dubin JA et al (2021) More-2-Eat implementation demonstrates that screening, assessment and treatment of malnourished patients can be spread and sustained in acute care; a multi-site, pretest post-test time series study. Clin Nutr 40:2100
23. Volkert D, Beck AM, Cederholm T, Cruz-Jentoft A, Goisser S, Hooper L et al (2019) ESPEN guideline on clinical nutrition and hydration in geriatrics. Clin Nutr 38(1):10–47

7

Geriatrics and Orthogeriatrics: Hydration and Dehydration

Vilborg Kolbrún Vilmundardóttir
and Sigrún Sunna Skúladóttir

Abstract

Previous chapters have described nutritional care in geriatrics and orthogeriatrics in detail, including special focus on malnutrition and best practice in nursing care. This chapter will focus on recommendations and guidelines for hydration, fluid intake and intravenous fluid therapy in geriatrics and orthogeriatrics.

Keywords

Fluid therapy · Water-electrolyte balance · Dehydration · Practice guidelines · Older adults

This chapter is a component of Part I: Nutritional Care in Old Age.
For an explanation of the grouping of chapters in this book, please see Chap. 1: 'Geriatrics and Orthogeriatrics: Providing Nutrition Care'.

V. K. Vilmundardóttir (✉)
The Faculty of Food Science and Nutrition, School of Health Sciences, University of Iceland, Reykjavik, Iceland
e-mail: vkv2@hi.is

S. S. Skúladóttir
The Faculty of Food Science and Nutrition, School of Health Sciences, University of Iceland, Reykjavik, Iceland

The Faculty of Nurse, School of Health Sciences, University of Iceland, Reykjavik, Iceland
e-mail: sss37@hi.is

Learning Outcomes
By the end of this chapter, you will be able to:

- Recognise and apply evidence-based recommendations and guidelines for hydration, fluid intake and intravenous fluid therapy for geriatric and orthogeriatric patients in hospital and outpatient settings, residential aged care and community living.
- Recognise age-related changes that influence hydration and fluid intake in older adults.
- Distinguish between the two subcategories of dehydration (low-intake dehydration and volume depletion).
- Implement best practice to screen for, assess and reassess dehydration and fluid balance at all stages in hospital.
- Implement best practice to treat dehydration and other hydration disturbances at all stages in hospital.

7.1 Geriatric Orthopaedic Patients

Geriatric orthopaedic patients are an especially frail and vulnerable group, considered at risk of being both dehydrated and malnourished [1–3]. Dehydration can have adverse health outcomes [4–7] (Table 7.1).

Adverse health outcomes (Table 7.1) can increase hospital-acquired complications and adverse events as well as the risk for readmission to hospital [4, 7]. This in turn can contribute to adverse outcomes and increased healthcare costs [4, 7, 8].

7.2 Hydration in Geriatrics

Proper hydration, where fluid intake and fluid losses are balanced, is a crucial component in maintaining bodily functions [9]. Hence, ensuring fluid intake that accounts for losses via urine, faeces, evaporation (lung and skin), wounds, surgery and medical procedures is essential. Fluid requirements are individualised, mainly based on caloric consumption, water losses and kidney capacity [6, 9]. In all settings, providing adequate amounts of fluid with drinks, nasogastrically,

Table 7.1 Adverse health outcomes commonly associated with dehydration

• Confusion	• Infections
• Constipation	• Longer stay in hospital
• Decreased quality of life	• Morbidity and mortality
• Delirium	• Pain
• Disability	• Pressure ulcers
• Drug toxicity	• Renal failure
• Falls and fractures	• Urinary tract infection
• Heart disease	

subcutaneously or intravenously to prevent dehydration whilst averting excessive amounts should be considered a priority.

7.2.1 Recommendations for Older Adults

Generally, an adequate intake (AI) of fluid for older adults is defined as 2.0 L/day for women and 2.5 L/day for men [6, 9]. Assuming 20% of fluids come from eating foods, this means women need at least 1.6 L/day of drinks and men 2.0 L/day. Clinical situations and environmental factors (i.e. higher temperatures) can change individual fluid needs, and in some patient groups, fluid restriction might be needed, e.g. those with heart failure or renal failure [5, 6]. For older adults that possibly need fluid restriction, an interdisciplinary approach is crucial to configure fluid requirements and timeframes of restrictions. It is important that older adults and interdisciplinary healthcare providers are able to identify fluids in both drinks and also foods (Table 7.2).

Drinks for older adults should include a range of different options, based on individual preferences [6]. There are many diverse drinks that provide fluids to the body, ranging from water, juices, milk-based supplements, smoothies, sports drinks, soups, tea or coffee and alcoholic beverages.

Offering a range of preferred drinks frequently during the day can improve total fluid intake and thus minimise the risk of dehydration [6]. Those at risk of malnutrition or malnourished should be offered energy- and/or protein-dense drinks, e.g. milk, milk-based drinks, smoothies or oral nutritional support (Chap. 5). Energy- and protein-dense drinks provide fluid as well as being an important source of energy, protein and nutrients. It is worthy to note that tea and coffee are both sources of fluid, but older patients should be encouraged to include other drinks throughout the day, thus possibly providing energy, protein and nutrients.

7.2.2 Age-Related Changes Associated with Hydration

Research indicates lower fluid intakes in older adults compared to younger groups, with different and interrelated causes [6, 8, 9]. Lower intakes are possibly explained

Table 7.2 Examples of amounts of fluid found in common drinks/foods

Food product	Portion size	Fluid (mL)
Whole milk (3.9%)	1 cup (250 mL)	220
Coffee/tea	1 cup (250 mL)	250
Apple juice	1 cup (250 mL)	220
Porridge	1 bowl (200 g)	180
Oral nutritional supplement drink	1 bottle (200 mL)	140
Yogurt	1 tub (200 g)	180
Boiled pasta/rice	1 bowl (200 g)	140
Boiled potatoes	3 small sized (150 g)	120

by physiological changes that occur with higher age, including decreases in kidney capacity and sense of thirst [6, 8]. Furthermore, total body water reduces with higher age, resulting in smaller fluid reserves. Medications also need consideration in this context, as many commonly used medications among older adults can encourage water losses, including diuretics and laxatives. Other potential causes include choosing to reduce drinking due to fear of incontinence and problems with getting to the bathroom; memory problems, i.e. forgetting to drink; social isolation; physical access to drinks; and problems with swallowing. Thus, all older adults are considered at risk of being dehydrated, needing special attention and encouragement when it comes to fluid intake [6, 9].

7.3 Dehydration and Other Hydration Disturbances

Undoubtedly, the main concern regarding hydration in older adults is dehydration, a commonly encountered problem in clinical situations, with reported prevalence among older adults in hospitals ranging from 4% to 58% [6].

Diagnosing dehydration is complex, due to differences in definitions and a wide range of possible causes [4, 6]. Generally, dehydration can be defined into two subcategories, based on whether a shortage of water is caused by low intake or excessive loss (Table 7.3).

Dehydration is associated with adverse outcomes in older adults, including increased morbidity and mortality, longer stay in hospital and increased risk of disability [4, 6]. Early diagnosis of dehydration in clinical settings is crucial, allowing for timely interventions and possibly prevention. Screening for low-intake dehydration and volume depletion (volume status) is recommended for all geriatric patients upon admission into hospital (Fig. 7.1).

7.3.1 Screening and Assessment of Dehydration

Underlying causes of dehydration can vary greatly, making screening and assessment in older adults complex [4, 6]. First and foremost assessment (and reassessment) should include detailed information on [4, 5]:

Table 7.3 Dehydration, as defined by ESPEN (the European Society for Clinical Nutrition and Metabolism) [6]

Dehydration: a shortage of water (fluid) in the body, caused by either insufficient intake of water (*low-intake dehydration*) or excessive loss of water (*volume depletion*) or combination of both
Low-intake dehydration: a shortage of water caused by low intake. Leads to loss of both intracellular and extracellular fluid, raises osmolality
Volume depletion: an excessive loss of water and salts caused by bleeding, fever, vomiting, diarrhoea or other causes. Leads to loss of extracellular fluid but not intracellular fluid, keeps osmolality normal or low

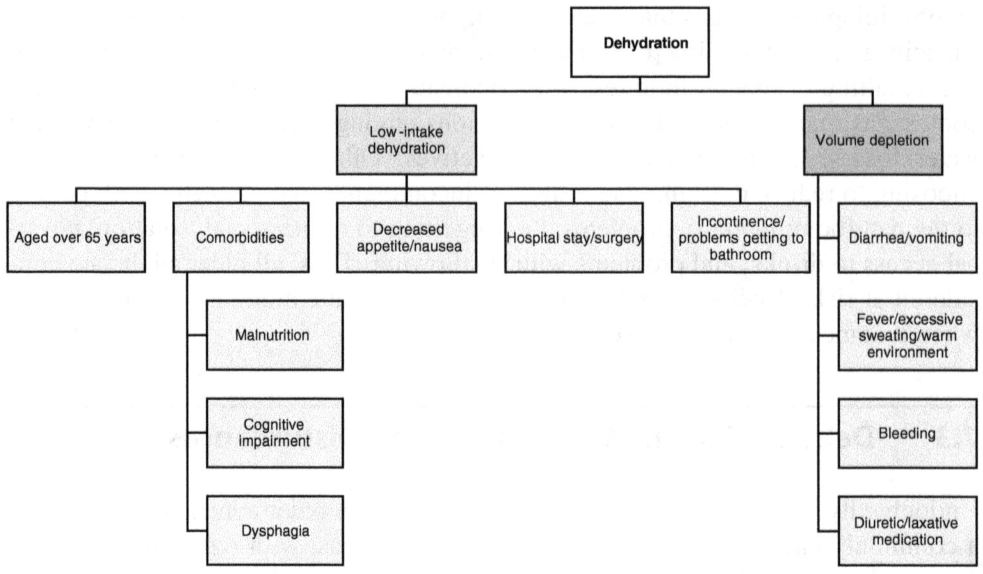

Fig. 7.1 Looking out for dehydration in older adults—red flags for nurses [1, 7, 10]

- Fluid intake history and abnormal losses
- Comorbidities (including malnutrition and refeeding syndrome)
- Clinical examination (pulse, blood pressure, capillary refill, jugular venous pressure, pulmonary or peripheral oedema, postural hypotension)
- Current medication
- Clinical measures (National Early Warning Score (NEWS), fluid balance charts and weight)
- Laboratory results (full blood count, urea, creatinine, electrolytes and osmolarity)

Systematically looking at the abovementioned factors, nurses can evaluate if older adults are at risk of dehydration/dehydrated and in turn consult with other healthcare providers, including but not limited to medical professionals and dietitians [4, 6].

7.3.1.1 Assessing Low-Intake Dehydration

In low-intake dehydration, the osmolality of fluid in the body is raised, as fluids are not replaced, whilst electrolytes are maintained [4, 6]. Based on this knowledge, the gold standard to both screen for and diagnose low-intake dehydration is direct measurement of serum/plasma osmolality (pOsm), using a threshold of >300 mOsm/kg. When direct measurement of osmolality is not available, the osmolarity equation ($pOsmc = 1.86 \times (Na^{+} + K^{+}) + 1.15 \times glucose + urea + 14$, all measured in mmol/L) should be used for diagnosis, using a threshold of >295 mmol/L [11].

Traditionally a diagnosis of low-intake dehydration has been based on clinical assessment; however, in a recently published consensus on dehydration, Lacey et al. point out a lack of evidence for this approach in the literature [4]. Thus, using simple measures such as skin turgor, mouth dryness, weight change, urine colour or specific gravity to assess dehydration is not recommended, due to the inaccurate nature of these measures [4, 6]. Measures shown to mildly correlate to low-intake dehydration, although having low diagnostic value, include expressions of fatigue, observed reduction in fluid oral intake and bioelectrical impedance analysis.

7.3.1.2 Assessing Volume Depletion

Irrespective of measured serum/plasma osmolality, all patients should be assessed for volume status [4, 5]. According to NICE (National Institute for Health and Care Excellence) guidelines on intravenous fluid therapy in adults in hospital, using the following indicators of volume depletion to assess the need for intravenous fluid therapy is recommended:

- Systolic blood pressure <100 mmHg
- Heart rate >90 beats per minute
- Capillary refill time >2 s/peripheries cold to touch
- Respiratory rate >20 breaths per minute
- National Early Warning Score (NEWS) ≥5
- Passive leg raising, suggesting fluid responsiveness

Volume depletion following excessive blood loss can be assessed using postural pulse change from lying to standing of ≥30 beats per minute or by observing severe dizziness, resulting in inability to stand [4, 6]. Volume depletion in patients suffering from vomiting or diarrhoea can be assessed using the following set of signs (with ≥4 out of 7 indicating depletion):

- Confusion
- Non-fluent speech
- Extremity weakness
- Dry mucous membranes
- Dry tongue
- Furrowed tongue
- Sunken eyes

7.3.2 Prevention and Treatment of Dehydration

7.3.2.1 Low-Intake Dehydration

Geriatric patients at risk or diagnosed with low-intake dehydration should be encouraged to increase fluid intake by offering drinks of different choices frequently, and fluid balance should be reassessed frequently [2, 4, 6]. For patients having difficulties with drinking, subcutaneous or intravenous fluids should be considered along with encouraging increased fluid intake. As for patients unable to drink, intravenous fluids should be considered.

Important factors in increasing fluid intake include:

- Goal setting and policies by hospitals and geriatric wards regarding fluid intake.
- Staff awareness and support for drinking.
- Educating patients on the importance of drinking.
- Recording individual preferences for drinks.
- Proactive offering of preferred drinks to patients.
- Taking patients to the toilet as quickly as possible when needed.
- Considering physical and visual limitations of patients (e.g. sport bottles to prevent spilling or using bright-coloured cups for visibility).
- Assessment of swallowing, providing relevant treatment to patients with signs of dysphagia.

7.3.2.2 Volume Depletion

Whilst focusing on underlying causes and trying to minimise fluid loss, geriatric patients at risk or diagnosed with volume depletion should routinely receive isotonic fluids orally (via rehydration therapy), nasogastrically, subcutaneously or intravenously [4–6]. Aiming to replace lost water and electrolytes, patients with severe depletion should routinely receive intravenous fluid therapy immediately, whilst those with milder depletion should have their needs met orally or enterally when possible and appropriate.

7.3.3 Fluid Overload

Excessive fluid intake can result in fluid overload, a state where intake exceeds renal or cardiac capacity, possibly resulting in life-threatening hyponatremia, renal failure and/or heart failure [2, 5]. Main risk factors for fluid overload include decreased renal and/or cardiac function, surgery and receiving intravenous fluid therapy. Thus, fluid intake and output should be closely monitored, especially in patients receiving intravenous fluid therapy.

7.3.4 Electrolyte Imbalances

Imbalances in serum sodium levels are commonly diagnosed in geriatric and especially orthogeriatric patients and should be monitored [5, 12]. Both hyponatremia (low sodium levels, <135 mmol/L) and hypernatremia (high sodium levels, >145 mmol/L) can have severe consequences and have been associated with falls, delirium, increased length of stay and increased 30-day mortality.

Serum potassium levels should be monitored in patients receiving intravenous fluid therapy, due to increased risk of either hypokalaemia (<3.0 mmol/L) or hyperkalaemia (>5.5 mmol/L) [5].

7.4 Hospitalisation After Fall

7.4.1 Arriving at the Emergency Department

Joe is an 84-year-old man who slipped when he was walking in his apartment this morning. He couldn't stand up, so his wife Julie called an ambulance. Physical examination shows his left leg to be shorter and externally rotated and he is in a lot of pain. Arriving at the ED, he is categorised as possibly having a hip fracture and therefore he is instructed to fast.

In many settings, including this case example hospital, older orthopaedic patients arriving at the emergency department (ED) after falling are fasted until diagnosis is established, in case an operation is needed [13].

As soon as diagnosis is established, assessment of fluid needs, fluid balance and the need of intravenous fluid therapy is needed; these should be guided by local procedural documentation considerate of recommendations and guidelines such as those described above. Any signs of volume depletion indicate that urgent fluid is needed, and recommendations highlight the importance of starting intravenous fluid therapy as soon as possible after arrival at the ED or possibly in the ambulance [3, 5, 13]. According to A Guide to Improving the Care of Fragility Fractures, it is critical to start early rehydration at the ED, using isotonic crystalloids [3]. Starting dehydration prevention at the beginning of the stay at the ED is a crucial component of treatment and has been shown to increase survival rates.

Joe has been at the ED for 2 h and has already gone to radiography, after which he was diagnosed with a hip fracture. Joe thinks he is lucky because he has a lovely nurse, Margareth, who has given him morphine for the pain. She has told him that he needs an operation to fix his fracture. Before Joe fell this morning, he hadn't eaten breakfast, and now Margareth has told him he can't eat before the operation and he will need intravenous fluid. However, due to Margareth having five other patients, she has not yet managed to put up his fluid.

7.4.2 Preoperation Nursing at the Ward

After a decision has been made according to admission and the patient is moved to a ward, fluid balance should be reassessed and appropriate treatment ensured [13]; again these should be informed by local processes considerate of recommendations and guidelines such as those described above (Sects. 7.3.1 and 7.3.2). When an operation is needed, knowing approximately at what time the operation will be is important as decreasing the fasting time of the patient as much as possible is recommended [13].

Joe doesn't feel so bad now that the morphine is working and he can even fall asleep from time to time. Margareth has told him that he will be moved to the orthopaedic ward, where she hands him over to the nurses and forgets to talk about his need for fluid therapy.

Geriatric patients are commonly dehydrated, and the risk of dehydration is increased during hospital stay [3, 6, 13]. Thus, when drinking is allowed, nurses and nursing staff should create an opportunity for the patient to drink, offering preferred drinks proactively at each contact with the patient. Generally, across many settings patients may have solids until 6 h before surgery and approved preoperative oral fluids until 2 h before surgery and then be placed nil by mouth until surgery [13, 14]. However, fasting guidelines vary according to types of surgery performed, different patient cohorts and the patient's individual circumstances, and we recommend local interdisciplinary teams work together to implement procedures and processes to safely minimise fasting times.

The nurse who is now taking care of Joe also has a lot of tasks to do, but it suddenly crosses her mind why he doesn't have intravenous fluid. Joe hasn't called the nurse, as he doesn't feel so bad when lying completely still in bed. The nurse previously told him that the operation would be soon. Finally, the theatre call the ward and say that they are ready to operate on Joe. The nurse now hangs up intravenous fluid, but it's now been 8 h since he fell and almost 16 h since he last ate or drank.

Correcting/preventing fluid imbalance, such as volume depletion and electrolyte disturbances that can affect comorbidities, is crucial before operation [5]. For this patient group, fluid overload is also a risk, possibly causing heart failure, peripheral oedema and hemodynamic imbalance, increasing the risk of delaying operation and/or complications post-operation.

7.4.3 Post-operation Nursing at the Ward

When a patient is moved from theatre to the ward, fluid balance should be reassessed and appropriate treatment ensured [15]; again this should be guided by locally developed, evidence-informed procedures and processes.

After operation, oral hydration and nutrition should be started as soon as possible, aiming to fulfil both fluid and nutritional needs [2, 4, 5, 15]. Regular reassessment of fluid balance should be provided during hospital stay.

Case example: Joe's operation went well, but when he arrives back at the orthopaedic ward, he is having hallucinations. He is in delirium and refuses to drink because he thinks the nurses are trying to poison him. He then tries to take the IV catheter from his hand. At further examination Joe is also diagnosed with acute kidney injury, and his vital signs show low blood pressure and a high pulse.

Special considerations post-operation should be given to:

Delirium: a threatening risk factor for geriatric and orthogeriatric patients, who are at high risk of delirium as they are older than 65 years and some have current hip fracture, two of the major risk factors for delirium [13, 16] (Chap. 19). Interventions to prevent delirium are recommended, including prevention and treatment of dehydration and frequent assessment of fluid balance.

Acute kidney injury (AKI): a major complication, sometimes associated with dehydration [4, 5]. Risk factors for AKI include age higher than 65 years, having acute surgery (i.e. orthopaedic surgery) and use of NSAIDs medicine. Monitoring signs of oliguria is recommended (less than 0.5 mL/kg/h of urine in more than 6 h, raised serum creatinine and 25% fall in glomerular filtration rate).

7.4.4 Best Practice at the Ward

Nurses and other staff members should follow recommendations and clinical guidelines regarding hydration, fluid balance and intravenous fluid therapy at all stages in hospital, including rehabilitation and at hospital discharge [2, 5, 15]. Preoperative carbohydrate drinks are considered to be harmless and have possible benefits on fluid balance; such drinks can be used up to 2 h before operation, thus possibly preventing dehydration, as well as allowing for early treatment, minimising the risk of adverse outcomes [17, 18].

Rewriting Joe's story in the best way, he would have been given an IVF in the ambulance the way to the hospital. Margareth, the ED nurse, would have screened for risk of dehydration, set up fasting clock to manage his fasting time and put up a fluid therapy plan for him as well as evaluated his fluid balance. The orthopaedic nurse would have checked the time plan in theatre for Joe and re-evaluated his fluid balance when he arrived at the ward and accordingly constructed a treatment plan, as well as given him a pre-op carbohydrate drink. Would this be the case, Joe may have been less likely to have developed delirium and avoided consequent preventable harm.

7.5 Summary

All hospitalised geriatric patients should be screened and assessed for dehydration, and frequent reassessment of fluid balance is recommended. Dehydration can be defined into two subcategories, based on whether a shortage of water is caused by low intake or excessive loss. Offering preferred drinks frequently to patients in a proactive way is encouraged at all stages in hospital, and fasting time before operation should be minimised. Frequent reassessment of fluid balance is key to assessing the need for fluid intake and/or intravenous fluid therapy at all stages.

Take-Home Points

- Geriatric and orthogeriatric patients are at high risk of dehydration.
- Dehydration and fluid balance should be assessed frequently during hospital stay, allowing for early detection, treatment and possibly prevention.
- Evidence-based recommendations and guidelines for hydration, fluid intake and intravenous fluid therapy should be applied at all stages in hospital.

References

1. Volkert D, Beck AM, Cederholm T, Cruz-Jentoft A, Goisser S, Hooper L et al (2019) ESPEN guideline on clinical nutrition and hydration in geriatrics. Clin Nutr 38(1):10–47
2. Meehan AJ, Maher AB, Brent L, Copanitsanou P, Cross J, Kimber C et al (2019) The International Collaboration of Orthopaedic Nursing (ICON): best practice nursing care standards for older adults with fragility hip fracture. Int J Orthop Trauma Nurs 32:3–26
3. Mears SC, Kates SL (2015) A guide to improving the care of patients with fragility fractures, Edition 2. Geriatr Orthop Surg Rehabil 6(2):58–120
4. Lacey J, Corbett J, Forni L, Hooper L, Hughes F, Minto G et al (2019) A multidisciplinary consensus on dehydration: definitions, diagnostic methods and clinical implications. Ann Med 51(3–4):232–251
5. National Institute for Health and Care Excellence (2013) Intravenous fluid therapy in adults in hospital [CG174]. https://www.nice.org.uk/guidance/cg174
6. Volkert D, Beck AM, Cederholm T, Cruz-Jentoft A, Goisser S, Hooper L et al (2019) ESPEN guideline on clinical nutrition and hydration in geriatrics. Clin Nutr 38(1):10–47
7. Hooper L, Abdelhamid A, Attreed NJ, Campbell WW, Channell AM, Chassagne P et al (2015) Clinical symptoms, signs and tests for identification of impending and current water-loss dehydration in older people. Cochrane Database Syst Rev (4):CD009647
8. Edmonds CJ, Foglia E, Booth P, Fu CHY, Gardner M (2021) Dehydration in older people: a systematic review of the effects of dehydration on health outcomes, healthcare costs and cognitive performance. Arch Gerontol Geriatr 95:104380
9. EFSA Panel on Dietetic Products N (2010) Allergies. Scientific opinion on dietary reference values for water. EFSA J 8(3):1459
10. Thomas DR, Cote TR, Lawhorne L, Levenson SA, Rubenstein LZ, Smith DA et al (2008) Understanding clinical dehydration and its treatment. J Am Med Dir Assoc 9(5):292–301

11. Hooper L, Abdelhamid A, Ali A, Bunn DK, Jennings A, John WG, Kerry S, Lindner G, Pfortmueller CA, Sjöstrand F, Walsh NP, Fairweather-Tait SJ, Potter JF, Hunter PR, Shepstone L (2015) Diagnostic accuracy of calculated serum osmolarity to predict dehydration in older people: adding value to pathology laboratory reports. BMJ Open. Oct 21;5(10):e008846. https://doi.org/10.1136/bmjopen-2015-008846. PMID: 26490100; PMCID: PMC4636668.
12. Madsen CM, Jantzen C, Lauritzen JB, Abrahamsen B, Jorgensen HL (2016) Hyponatremia and hypernatremia are associated with increased 30-day mortality in hip fracture patients. Osteoporos Int 27(1):397–404
13. Mohanty S, Rosenthal RA, Russell MM, Neuman MD, Ko CY, Esnaola NF (2016) Optimal perioperative management of the geriatric patient: a best practices guideline from the American College of Surgeons NSQIP and the American Geriatrics Society. J Am Coll Surg 222(5):930–947
14. Australian and New Zealand College of Anaesthetists (2017) Guideline on pre-anaesthesia consultation and patient preparation. https://www.anzca.edu.au/resources/professional-documents/guidelines/ps07-guidelines-on-pre-anaesthesia-consultation-an
15. Powell-Tuck J, Gosling P, Lobo D, Allison S, Carlson G, Gore M, et al (2011) British consensus guidelines on intravenous fluid therapy for adult surgical patients. https://www.bapen.org.uk/pdfs/bapen_pubs/giftasup.pdf
16. National Institute for Health and Care Excellence (2010) Delirium: prevention, diagnosis and management [CG103]. https://www.nice.org.uk/guidance/cg103
17. Lobo DN, Gianotti L, Adiamah A, Barazzoni R, Deutz NEP, Dhatariya K et al (2020) Perioperative nutrition: recommendations from the ESPEN expert group. Clin Nutr (Edin, Scot) 39(11):3211–3227
18. Hellström PM, Samuelsson B, Al-Ani AN, Hedström M (2017) Normal gastric emptying time of a carbohydrate-rich drink in elderly patients with acute hip fracture: a pilot study. BMC Anesthesiol 17(1):23

8

Health Impacts of Sarcopenia, Physical Dysfunction, Malnutrition and Cachexia

Carla M. Prado, Jack J. Bell and M. Cristina Gonzalez

Abstract

Malnutrition, sarcopenia, frailty and cachexia are different conditions but have overlapping characteristics and consequences for older adults. These conditions are especially prevalent in hospitalised patients affecting almost two thirds of older adults. They can often be hidden conditions; hence multidisciplinary awareness is needed for optimal identification and management. This chapter provides an overview of the definitions of each of these syndromes, its detrimental impact on health outcomes of older adults and tips for clinical practice implementation.

Keywords

Definitions · Muscle mass · Malnutrition · Sarcopenia · Frailty · Physical function Cachexia

C. M. Prado (✉)
Nutrition, Food and Health, University of Alberta, Edmonton, AB, Canada

Faculty of Agricultural, Life and Environmental Science - Agricultural, Food & Nutri Science Department, University of Alberta, Edmonton, AB, Canada
e-mail: carla.prado@ualberta.ca

J. J. Bell
Allied Health, The Prince Charles Hospital, Chermside, Queensland, Australia

School of Human Movement and Nutrition Sciences, The University of Queensland, St Lucia, QLD, Australia
e-mail: jack.bell@health.qld.gov.au

M. C. Gonzalez
Post-graduate Program in Health and Behavior, Catholic University of Pelotas, Pelotas, RS, Brazil

Learning Outcomes
By the end of this chapter, you will be able to:

- Recognise the commonalities and differences among malnutrition, physical dysfunction, sarcopenia, frailty and cachexia.
- Report prevalence and consequences of these conditions in older adults.
- Justify nutritional interventions and tips for clinical practice implementation.

8.1 Preface

A 65-year-old male presenting with excess body weight (body mass index (BMI) = 31 kg/m^2) and reporting no concerns is at your clinic today for annual check-up. During the consultation, the patient casually mentions he often needs help with opening jars noting he 'is not as strong as he used to be'. Physical examination, blood pressure and laboratory results are normal.

This patient is likely suffering from sarcopenia, a condition often observed with ageing, and that associates with functional decline, among other outcomes. Low muscle mass is a defining feature of sarcopenia, also associated with other conditions discussed in this chapter: malnutrition, frailty and cachexia (Table 8.1). In fact, these syndromes may overlap, and almost two thirds of older medical inpatients would show at least one of these conditions [1].

8.2 Definitions, Diagnosis, Prevalence and Relevance

8.2.1 Malnutrition

According to the World Health Organization (WHO), malnutrition is a condition associated with deficiencies, excesses or imbalances in a person's intake of energy and/or nutrients. It includes undernutrition, micronutrient-related malnutrition, excess body weight and diet-related communicable disease [2]. Although different

Table 8.1 Malnutrition, sarcopenia, frailty and cachexia: differences and similarities

	Malnutrition	Sarcopenia	Frailty	Cachexia
Weight loss	X	?	X	X
Low body mass index (BMI)	X	?	X	X
Muscle loss/weakness	X	X	X	X
Fat loss	?	?	?	?
Inflammation	X	?	?	X
Loss of appetite/nutrition impact symptoms	X	–	?	X
Low food intake	X	–	Sometimes	X

X = yes/usually present, ? = not necessarily present

criteria have been proposed for the diagnosis of undernutrition or protein-energy malnutrition (malnutrition), a global consensus was recently commissioned by major scientific societies, launching the Global Leadership Initiative on Malnutrition (GLIM) empirical diagnostic consensus [3]. According to the GLIM criteria, the diagnosis of malnutrition is divided into phenotypic and etiologic criteria, with two stages of severity (moderate and severe) (Table 8.2). These, and other well-recognised malnutrition diagnostic tools, ensure the diagnosis of malnutrition is not reliant on single-point measures such as BMI, albumin, identification of less than expected fat mass and/or reduced muscle mass or function alone. Suitable diagnostic tools should consider evidence of weight loss, low BMI or reduced muscle mass in combination with either inadequate intake or uptake of protein and/or energy sources or increased requirements for protein and energy. For example, an individual may have experienced weight loss and muscle depletion as a result of stroke-related inactivity. However, unless protein or energy intake is deficient or the subject has a co-morbid condition increasing metabolic requirements, these would not be diagnosed as malnutrition. Conversely, a high BMI alone does not preclude malnutrition, for example, in a person with obesity with sustained inadequate protein intake and consequent muscle loss [17].

Older adults are at risk for malnutrition. Malnutrition in this population may be associated with physiological, disease- or age-related changes, socio-economic or cultural factors, in addition to misinformation or misconceptions which can impact accessibility to food or adequacy of protein/energy intake [18]. These are detailed in Chaps. 3 and 4.

Malnutrition may go unrecognised in older adults due to a broad variety of factors, including failure to screen for malnutrition; poor screening tool sensitivity; reliance on inappropriate diagnostic measures, for example, albumin; and the misconception that malnutrition is only present in patients who are thin. With increasing prevalence of obesity globally, observing a diagnosis of overweight or obese malnutrition (DOOM) in older hospitalised patients is not uncommon and increases the likelihood of hospital-acquired complications, reduced mobility and 12-month mortality [17, 19]. A misdirected healthy self-image, association of unintentional weight loss as a perceived positive benefit or a denial of reducing intake or unintentional weight loss to maintain a positive effect leads many malnourished patients to report their nutrition status as good to excellent [18, 20].

As mentioned in previous chapters, a 2016 systematic review of 54 studies using validated tools to screen for malnutrition in community-living adults concluded that up to 83% of adults age 65 and older are at risk for malnutrition [21]. A multinational effort to describe the prevalence of malnutrition [22] in 12 countries has reported this condition to be present in approximately 50% of those in rehabilitation, 39% in those hospitalised, 14% in residential care and 6% in community-living older adults. Malnutrition in older adults leads to detrimental impacts on health, cognitive and physical functioning and quality of life [23]. It has been associated with increased healthcare costs and short time survival [18].

Table 8.2 Overview of screening, assessment and nutritional management of malnutrition, sarcopenia, frailty and cachexia

Considerations	Screening[a]	Assessment[a]	Nutritional management
Malnutrition	Validated screening tools	Phenotypic	
	• Malnutrition Screening Tool (MST)	• Non-volitional weight loss	• Nutritional education or counselling targeted to patient's needs and preferences
	• Mini Nutritional Assessment Short Form Revised (MNA-SF)	• Low body mass index	• Oral nutritional supplements
	• Nutrition Risk Screening 2002 (NRS®-2002)	• Reduced muscle mass	• Meal delivery programmes
	• Malnutrition Universal Screening Tool (MUST)	Etiologic	
	• Mini Nutritional Assessment (MNA)[b]	• Reduced food intake or assimilation	
		• Disease burden/inflammatory condition	
Sarcopenia		Different options proposed combining:	
	• SARC-F questionnaire	Function/strength assessment	• High-protein diet (minimum of 1, optimal 1.5 g/kg body weight/day)
	• SARC-CalF questionnaire (SARC-F combined with calf circumference)	• Short Physical Performance Battery (SPPB)	• Optimal caloric intake
	• Ishii score [4]	• Grip strength	• Physical activity (resistance exercises)
		• Gait speed	
		• Chair stand	
		Muscle mass assessment	
		• Bioelectrical impedance analysis	
		• Dual-energy X-ray absorptiometry	
		• Computerised tomography	
		• Calf circumference	

Frailty	• Frail Scale [5–7]		Adequate protein, energy, micronutrients where deficient
	• Clinical Frailty Scale [8]		Physical activity/exercise
	• Rockwood-Mitnitski Frailty Index [9]		Comorbidity management
	• Fried's Frailty Phenotype Approach [10]		Shared goal setting/decision-making
	• Reported Edmonton Frail Scale [11]		
Cachexia	Underlying catabolic disease (e.g. cancer, heart failure, chronic obstructive pulmonary disease)	Overall [12]	
	• The cachexia score (CASCO), miniCASCO [13, 14]	• Unintentional weight loss	• Nutritional counselling
	• CASC-IN [15]	• Low body mass index (BMI)	• Oral nutritional supplements with anti-inflammatory ingredients
		• Low albumin	• Enteral feeding
		• Low muscle or fat-free mass	
		• Evidence of cytokine excess	
		One of the following for cancer cachexia:	
		Weight loss	
		• >5% with any BMI	
		• Weight loss >2% with BMI <20 kg/m^2	
		• Sarcopenia with weight loss >2% [16]	

[a]Suggested tools only; local treating teams should identify and select tools with consideration to populations and context
[b]Screening and assessment tool

8.2.2 Low Muscle Mass, Physical Dysfunction and Sarcopenia

The loss of muscle mass and strength in ageing is studied in the context of sarcopenia. Although muscle mass and strength decline progressively after the age of 40, this loss is accelerated with advancing age (65 and older), becoming even more pronounced in individuals aged 85 and older. Estimates indicate that approximately 45% of older adults in the United States are affected by sarcopenia. Furthermore, sarcopenia has been reported to affect 30% of individuals over 60 years of age and more than 50% of people over 80 years [24]. A recent systematic review and meta-analysis of general population studies including 58,404 individuals found that 10% of men (95% CI 8–12%) and 10% of women (95% CI 8–13%) had sarcopenia [25]. Notably, prevalence rates are widely variable depending on the diagnostic criteria used.

Similar to malnutrition, there is no gold standard for screening or diagnosing sarcopenia. A well-recognised screening tool for sarcopenia is the SARC-F questionnaire [26] which measures **s**trength, **a**ssistance needed in walking across a room, **r**ising from chair/bed difficulty, **c**limbing stars and **f**alls. The addition of calf circumference to this questionnaire has been found to improve the sensitivity of SARC-F [27].

Several approaches are available for the diagnosis of sarcopenia such as the European Working Group on Sarcopenia in Older People (EWGSOP-2) [28], the Foundation for the National Institutes of Health (FNIH) initiative [29] and the Asian Working Group for Sarcopenia (AWGS) [30]. Notably, cut-off points for sarcopenia diagnosis should be race- and most often sex-specific. For a description of approaches and cut-offs, we refer the reader to Landi et al. [31], which includes the most commonly used definitions, with the exception of the EWGSOP which has been recently updated. The EWGSOP-2 now defines low muscle strength as a key criterion, followed by low muscle mass to confirm the sarcopenia diagnosis and gait speed to diagnose the severity of the condition [28].

The use of mass versus function conundrum is an ongoing source of debate related to sarcopenia diagnosis. Sarcopenia of ageing is considered *primary sarcopenia*, but in the context of a chronic disease (i.e. independent of ageing), sarcopenia is considered *secondary sarcopenia* as observed in the context of cancer, pulmonary diseases, heart failure and kidney disease, among others [32]. Patients may have both but the difference is that the diagnosis of secondary sarcopenia is widely pursued using measures of muscle mass alone. Therefore, secondary sarcopenia can be identified by low muscle mass.

Body composition techniques commonly used to diagnose low muscle mass include dual-energy X-ray absorptiometry (DXA), bioelectrical impedance analysis (BIA), computerised tomography and magnetic resonance imaging [28], although the latter is extremely limited and solely used in research settings. We refer the reader to a more in-depth discussion of the pros and cons of each body composition assessment technique [33, 34] and available cut-offs. Of increasing interest is the use of calf circumference, which correlates well with muscle mass, but has been primarily studied in older adults. Although calf circumference is only a proxy of muscle mass, it is the most commonly used tool for muscle mass assessment in clinical practice [35].

Sarcopenia in ageing occurs at any body weight and BMI; in individuals with obesity, it is termed sarcopenic obesity, a condition related to worse health outcomes than either in isolation. The prevalence of sarcopenic obesity is on the rise due to the ageing of the population and the obesity epidemic [36]. Diagnostic criteria are as variable for this condition as is the diagnosis of sarcopenia and obesity in isolation, although a consensus proposal is in the works by an international expert panel [37].

Criteria included in screening and diagnostic tools for sarcopenia (versus malnutrition) are shown in Table 8.2. Sarcopenia is a debilitating syndrome associated with disability, physical impairments, falls and fractures, decreased quality of life, hospitalisations and death [28]. Its related direct healthcare costs in the Unites States are estimated to be greater than $18 billion per year, with a total estimated cost of hospitalisation of $40 billion per year [38]. A 10% reduction in the prevalence of sarcopenia could translate to $1.1 billion cost savings [39]. Due to the importance of sarcopenia, the WHO recently released the International Classification of Diseases code for sarcopenia (ICD-10 under the code M62.84; sarcopenia related to age), a major advancement for clinical practice and research.

8.2.3 Frailty

Definitions of frailty syndrome generally consider a combination of age- or disease-related physiological decline [40, 41] across multiple physiological systems, weakness or fatigue, reduced likelihood of positive outcome from healthcare interventions and/or increased susceptibility to adverse health outcomes.

There is no gold standard for the diagnosis of frailty, with a perhaps an overwhelming selection of screening or diagnostic options to consider [40]. Tools are commonly aligned to either a 'phenotypic' or 'deficit accumulation' framework. The former of these targets observable characteristics, for example, reduced activity, function, strength or energy levels, whilst the latter focusses on cumulative totals of co-morbidities or conditions. Some suggested frailty screening and assessment tools recommended by the Agency for Clinical Innovation are listed in Table 8.2; however which tools to apply should be considerate of contextual factors. A detailed overview of commonly used frailty instruments is provided elsewhere [40, 41]. As such local treating teams are encouraged to carefully consider which tool is most likely to assist appropriate frailty identification and interventions.

The pathophysiology of frailty is complex, ranging from endocrine or immunological dysregulation, disease states and environmental, physiological or physical stressors, all of which may also contribute to sarcopenia, malnutrition or inflammatory processes. In fact, there is a close relationship between sarcopenia and physical frailty, and sarcopenia can be considered as the biological substrate for physical frailty [42].

A diagnosis of frailty is not inconsequential. Estimates of pre-frailty and frailty vary according to both screening and diagnostic tools applied, and genuine population differences, although many studies suggest prevalence between 10% and 40% of older populations [41, 43]. Regardless of the tools applied, frailty is routinely associated with functional decline, falls and fractures, hospital-acquired complications, hospitalisations and institutionalisation, reduced quality of life and increased mortality. The healthcare costs of frailty are increased at any level of care, including greater healthcare use and increased hospitalisation costs [43].

8.2.4 Cachexia

Cachexia is the most severe condition discussed in this chapter. It is associated with an underlying condition that leads to excessive catabolism [44] and has been studied in the context of cancer, congestive heart failure, chronic obstructive pulmonary disease and chronic kidney disease, among others [12, 45]. Together with precachexia, its prevalence across disease conditions has been estimated at 10–40%, affecting more than 30 million people in the United States, based on a 2008 publication [12, 46].

Cachexia is a multimodal problem, where the presence of inflammatory cytokines, reduced food intake and metabolic dysfunction, including in energy metabolism, may contribute to its development and progression [47]. A multimodal intervention is now recognised ideal where nutrition, exercise and pharmacological interventions are included as part of optimal cancer care. A key element for successful treatment is the identification of cachexia in its earlier phase (precachexia), where inflammation is not so impactful, and nutritional counselling and protein supplements may prevent or decrease weight loss.

A defining feature of cachexia is muscle loss that occurs unrelated to changes in fat mass. Additionally, it has been associated with substantial inflammatory process, insulin resistance and an imbalance between protein synthesis and degradation, favouring the latter. Anorexia, weight loss and weakness are all associated with cachexia and of obvious unfavourable consequences to older adults. Patients with cancer cachexia have a poor prognosis; they present with poor physical function, poor quality of life and shorter survival.

Cachexia has been primarily studied in the context of cancer with an estimated prevalence at the European Union of 30% [48]. The most commonly used criteria for cancer cachexia is shown in Table 8.2 and is based on an international consensus group [16]. Sarcopenia in the context of cachexia is defined as secondary sarcopenia, and hence, only measures of muscle mass have been used in the great majority of publications assessing sarcopenia in cachexia. This is also endorsed by the consensus group [16]. Definitions of sarcopenia of ageing (primary sarcopenia) that include measures of muscle strength/function have generally not been validated in the context of chronic diseases, including cancer. The diagnosis of low muscle mass (or sarcopenia) in cancer cachexia can be done using the body composition techniques or surrogate assessments described in Sect. 8.2.2. Based on the consensus group [16], physical examination including anthropometry can be used to estimate or evaluate muscle mass status, although they are not as accurate as body composition assessment techniques. Bioelectrical impedance analysis and computerised tomography scans are among the most popular bedside tools for the estimation and measurement (respectively) of body composition in cancer cachexia publications.

8.3 Nutritional Treatment and Management Approaches

Nutrition is a powerful therapy. Every other therapeutic approach is likely to fail if essential nutrients are not provided for optimal energy intake and muscle anabolism. An overview of nutritional management approaches for the conditions discussed in this chapter is shown in Table 8.2. Additional details on nutrition support are provided in Chap. 5.

In the context of malnutrition, common dietary approaches include multidisciplinary nutritional interventions, dietary intensive treatment, medical treatment and meal delivery service (e.g. Meals on Wheels) [49]. Individuals with poor nutrition knowledge are at greater risk to develop malnutrition [50]; hence nutritional education has the potential to improve nutritional status although knowledge does not necessarily translate in healthy eating habits [51]. Helping with meal planning and use of social programmes during mealtimes may positively influence meal choices. Nutrient-rich, flavour-enhanced meals (with herbs and spices) and the addition of nutritional supplements are helpful strategies [52] (Chaps. 3–5).

In the context of sarcopenia, both the quantity and quality of nutrients are essential to sustain muscle mass as shown in Fig. 8.1. These nutrients are important to several conditions hereby discussed, and they have an important role to be explored

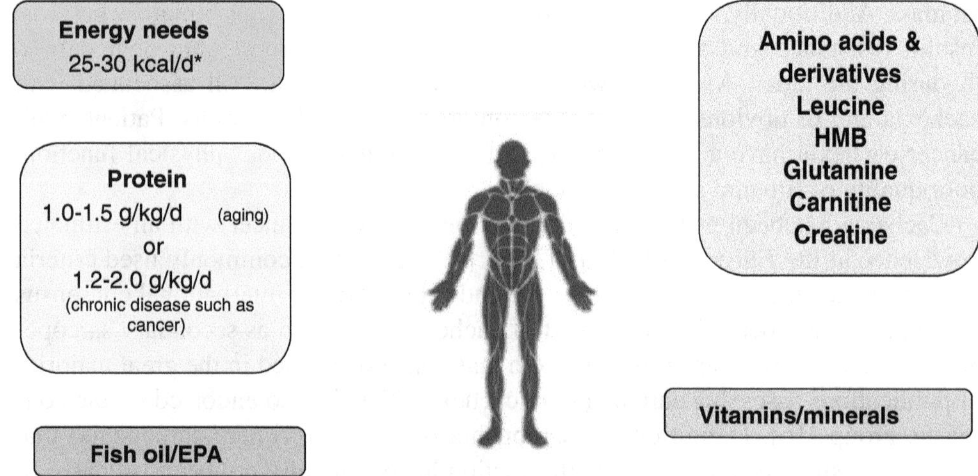

Fig. 8.1 Nutrients under consideration for the treatment of low muscle mass. *HMB* beta-hydroxy beta-methylbutyrate, *EPA* eicopentaenoic acid. (Adapted from Prado et al. J Cachexia Sarcopenia Muscle. 2020; 11: 366–380 [53] and Prado et al. Ann Med. 2018;50:675–693)

in the context of prevention and treatment of muscle wasting. However, with the exception of targeted energy and protein needs, there is insufficient evidence to support additional supplementation of nutrients shown in Fig. 8.1. Furthermore, vitamins and minerals should be provided at Dietary Reference Intake levels. More research is needed to explore the impact of these nutrients alone or as part of a multimodal approach to maximise patient's anabolic potential [32, 53, 54].

With respect to frailty, evidence supports ensuring adequate protein, energy and micronutrient intakes. Additional work is required to confirm whether multimodal approaches, combining nutrition care with physical activity [55, 56], comorbidity management and provision of advice on health behaviour improvements prevent or ameliorate frailty in the reversible phases of the condition [41, 43]. The available limited research on the effectiveness of system-level interventions is inconclusive (Table 8.1) [41, 43]. However, in the absence of adequate supporting evidence, we would suggest teams consider multi-model, interdisciplinary interventions at the individual and system levels across the continuum of care (Chaps. 1, 3–6, and 13). Treating teams should also ensure that chosen interventions are aligned with treatment intent, goal setting and shared decision-making processes (Chap. 21).

In the context of cachexia, nutrition therapy depends on individual patient's needs. Recently published guidelines for the management of cancer cachexia (which can be translated to other clinical settings) [57] acknowledge the importance of dietary counselling, fortified foods, oral nutritional supplements or enteral feds with adequate energy and protein (and potentially anti-inflammatory ingredients) as important nutritional strategies as outlined by Arends et al. [44]. In patients with less than 3-month life expectancy (i.e. refractory cachexia), nutrition is palliative, provided as needed to alleviate feelings of hunger and thirst [44]. Nutritional care should be adjusted according to patient's specific nutritional and metabolic requirements (Chap. 21).

In all the disease contexts, physical activity provides essential anabolic stimuli. Aerobic training may also help optimise fat mass. Pharmacological interventions have not been approved for the management of muscle wasting specifically but can be used to manage the underlying disease and unfavourable symptoms that can culminate in muscle loss. Therefore, this potentially offsets nutrition impact symptoms, optimising anabolism through increased food intake and anabolic potential.

8.4 Key Levels to Implement Change

An engaged multidisciplinary team can work collectively and collaboratively in the identification of malnutrition, physical dysfunction, sarcopenia, frailty or cachexia. Nurses are the frontline staff with most patient contact who can also be responsible for screening patients for these conditions. Dietitians provide the specialised assessment and support of patient's nutritional status, and medical professionals can support the holistic approach and ensure integration of the care process with all members of the healthcare team. Documentation of the diagnosis and care plan is essential and all are responsible (Chaps. 3, 4, and 6).

Accurate assessment of these conditions should be at the core of management pathway for at risk patients [58]. Creating an institutional culture on the relevance of these conditions helps to redefine priorities and advance assessment/interventions and monitoring of a quality improvement programme [59] targeting malnutrition, physical dysfunction, sarcopenia, frailty or cachexia. Patient engagement is key to advancing care, and the use of animated videos, infographics and other patient resources can be instrumental to achieve that [60, 61]. Selected examples can be watched using the following links provided below (see recommended viewing).

8.5 Conclusion

The syndromes hereby discussed are distinct yet interrelated. As such, their components should be considered as interlinked factors, one leading to another and on a potentially vicious cycle manner. A perfect diagnosis can be challenging for the healthcare team, especially as some of the conditions may be hidden, requiring an in-depth assessment of nutritional status. Optimisation of assessment and treatment can support timely and comprehensive care to older adults involving multimodal care across the continuum of care.

References

1. Gingrich A, Volkert D, Kiesswetter E, Thomanek M, Bach S, Sieber CC et al (2019) Prevalence and overlap of sarcopenia, frailty, cachexia and malnutrition in older medical inpatients. BMC Geriatr 19(1):120. https://doi.org/10.1186/s12877-019-1115-1
2. World Health Organization (2020) Malnutrition. https://www.who.int/news-room/fact-sheets/detail/malnutrition#:~:text=Malnutrition%20refers%20to%20deficiencies%2C%20excesses,low%20weight%2Dfor%2Dage)%3B. Accessed 28 Oct 2020
3. Cederholm T, Jensen GL, Correia M, Gonzalez MC, Fukushima R, Higashiguchi T et al (2019) GLIM criteria for the diagnosis of malnutrition - a consensus report from the global clinical nutrition community. Clin Nutr (Edin, Scot) 38(1):1–9. https://doi.org/10.1016/j.clnu.2018.08.002
4. Ishii S, Tanaka T, Shibasaki K, Ouchi Y, Kikutani T, Higashiguchi T et al (2014) Development of a simple screening test for sarcopenia in older adults. Geriatr Gerontol Int 14(Suppl 1):93–101. https://doi.org/10.1111/ggi.12197
5. Agency for Clinical Innovation NG. Frailty screening and assessment tools. https://www.aci.health.nsw.gov.au/resources/frailty-taskforce/reports/frailty-screening-and-assessment-tools
6. Victoria State Government hv. Identifying frailty. https://www2.health.vic.gov.au/hospitals-and-health-services/patient-care/older-people/frailty/frailty-identifying
7. Woo J, Leung J, Morley JE (2012) Comparison of frailty indicators based on clinical phenotype and the multiple deficit approach in predicting mortality and physical limitation. J Am Geriatr Soc 60(8):1478–1486. https://doi.org/10.1111/j.1532-5415.2012.04074.x

8. Rockwood K, Song X, MacKnight C, Bergman H, Hogan DB, McDowell I et al (2005) A global clinical measure of fitness and frailty in elderly people. Can Med Assoc J 173(5):489–495. https://doi.org/10.1503/cmaj.050051
9. Mitnitski AB, Song X, Rockwood K (2004) The estimation of relative fitness and frailty in community-dwelling older adults using self-report data. J Gerontol A Biol Sci Med Sci 59(6):M627–M632. https://doi.org/10.1093/gerona/59.6.m627
10. Fried LP, Tangen CM, Walston J, Newman AB, Hirsch C, Gottdiener J et al (2001) Frailty in older adults: evidence for a phenotype. J Gerontol A Biol Sci Med Sci 56(3):M146–M156. https://doi.org/10.1093/gerona/56.3.m146
11. Rolfson DB, Majumdar SR, Tsuyuki RT, Tahir A, Rockwood K (2006) Validity and reliability of the Edmonton Frail Scale. Age Ageing 35(5):526–529. https://doi.org/10.1093/ageing/afl041
12. Morley JE, Thomas DR, Wilson M-MG (2006) Cachexia: pathophysiology and clinical relevance. Am J Clin Nutr 83(4):735–743. https://doi.org/10.1093/ajcn/83.4.735
13. Argilés JM, Betancourt A, Guàrdia-Olmos J, Peró-Cebollero M, López-Soriano FJ, Madeddu C et al (2017) Validation of the CAchexia SCOre (CASCO). Staging cancer patients: the use of miniCASCO as a simplified tool. Front Physiol 8:92. https://doi.org/10.3389/fphys.2017.00092
14. Argilés JM, López-Soriano FJ, Toledo M, Betancourt A, Serpe R, Busquets S (2011) The cachexia score (CASCO): a new tool for staging cachectic cancer patients. J Cachexia Sarcopenia Muscle 2(2):87–93. https://doi.org/10.1007/s13539-011-0027-5
15. Argilés JM, López-Soriano FJ, Castillejo M, Moreno C, Madeddu C, Serpe R, Busquets S (2019) CASC-IN: a new tool to diagnose pre-cachexia in cancer patients. Ann Clin Oncol. https://doi.org/10.31487/j.ACO.2019.04.03
16. Fearon K, Strasser F, Anker SD, Bosaeus I, Bruera E, Fainsinger RL et al (2011) Definition and classification of cancer cachexia: an international consensus. Lancet Oncol 12(5):489–495. https://doi.org/10.1016/s1470-2045(10)70218-7
17. Bell JJ, Pulle RC, Lee HB, Ferrier R, Crouch A, Whitehouse SL (2021) Diagnosis of overweight or obese malnutrition spells DOOM for hip fracture patients: a prospective audit. Clin Nutr (Edin, Scot) 40:1905. https://doi.org/10.1016/j.clnu.2020.09.003
18. Mangels AR (2018) CE: malnutrition in older adults. Am J Nurs 118(3):34–41. https://doi.org/10.1097/01.NAJ.0000530915.26091.be
19. Ness SJ, Hickling DF, Bell JJ, Collins PF (2018) The pressures of obesity: the relationship between obesity, malnutrition and pressure injuries in hospital inpatients. Clin Nutr (Edin, Scot) 37(5):1569–1574. https://doi.org/10.1016/j.clnu.2017.08.014
20. Federal Interagency Forum on Aging-Related Statistics (2016) Older Americans 2016: key indicators of well-being. Federal Interagency Forum on Aging-Related Statistics, Washington, DC
21. Hamirudin AH, Charlton K, Walton K (2016) Outcomes related to nutrition screening in community living older adults: a systematic literature review. Arch Gerontol Geriatr 62:9–25. https://doi.org/10.1016/j.archger.2015.09.007
22. Kaiser MJ, Bauer JM, Rämsch C, Uter W, Guigoz Y, Cederholm T et al (2010) Frequency of malnutrition in older adults: a multinational perspective using the mini nutritional assessment. J Am Geriatr Soc 58(9):1734–1738. https://doi.org/10.1111/j.1532-5415.2010.03016.x
23. Corish CA, Bardon LA (2019) Malnutrition in older adults: screening and determinants. Proc Nutr Soc 78(3):372–379. https://doi.org/10.1017/s0029665118002628
24. Baumgartner RN, Koehler KM, Gallagher D, Romero L, Heymsfield SB, Ross RR et al (1998) Epidemiology of sarcopenia among the elderly in New Mexico. Am J Epidemiol 147(8):755–763. https://doi.org/10.1093/oxfordjournals.aje.a009520
25. Shafiee G, Keshtkar A, Soltani A, Ahadi Z, Larijani B, Heshmat R (2017) Prevalence of sarcopenia in the world: a systematic review and meta- analysis of general population studies. J Diab Metab Disord 16:21. https://doi.org/10.1186/s40200-017-0302-x
26. Malmstrom TK, Morley JE (2013) SARC-F: a simple questionnaire to rapidly diagnose sarcopenia. J Am Med Dir Assoc 14(8):531–532. https://doi.org/10.1016/j.jamda.2013.05.018

27. Barbosa-Silva TG, Menezes AM, Bielemann RM, Malmstrom TK, Gonzalez MC (2016) Enhancing SARC-F: improving sarcopenia screening in the clinical practice. J Am Med Dir Assoc 17(12):1136–1141. https://doi.org/10.1016/j.jamda.2016.08.004
28. Cruz-Jentoft AJ, Bahat G, Bauer J, Boirie Y, Bruyère O, Cederholm T et al (2019) Sarcopenia: revised European consensus on definition and diagnosis. Age Ageing 48(1):16–31. https://doi.org/10.1093/ageing/afy169
29. Studenski SA, Peters KW, Alley DE, Cawthon PM, McLean RR, Harris TB et al (2014) The FNIH sarcopenia project: rationale, study description, conference recommendations, and final estimates. J Gerontol A Biol Sci Med Sci 69(5):547–558. https://doi.org/10.1093/gerona/glu010
30. Chen LK, Lee WJ, Peng LN, Liu LK, Arai H, Akishita M (2016) Recent advances in sarcopenia research in Asia: 2016 Update From the Asian Working Group for Sarcopenia. J Am Med Dir Assoc 17(8):767.e1–767.e7. https://doi.org/10.1016/j.jamda.2016.05.016
31. Landi F, Calvani R, Cesari M, Tosato M, Martone AM, Ortolani E et al (2018) Sarcopenia: an overview on current definitions, diagnosis and treatment. Curr Protein Pept Sci 19(7):633–638. https://doi.org/10.2174/1389203718666170607113459
32. Bauer J, Morley JE, Schols A, Ferrucci L, Cruz-Jentoft AJ, Dent E et al (2019) Sarcopenia: a time for action. An SCWD position paper. J Cachexia Sarcopenia Muscle 10(5):956–961. https://doi.org/10.1002/jcsm.12483
33. Prado CM, Heymsfield SB (2014) Lean tissue imaging: a new era for nutritional assessment and intervention. JPEN J Parenter Enteral Nutr 38(8):940–953. https://doi.org/10.1177/0148607114550189
34. Sheean P, Gonzalez MC, Prado CM, McKeever L, Hall AM, Braunschweig CA (2020) American Society for Parenteral and Enteral Nutrition Clinical Guidelines: the validity of body composition assessment in clinical populations. JPEN J Parenter Enteral Nutr 44(1):12–43. https://doi.org/10.1002/jpen.1669. Epub 2019 Jun 19. PMID: 31216070
35. Bruyère O, Beaudart C, Reginster J-Y, Buckinx F, Schoene D, Hirani V, Cooper C, Kanis JA, Rizzoli R, McCloskey E, Cederholm T, Cruz-Jentoft A, Freiberger E (2016) Assessment of muscle mass, muscle strength and physical performance in clinical practice. Eur Geriat Med 7(3):243–246. https://doi.org/10.1016/j.eurger.2015.12.009
36. Roubenoff R (2004) Sarcopenic obesity: the confluence of two epidemics. Obes Res 12(6):887–888. https://doi.org/10.1038/oby.2004.107
37. Donini LM, Busetto L, Bauer JM, Bischoff S, Boirie Y, Cederholm T et al (2020) Critical appraisal of definitions and diagnostic criteria for sarcopenic obesity based on a systematic review. Clin Nutr (Edin, Scot) 39(8):2368–2388. https://doi.org/10.1016/j.clnu.2019.11.024
38. Goates S, Du K, Arensberg MB, Gaillard T, Guralnik J, Pereira SL (2019) Economic impact of hospitalizations in US adults with sarcopenia. J Frailty Aging 8(2):93–99. https://doi.org/10.14283/jfa.2019.10
39. Janssen I, Shepard DS, Katzmarzyk PT, Roubenoff R (2004) The healthcare costs of sarcopenia in the United States. J Am Geriatr Soc 52(1):80–85. https://doi.org/10.1111/j.1532-5415.2004.52014.x
40. Buta BJ, Walston JD, Godino JG, Park M, Kalyani RR, Xue QL et al (2016) Frailty assessment instruments: systematic characterization of the uses and contexts of highly-cited instruments. Ageing Res Rev 26:53–61. https://doi.org/10.1016/j.arr.2015.12.003
41. Dent E, Martin FC, Bergman H, Woo J, Romero-Ortuno R, Walston JD (2019) Management of frailty: opportunities, challenges, and future directions. Lancet (Lond, Engl) 394(10206):1376–1386. https://doi.org/10.1016/s0140-6736(19)31785-4
42. Cruz-Jentoft AJ, Sayer AA (2019) Sarcopenia. Lancet (Lond, Engl) 393(10191):2636–2646. https://doi.org/10.1016/s0140-6736(19)31138-9

43. Hoogendijk EO, Afilalo J, Ensrud KE, Kowal P, Onder G, Fried LP (2019) Frailty: implications for clinical practice and public health. Lancet (Lond, Engl) 394(10206):1365–1375. https://doi.org/10.1016/s0140-6736(19)31786-6
44. Arends J, Baracos V, Bertz H, Bozzetti F, Calder PC, Deutz NEP et al (2017) ESPEN expert group recommendations for action against cancer-related malnutrition. Clin Nutr (Edin, Scot) 36(5):1187–1196. https://doi.org/10.1016/j.clnu.2017.06.017
45. Yoshida T, Delafontaine P (2015) Mechanisms of cachexia in chronic disease states. Am J Med Sci 350(4):250–256. https://doi.org/10.1097/maj.0000000000000511
46. Tan BH, Fearon KC (2008) Cachexia: prevalence and impact in medicine. Curr Opin Clin Nutr Metab Care 11(4):400–407. https://doi.org/10.1097/MCO.0b013e328300ecc1
47. Del Fabbro E (2019) Combination therapy in cachexia. Ann Palliat Med 8(1):59–66. https://doi.org/10.21037/apm.2018.08.05
48. Anker MS, Holcomb R, Muscaritoli M, von Haehling S, Haverkamp W, Jatoi A et al (2019) Orphan disease status of cancer cachexia in the USA and in the European Union: a systematic review. J Cachexia Sarcopenia Muscle 10(1):22–34. https://doi.org/10.1002/jcsm.12402
49. Young C, Argáez C (2019) Interventions for malnutrition in older adults: a review of clinical effectiveness. CADTH rapid response report. Canadian Agency for Drugs and Technologies in Health (CADTH), Ottawa, ON, p 4
50. Smith ML, Bergeron CD, Lachenmayr S, Eagle LA, Simon JR (2020) A brief intervention for malnutrition among older adults: stepping up your nutrition. Int J Environ Res Public Health 17(10):3590. https://doi.org/10.3390/ijerph17103590
51. Turconi G, Rossi M, Roggi C, Maccarini L (2013) Nutritional status, dietary habits, nutritional knowledge and self-care assessment in a group of older adults attending community centres in Pavia, Northern Italy. J Hum Nutr Dietet 26(1):48–55. https://doi.org/10.1111/j.1365-277X.2012.01289.x
52. Mayo Clinic (2019) Senior health: how to prevent and detect malnutrition. https://www.mayoclinic.org/healthy-lifestyle/caregivers/in-depth/senior-health/art-20044699. Accessed 28 Oct 2020
53. Prado CM, Purcell SA, Laviano A (2020) Nutrition interventions to treat low muscle mass in cancer. J Cachexia Sarcopenia Muscle 11(2):366–380. https://doi.org/10.1002/jcsm.12525. Epub 2020 Jan 8. PMID: 31916411; PMCID: PMC7113510
54. Prado CM, Anker SD, Coats AJS, Laviano A, von Haehling S (2021) Nutrition in the spotlight in cachexia, sarcopenia and muscle: avoiding the wildfire. J Cachexia Sarcopenia Muscle 12(1):3–8. https://doi.org/10.1002/jcsm.12673. Epub 2020 Dec 31. PMID: 33382196; PMCID: PMC7890147
55. Hernández Morante JJ, Gómez Martínez C, Morillas-Ruiz JM (2019) Dietary factors associated with frailty in old adults: a review of nutritional interventions to prevent frailty development. Nutrients 11(1):102. https://doi.org/10.3390/nu11010102
56. Lorenzo-López L, Maseda A, de Labra C, Regueiro-Folgueira L, Rodríguez-Villamil JL, Millán-Calenti JC (2017) Nutritional determinants of frailty in older adults: a systematic review. BMC Geriatr 17(1):108. https://doi.org/10.1186/s12877-017-0496-2
57. Roeland EJ, Bohlke K, Baracos VE, Bruera E, Del Fabbro E, Dixon S et al (2020) Management of cancer cachexia: ASCO guideline. J Clin Oncol Off J Am Soc Clin Oncol 38(21):2438–2453. https://doi.org/10.1200/jco.20.00611
58. Deutz NEP, Ashurst I, Ballesteros MD, Bear DE, Cruz-Jentoft AJ, Genton L et al (2019) The underappreciated role of low muscle mass in the management of malnutrition. J Am Med Dir Assoc 20(1):22–27. https://doi.org/10.1016/j.jamda.2018.11.021
59. Tappenden KA, Quatrara B, Parkhurst ML, Malone AM, Fanjiang G, Ziegler TR (2013) Critical role of nutrition in improving quality of care: an interdisciplinary call to action to address adult hospital malnutrition. JPEN J Parenter Enteral Nutr 37(4):482–497. https://doi.org/10.1177/0148607113484066
60. George S, Moran E, Duran N, Jenders RA (2013) Using animation as an information tool to advance health research literacy among minority participants. AMIA Annu Symp Proc 2013:475–484

61. Keselman A, Logan R, Smith CA, Leroy G, Zeng-Treitler Q (2008) Developing informatics tools and strategies for consumer-centered health communication. J Am Med Inform Assoc 15(4):473–483. https://doi.org/10.1197/jamia.M2744

9

Skeletal Health in Older Adults

Helen Wilson, Diana Calcraft, Cai Neville,
Susan Lanham-New and Louise R. Durrant

Abstract

Achieving and maintaining skeletal health throughout the life trajectory is essential for the prevention of bone diseases such as rickets, osteomalacia and osteoporosis. Rickets and osteomalacia are usually a result of calcium and/or vitamin D deficiency, causing softening of bones and bone pain, and both conditions are treatable with calcium and vitamin D supplementation. Osteoporosis is a multifaceted disease mainly affecting older people, and its pathogenesis (and hence treatment) is more complex. Untreated osteoporosis results in fragility fractures causing morbidity and increased mortality.

Nutrition is one of many factors that influence bone mass and risk of bone disease. Developing a nutritional sciences approach is a feasible option for improving bone health.

The importance of adequate calcium and vitamin D in ensuring skeletal integrity throughout the life course has a sound evidence base. Poor vitamin D status in population groups of all ages is widespread across many countries (including affluent and non-affluent areas). Public health approaches are required to correct

This chapter is a component of Part I: Nutritional Care in Old Age.
For an explanation of the grouping of chapters in this book, please see Chap. 1: 'Geriatrics and Orthogeriatrics: Providing Nutrition Care'.

H. Wilson (✉) · D. Calcraft · C. Neville
Royal Surrey Foundation NHS Trust, Surrey, UK
e-mail: hwilson6@nhs.net; diana.calcraft@nhs.ne; c.neville@nhs.net

S. Lanham-New · L. R. Durrant
Nutrition, Food & Exercise Sciences Department, Faculty of Health & Medical Sciences, University of Surrey, Surrey, UK
e-mail: s.lanham-new@surrey.ac.uk; Durrant@yakult.co.uk

this given the fact that vitamin D is not just required for musculoskeletal health but also for other health outcomes.

Dietary protein may be beneficial for bone due to its effect of increasing insulin-like growth-factor-1 (IGF-1). Recent meta-analyses show that dietary protein has a beneficial role to play in bone health at all ages.

Other nutritional factors and nutrients (such as potassium, magnesium, vitamin K and acid-base balance) are also likely to have an important role in bone health, though the literature is less clear in terms of the association/relationship and more research is required.

Keywords

Bone health · Osteoporosis · Fragility fractures · Frailty · Vitamin D

Learning Outcomes
By the end of this chapter, you will be able to:

- Explain the role of key nutrients and other factors that influence bone mass and risk of bone disease.
- Apply knowledge learned and tools to identify older adults with or at risk of musculoskeletal frailty and fractures.
- Apply multicomponent strategies to prevent and manage frailty, fragility, fractures and osteoporosis.

9.1 Introduction

9.1.1 Bone

Bone is a complex living tissue. It provides structure, support and protection for the body. It is formed from collagen reinforced by minerals. There are two types of bone in the skeleton: cortical and trabecular. Cortical bone is smooth, dense and strong and is found at the surface of bone. Trabecular bone has a honeycomb structure and is found inside the bones, making bone strong, light and slightly flexible. Bone is built and develops its strength through the early years.

9.1.2 Normal Bone Metabolism

Bone metabolism is a continual cycle of bone formation and bone resorption undertaken by cells called osteoclasts and osteoblasts [1]. The bone matrix created requires mineralisation with calcium phosphate. Bone metabolism is influenced by hormones and other regulatory factors.

Think of the bones like an enormous house, constantly in need of maintenance and updating. Bone cells are like groups of workmen, ones that pull down the old walls (cells called osteoclasts) and ones that build up new walls (cells called osteoblasts). This process continues constantly, and slowly, over time, and the house (or the skeleton) is renewed. Ageing causes the groups of workmen building up new walls (the osteoblasts) to get slower and slower and fall behind their destructive colleagues. This leads to crumbling walls in the house making it more likely to fall down or the bone to fracture.

9.1.3 Peak Bone Mass (PBM)

The skeleton usually reaches maximum growth between the late second and early third decades and mineralises during this time as well. During this time, bone is being laid down faster than it is being absorbed, gradually increasing in density. Peak bone mass is achieved in the early fourth decade when bone is at its most robust. Genetic factors play a key role in the population variation of PBM, with estimates around 70–75% [2]. However, this still leaves plenty of room for key modifiable exogenous factors such as the effects of diet (including calcium, vitamin D, protein and other essential minerals) hormones and physical activity. After the fourth decade, bone mass declines, more gradually in men than women as a result of the menopause [3, 4].

9.2 Nutrients and Bone Health

9.2.1 Calcium

Calcium is an important component of the skeleton and is one of the predominant minerals found in bone. Over 99% of the body's total calcium is found in bones and teeth in the form of hydroxyapatite. The remaining 1% of calcium circulates in the blood. Phosphorus and magnesium also make up a large percentage of the bone matrix, with over 88% and 60% of the body's content of these minerals deposited in bone. There is no functional marker for calcium nutritional status, since serum/plasma calcium levels are homeostatically controlled by the body [5].

Inadequate calcium intake is a worldwide problem, having been reported in children, adolescents and adults across Europe, North America, Asia and Oceania [6]. In older adults, calcium intake varies between countries [6]. In the UK, preschool children [7] and adolescents aged 11–18 years [8] have been reported to have dietary calcium intakes below the relative UK Department of Health reference nutrient intake (RNI), whereas younger and older adults are meeting the UK RNI [8, 9].

The evidence that calcium supplementation improves attainment of bone density in childhood and prevents fractures in older age is weak and inconsistent [10, 11]. Thus, calcium supplementation is not recommended for fracture prevention at a population level.

There is however good data to show that calcium supplements are effective in reducing bone loss in late menopausal women (>5 years postmenopause), particularly in those with low habitual calcium intake (<400 mg/day) [12]. In the key study by [13], late postmenopausal women were found to have a significant reduction in lumbar spine and femoral neck bone loss following supplementation with 500 mg calcium per day, but no such effect was seen in early postmenopausal women (<5 years postmenopause). Reviews of over 20 studies have shown that calcium supplementation can decrease bone loss by approximately 1% per year. There are some data to suggest that the effect of calcium supplementation may be greater at skeletal sites with more cortical bone. There are also data to suggest that calcium supplementation improves the efficacy of antiresorptive therapy on bone mass [14].

9.2.2 Vitamin D

Vitamin D is the generic term for two molecules: ergocalciferol and cholecalciferol. Ergocalciferol (vitamin D_2) is derived by ultraviolet (UV) irradiation of ergosterol, which is found in fungi and plants [15]. Cholecalciferol (vitamin D_3) is formed from the effect of UV irradiation on the skin. The action of sunlight on the skin converts 7-dehydrocholesterol to previtamin D, which is metabolised to vitamin D by a temperature-dependent isomerisation. Vitamin D is then transported via the general circulation to the liver, where the enzyme 25-hydroxylase converts it to 25-hydroxy-vitamin D (25-OHD). This is the key circulating vitamin D metabolite and the best indicator of clinical status [15]. The kidney is the site for further conversion to calcitriol or $1,25(OH)_2D_3$.

Calcitriol ($1,25(OH)_2D_3$), the active form of vitamin D, helps to maintain normal blood levels of calcium and phosphate. It promotes calcium absorption and bone mineralisation. It also enhances osteoclastic activity (bone turnover). Together with parathyroid hormone (PTH), it regulates calcium and phosphorus metabolism by promoting calcium absorption from the gut and kidney tubules [15].

25-Hydroxy-vitamin D (25-OHD) is the major circulating vitamin D metabolite and can be measured in the blood, considered the gold standard method for establishing vitamin D status [16]. However, there is a lack of consensus and definition regarding the suggested thresholds of 25-OHD used to define vitamin D deficiency or optimal levels, and the range of terminology and associated values used make comparisons of reported prevalence difficult.

The World Health Organization and the UK's Scientific Advisory Committee on Nutrition (SACN) state that 25-OHD levels <25 nmol/L (10 mg/mL) is the deficiency threshold [17–19] with regard to the prevention of rickets and osteomalacia, and the WHO also defines vitamin D insufficiency as 25-OHD levels <50 nmol/L. However, the US Institute of Medicine (IOM) defines 25-OHD levels <30 nmol/L as deficiency, 30–50 nmol/L as inadequacy and >50 nmol/L as sufficient [20].

The UK National Osteoporosis Society has agreed with the IOM thresholds and proposed that the UK practitioners should also adopt these [21]. Commonly, vitamin D deficiency is defined by a 25-OHD threshold of <25–30 nmol/L, with insufficiency defined by 25-OHD levels in the range of 25–49 nmol/L [22]. Conversely, the Endocrine Society Task Force (USA/Canada) define deficiency as 25-OHD levels <50 nmol/L and advocate that 25-OHD levels should exceed 75 nmol/L [23].

> Vitamin D deficiency has been associated with skeletal conditions and other musculoskeletal health outcomes. Low 25-OHD levels of <12 nmol/L in children often result in rickets [19]. In adults, 25-OHD levels ≤20 nmol/L result in osteomalacia [19].

In addition, epidemiological studies and randomised controlled trials have reported associations between vitamin D levels and muscle strength and function [24, 25], fracture risk [26, 27] and risk of falls [28]. Specifically, supplementation with vitamin D has been shown to have a positive effect on bone mineral density [26, 27, 29] with a recent meta-analysis of 23 studies showing a small benefit on femoral neck bone mineral density [30].

Our main source of vitamin D is the ultraviolet (UV) in sunlight. Much of the UV in sunlight is absorbed by clouds, ozone and other forms of atmospheric pollution. UV sunlight varies daily, seasonally and depending on latitude. In the UK, there is no UV radiation of the appropriate wavelength (280–310 mm) from the end of October to the end of March. For the remaining months of the year, the main percentage of the effective UV radiation occurs between 11.00 am and 3.00 pm [31].

A number of factors reduce the vitamin D production from UV exposure. Sunscreens absorb UVB radiation when applied to the skin, thereby reducing the production of previtamin D3. Glass absorbs all UVB photons, and hence sunlight that has passed through glass will not promote vitamin D3 synthesis in the skin. Clothing also absorbs UVB radiation; this is particularly relevant for women who cover up for cultural reasons.

There are few dietary sources of vitamin D. The major providers are fat spreads (which are often fortified with vitamin D), fish, eggs, pastry products, fortified breakfast cereals and meat [18].

9.2.3 Vitamin K

Vitamin K ('koagulation vitamin') was first described in Denmark by Dam (1935) as a dietary-derived coagulation factor [32]. He noted that a bleeding disorder in chickens was corrected by feeding a variety of vitamin K-rich foods. The fat-soluble vitamin was finally isolated in 1939. Vitamin K refers to a family of compounds with a common chemical structure, 2-methyl-1,4-naphthoquinone. Phylloquinone (vitamin K1) is present in plant-based foods, particularly green leafy vegetables.

Menaquinones (vitamin K2) are derived from bacterial fermentation of foods such as cheese [33].

Vitamin K has an important function for the skeleton. There are data to show that low serum concentrations of vitamin K are associated with low bone mineral density and increased risk for osteoporotic fracture [34].

The results of randomised controlled trials looking at the effects of vitamin K supplementation and markers of bone health have been very disappointing, and the most recent vitamin K/fracture prevention meta-analysis did not demonstrate a beneficial effect of this nutrient on markers of bone health or prevention of osteoporotic fracture [35].

9.2.4 Protein

Historically there has been much debate as to whether dietary protein is good or bad for bone health. Insulin-like growth factor-1 (IGF-1) is a hormone which builds up the bone. IGF-1 is stimulated by dietary protein intake. In terms of epidemiology, many studies have found a positive association between dietary protein intake and bone health [36, 37], but some have found no association [38]. In particular there is conflicting evidence as to whether protein intake is associated with hip fracture risk, with a recent systematic reviews and meta-analyses finding a positive association between dietary protein intake and bone mass density, but not fracture risk [39, 40]. Therefore, dietary protein may have beneficial effects on bone density, but this may not necessarily translate into reduced risk of fracture.

9.2.5 Other Nutrients

There are numerous studies looking at other nutrients including potassium, vitamin C, vitamin E and vitamin A. It is difficult to draw clear conclusions from the evidence available, and none of these supplements are routinely recommended in promoting bone health [41].

9.3 Other Factors Influencing Bone Health

Hormones are extremely important in bone health. Normal testosterone and normal menstruation are required in order for bone to reach peak bone mass. Cigarette smoking and excessive alcohol intake may further accelerate the loss of bone in both women and men [1].

The skeleton also needs to be used appropriately. Bone density is achieved by putting weight through it. Over 100 years ago, a German scientist called Julius Wolff suggested the theory that bone would adapt to the load under which it is placed and would remodel to become stronger to resist that sort of loading, now known as Wolff's law [42]. More recently, this concept has been refined to a general theory of bone mass regulation, known as the mechanostat model [43]. In the absence of weight-bearing exercise, bone loss will occur at both axial and appendicular skeletal sites. Early astronauts discovered that when they landed back on Earth, they had lost significant bone density and strength; it is the action of gravity through bones that gives them strength.

9.4 Osteoporosis

Osteoporosis is a term derived from osteo (bone) and porous (full of holes). This means that the bone is fragile and at increased risk of fracture. There are a pathological definition based on the appearance of bone under the microscope and a clinical definition where fracture type, mechanism of fracture and results of a bone density scan are used to define osteoporosis.

Osteoporosis is often diagnosed following a low trauma fracture typically affecting the wrist, a vertebral body in the spine or a hip (more specifically the neck of femur).

The most common and widely available bone density scan is the DEXA or dual-energy X-ray absorptiometry scan [44]. The result is described by a *T*-score and a *Z*-score. The *T*-score compares the result with that of a healthy 40-year-old. The *Z*-score compares the result to an age-matched average. The *T*-score is more widely used to diagnose osteoporosis. This score has been validated for use in different populations across the world. The measurements are ranked on a scale of normal distribution. Standard deviations of +1 or −1 are considered normal. This encompasses about 80% of the population. Scores from −1 to −2.5 are considered osteopenia ('thin' bone). A *T*-score of less than −2.5 is considered as osteoporotic. There are other ways to measure bone density including quantitative CT [45], but this is much less widely used.

Bone density is a strong predictor of fracture, yet many fragility fractures occur without osteoporosis as assessed by density criteria; this highlights the need to consider additional factors other than bone mineral density that may contribute to an older adult's risk of fracture [46].

9.4.1 Risk Factors for Osteoporosis

There are a range of conditions and factors that accelerate bone density decline. These are termed risk factors and may be used in diagnosing and directing management of osteoporosis.

Osteoporosis increases with age and is more common in women, largely because of menopause and the loss of the hormonal access. Premature menopause and treatments that bring on menopause or reduce testosterone increase risk. Amenorrhoea associated with multiple pregnancies or often seen in eating disorders is strongly associated with reduced bone density [46, 47].

Osteoporosis is more common in Caucasian or Asian individuals and in those with a family history of maternal or paternal hip fracture. Body mass index is important with osteoporosis being more common in those who are underweight due to

Table 9.1 Risk factors for fractures [46, 49]

Nutritional status	Deficiencies calcium, vitamin D, magnesium, protein. Low body weight
Lifestyle	Smoking, alcohol (>2 units/day), physical inactivity, lack of nutritious food
Falls	Previous falls
Skeleton 'diseases'	Family history of osteoporosis or fractures. History of low-impact fracture. Thoracic kyphosis, height loss (>4 cm), low BMD
Endocrine diseases	Type 2 diabetes, hyperthyroidism, hyperparathyroidism, Cushing's disease
Inflammatory diseases	Rheumatoid arthritis, connective tissue diseases, spondylitis, IBD
Respiratory diseases	Asthma, COPD
Neurological/ psychiatric diseases	Parkinson, multiple sclerosis, stroke, depression, dementia
Immune diseases/ cancer	HIV
Medications	Proton pump inhibitors, affecting gonadal hormone production. Some immunosuppressants, antidiabetic drugs, antipsychotics, anticonvulsants Excess thyroid hormone treatment

less basal bone mass and those with obesity. Both smoking and alcohol increase risk in a dose-dependent fashion [48].

Secondary osteoporosis occurs in those with other conditions associated with osteoporosis, e.g. rheumatoid arthritis, type 1 diabetes, untreated long-standing hyperthyroidism, hypogonadism or premature menopause (less than 45 years), chronic malnutrition (including eating disorders such as anorexia nervosa) or malabsorption, chronic liver disease and osteogenesis imperfecta in adults (Table 9.1) [50].

Medications associated with osteoporosis include steroids, low molecular weight heparin, proton pump inhibitors (e.g. omeprazole, lansoprazole), SSRIs (selective serotonin reuptake inhibitors; antidepressants), aromatase inhibitors for breast cancer and anti-epileptics. This list is by no means exhaustive. These are often dose-dependent, with longer exposure being more highly correlated with risk. In the context of steroids, a significant proportion of bone loss is thought to occur in the first 3 months of treatment. A clinically relevant dose is more than 3 months of at least 5 mg of prednisolone daily (Table 9.1) (Chap. 19) [51].

9.5 Fragility, Fractures and Falls

Fragility is defined as 'the quality of being easily broken or damaged' [52]. A fracture is a crack or break in a bone. Fragility fractures occur as a result of a fall from a standing height in someone with delicate or vulnerable bones. Fragility fractures are common and occur in one in three women and one in five men aged over 50 years. It is estimated that across the world a fragility fracture occurs every 3 s.

Falls are more common with age and one third of people over 65 years of age will fall each year. Falls are more likely to result in fractures, particularly in those with osteoporosis. A previous fracture is a strong predictor of future fractures [53]. This is often progressive with time; Fig. 9.1 highlights the progressive impact of osteoporosis, as commonly seen in ageing individuals.

Wrist fractures often occur in early stages of osteoporosis in mobile individuals who fall forwards onto an outstretched hand. They usually result in a temporary disability but heal well with most individuals regaining most of their previous level of function. Vertebral fragility fractures may occur insidiously without significant trauma and be attributed to an exacerbation of chronic back pain. Progressive vertebral fractures can occur over many years resulting in loss of height with significant curvature of the spine (kyphosis) leading to progressive problems with balance, mobility and breathing. Hip fractures are considered the most significant fragility fracture associated with increased morbidity and mortality. They usually occur in older adults with intracapsular fractures resulting from a sideways fall onto the hip. There has been a focus on hip fracture management in the UK over the last 12 years with year-on-year reduction in mortality with the latest figure of 6.1% at 30 days [55]. However the 1-year mortality remains around 22% [56].

A significant proportion of older adults presenting with hip fracture have frailty. One study identified that 17% had no frailty, 39% had mild frailty [4, 5] and 44% had moderate to severe frailty [57]. Frailty is a widely used term in healthcare and is associated with functional decline and mortality. It is often associated with multimorbidity and ageing but is not synonymous with either. The word frailty often conjures up an image of an older person such as that described above, with poor muscle mass, a curved spine and arthritic joints struggling with mobility and function [58, 59].

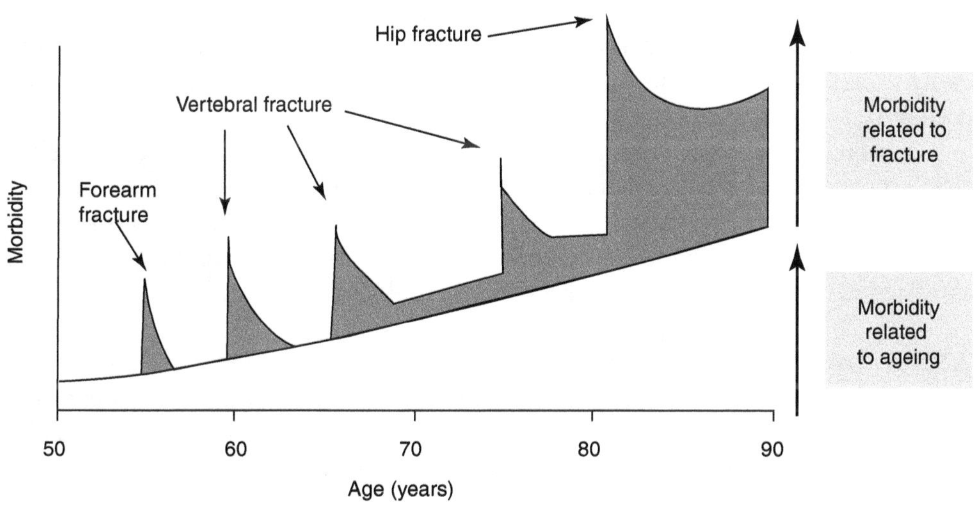

Fig. 9.1 The burden of osteoporosis [54]. (With permission of Kanis JA, Johnell O. The burden of osteoporosis. J Endocrinol Invest. 1999;22(8):583–8)

Key causes of frailty, prevalence, associated outcomes and preventative and interventional management strategies have been previously detailed (Chap. 8). We highlight here the concept of musculoskeletal frailty, which often includes a loss of muscle (sarcopenia), loss of collagen (osteoarthritis) and loss of bone (osteoporosis) [60]. All elements of musculoskeletal frailty can be significantly reduced by a life-course approach to healthy ageing [61] (Chaps. 4 and 14). This is important as musculoskeletal frailty is a key predictor of fall-related fractures.

9.5.1 Frailty, Falls and Bone Health Assessment

9.5.1.1 Frailty Assessment

The description of frailty using a phenotypical approach was first described by Fried [58] and colleagues requiring the presence of three or more out of five indicators: weakness (reduced grip strength), slowness (gait speed), weight loss, low physical activity and exhaustion. Whilst global consensus is lacking, a useful broad definition encompasses a loss of physiological reserve so that systems fail with minor stressors. Frailty can be classified in many ways; a practical and widely used tool for frailty identification is the Rockwood Clinical Frailty Scale. This scale can be applied for those with frailty as a result of physical or cognitive decline (Fig. 9.2) [62].

9.5.1.2 Falls Risk Assessment

In addition to advancing musculoskeletal frailty, other key factors influencing the incidence of falls include effects of polypharmacy, metabolic imbalances, cardiac events, related to alcohol intake, lack of a safe living environment, visual disturbances, reduced cognition (with poor safety awareness) and also reduced continence resulting in hurrying to the toilet or trying to manage incontinence [63]. A recent study has identified that malnourished inpatients were almost 8 times more likely to have a harmful fall than those not malnourished, independent of age and BMI [64].

Consequently, clinical care guidelines, for example, the UK's NICE Guideline [65], recommend that older people are asked about their history of falls whenever coming into contact with health or social care practitioners. Where falls (or risk of falls) have been identified, older adults should be offered a multifactorial risk assessment and interventions to prevent further falls.

9.5.1.3 Bone Health Assessment

Given the complexities within and across sarcopenia, osteoarthritis, osteoporosis and frailty and the diversity of factors that contribute to fracture risk, bone health assessment requires an individualised, comprehensive approach. In a number of settings, bone health assessment applies a personalised fracture risk assessment tool such as FRAX® (https://www.sheffield.ac.uk/FRAX/). The FRAX® tool uses clinical risk factors to establish an individual's fracture risk based on studying population-based cohorts from Europe, North America, Asia and Australia.

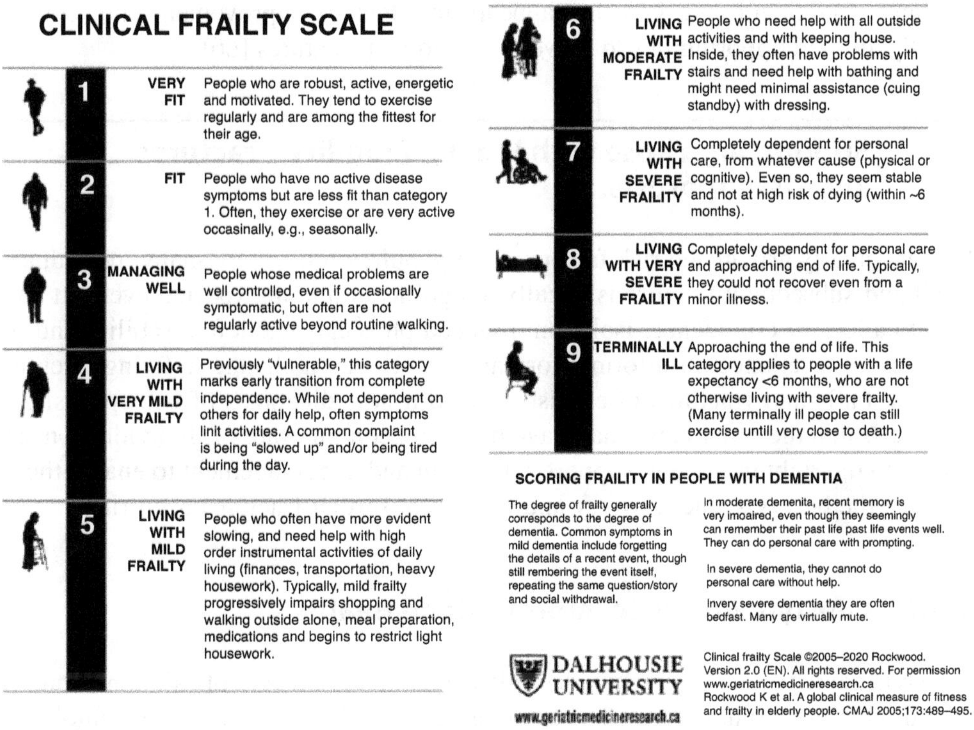

CLINICAL FRAILTY SCALE

1	VERY FIT	People who are robust, active, energetic and motivated. They tend to exercise regularly and are among the fittest for their age.
2	FIT	People who have no active disease symptoms but are less fit than category 1. Often, they exercise or are very active occasinally, e.g., seasonally.
3	MANAGING WELL	People whose medical problems are well controlled, even if occasionally symptomatic, but often are not regularly active beyond routine walking.
4	LIVING WITH VERY MILD FRAILTY	Previously "vulnerable," this category marks early transition from complete independence. While not dependent on others for daily help, often symptoms linit activities. A common complaint is being "slowed up" and/or being tired during the day.
5	LIVING WITH MILD FRAILTY	People who often have more evident slowing, and need help with high order instrumental activities of daily living (finances, transportation, heavy housework). Typically, mild frailty progressively impairs shopping and walking outside alone, meal preparation, medications and begins to restrict light housework.
6	LIVING WITH MODERATE FRAILTY	People who need help with all outside activities and with keeping house. Inside, they often have problems with stairs and need help with bathing and might need minimal assistance (cuing standby) with dressing.
7	LIVING WITH SEVERE FRAILITY	Completely dependent for personal care, from whatever cause (physical or cognitive). Even so, they seem stable and not at high risk of dying (within ~6 months).
8	LIVING WITH VERY SEVERE FRAILITY	Completely dependent for personal care and approaching end of life. Typically, they could not recover even from a minor illness.
9	TERMINALLY ILL	Approaching the end of life. This category applies to people with a life expectancy <6 months, who are not otherwise living with severe frailty. (Many terminally ill people can still exercise untill very close to death.)

SCORING FRAILITY IN PEOPLE WITH DEMENTIA

The degree of frailty generally corresponds to the degree of dementia. Common symptoms in mild dementia include forgetting the details of a recent event, though still rembering the event itself, repeating the same question/story and social withdrawal.

In moderate demenita, recent memory is very imoaired, even though they seemingly can remember their past life past life events well. They can do personal care with prompting.

In severe dementia, they cannot do personal care without help.

Invery severe dementia they are often bedfast. Many are virtually mute.

DALHOUSIE UNIVERSITY

www.geriatricmedicineresearch.ca

Rockwood K et al. A global clinical measure of fitness and frailty in elderly people. CMAJ 2005;173:489–495.

Fig. 9.2 The Rockwood Clinical Frailty Scale. *Source*: (Canadian Study on Health & Aging, Revised 2008. 2. K. Rockwood et al. A global clinical measure of fitness and frailty in elderly people. CMAJ 2005;173:489–495. © 2007–2009. Version 1.2. All rights reserved. Geriatric Medicine Research, Dalhousie University, Halifax, Canada. Permission granted to copy for research and educational purposes only. Participating Sites: Cape Breton District HEALTH AUTHORITY Making Healthier Choices Together Sponsors: © 2007–2009. Version 1.2. All rights reserved. Geriatric Medicine Research, Dalhousie University, Halifax, Canada. Permission granted to copy for research and educational purposes only)

The FRAX® algorithms are freely available on the website and give the 10-year probability of fracture. The National Osteoporosis Guideline Group graphs provide a visual guide for clinicians and patients in recommending treatment, further assessment with DXA scan or lifestyle advice.

An initial fragility fracture is a strong predictor of second fracture; the importance of secondary fracture prevention cannot be overemphasised. As an example, Hip Fracture Care Clinical Care Standards require that hip fracture patients are assessed for future fall and fracture risk by suitably qualified orthogeriatric healthcare professionals, with documented plans for management including assessment for risk of falls, fall history and risk factors for falls, including a medication review, and formulation of a plan to prevent further falls. Despite such recommendations, falls risk assessment and secondary prevention strategies such as prescription of bone protection medication are often not undertaken following identification of initial fragility fracture. Audit data continues to highlight substantial variation and an ongoing, significant care gap that appears resistant to improvement and, consequently, missed opportunities to prevent consequent fractures [66].

9.6 Supporting Those with Frailty, Fragility, Fractures and Osteoporosis

Despite clearly articulated risk factors at the population level, for many individuals a fall and subsequent fracture is usually a significant and unexpected event. It can lead to a loss of confidence, isolation, reduced physical function, disability and in some cases a reliance on informal/formal care or even a change in living circumstances. Falls and fractures often also lead to a new diagnosis of osteoporosis, a disease which the older adult may have hitherto been unaware of. Individuals need access to the right treatment, support, education and encouragement to enable them to make the best possible recovery and to prevent further fractures occurring.

9.6.1 Lifestyle Advice to Improve Bone Health

Lifestyle advice includes nutritional guidance including sources of calcium, vitamin D and other essential nutrients and minerals as described above. Ceasing smoking, avoiding alcohol excess and encouraging a balanced diet rich in fruit and vegetables and ensuring at least sufficient or increased protein intakes (as recommended in older adults) may also contribute to the prevention of osteoporosis, improved bone health and/or reduced complications [1, 53, 67, 68].

For older adults with conditions that affect nutrition, a dietitian review is advised. Suggesting exercise as a prescription rather than a casual activity can influence uptake (Chap. 14). It is important to support the older adult through the initial trauma recovery to the post-injury rehabilitation and ultimately to a regular exercise schedule to maintain their mobility and balance.

Physical activity and exercise plays [1] a key role in improving bone health as well as improving balance. The work carried out by the Royal Osteoporosis Society (ROS) in the recent 'strong, steady and straight campaign' is a helpful consensus document providing the evidence to encourage older adults to exercise and provides the healthcare provider some clarity around the use of exercise in those with osteoporosis [69]. Strategies to reduce the risk of falls are also recommended as a key lifestyle management approach [49].

Older adults with osteoporosis often experience loss of confidence following a low-impact fall resulting in fracture. Thus their fear of falling results in restriction of movement and lifestyle. This in turn results in deconditioning and an increase in their risk of further falls and fracture. This consensus document indicates that increased activity and weight-bearing exercise is likely to provide greater lifestyle benefits and reduce fracture risk.

9.6.2 Supplementation and Medications

For most patients, calcium and vitamin D supplements are recommended. Medication for established osteoporosis has a good evidence base, for example, antiresorptive therapy (e.g. bisphosphonates, denosumab). Hormonal treatments may also be appropriate for some individuals [1]. Consideration must be given to potential side effects and adverse outcomes, duration of treatments and monitoring processes for prescribed supplements and/or medications [12].

Long-term medication adherence however remains a challenge [70] with less than 30% of patients continuing to take medication at 2 years. The asymptomatic nature of osteoporosis requires careful attention to emphasise the risk of complications from untreated disease. There are many factors which affect patients' persistence [71].

These can be positively influenced by establishing a good relationship with the older adult, a medication regime to suit the individual and a clear understanding of the benefits. Negative influencers include the effect of negative press reports on long-term use of antiresorptive agents. As an example, the SCOOP trial in 2012 [72] identified that patients who underwent a DEXA scan and had the result explained to them were more likely to be adherent and persistent with medication.

Whether in relation to supplements or medications likely to adversely influence bone health and fracture risk, older adults should be supported to make an informed decision regarding medication by providing clear information about benefits and possible side effects. It is essential for older adults also to understand how to take medications to ensure they are effective and to minimise potential harm [49].

9.6.3 Education, Training and Sociopolitical Action

Valuable research by Yardley et al. [73] into designing and delivering advice about falls prevention indicated that if falls prevention education is given in a patronising way, where the individual is somehow seen to be negligent or they have done something 'stupid', they are less likely to engage in a falls prevention programme.

Listening to the older adult's experience of falling and placing falls education within an exercise/balance initiative can make the older person more likely to actively engage in both falls prevention and exercise [63, 73].

Training to support the management of osteoporosis should be integrated into training processes across medical, nursing and allied health disciplines [49]. Programme and political level action is the recognised fourth pillar for orthogeriatric care; advocating for change in healthcare policy and priorities by engaging and mobilising healthcare leaders, policymakers and other sociopolitical influencers is a key factor to realising better bone health for individuals and populations [49, 72, 74].

Across acute, rehabilitation and secondary prevention settings, the importance of education and training for older adults, their carers, healthcare providers and services, organisations and professional bodies should be considered a fundamental priority. This is perhaps best highlighted by the Fragility Fracture Network call to action [75] which highlights the need for engaged, educated healthcare stakeholders to support coordinated care for those with or at risk of fragility fracture across acute, rehabilitation and secondary prevention settings. Perhaps most importantly, this needs to be underpinned sociopolitical action to overcome the failure for uptake of key opportunities for care improvement.

9.6.3.1 Coordinated Care Opportunities to Optimise Bone Health, Fragility and Fractures in Older Adults

Example 1: Orthogeriatric Services

Orthogeriatric services have been developed as a result of a focus on hip fracture care. Best practice for hip fractures involves early surgery and standardised perioperative management with coordination between orthopaedic, anaesthetic and geriatric services [76].

A coordinated approach throughout the older adult's journey is imperative to ensure that individuals are optimised before surgery to reduce post-operative complications and have access to appropriate interdisciplinary rehabilitation. Falls and bone health assessment are key to future fracture prevention.

Care Example 2: Fracture Liaison Services

The 'Capture the Fracture' campaign led by the International Osteoporosis Foundation is a global resource supporting the implementation of a post-fracture coordination programme such as a fracture liaison service. This coordinated, multidisciplinary approach has a strong evidence base in preventing further fractures also resulting in significant cost saving for healthcare systems and has also been demonstrated to reduce mortality [55, 77]. Globally there are almost 600 fracture liaison services registered with the 'Capture the Fracture' campaign over 48 countries (https://www.capturethefracture.org/).

Example 3: Fracture Liaison Nurses

Advancing older adult understanding through education is the key to self-management of bone health. The approach must be adjusted to the individual, their abilities and experience. For older adults living with frailty, engagement with their family and carers is often required. In many settings, fracture liaison nurse (FLN) roles have been established to advance knowledge of falls and bone health in addition to skills in health promotion. The overarching roles of the FLN (or similar positions) often include supporting an individual in coming to terms with their injury, working through the stages of the illness experience, encouraging older adults to actively participate in rehabilitation and educating older adults to manage their own bone health [78].

Example 4: Audit and Feedback

The role of audit and feedback to improve outcomes is well established. Implementation of the National Hip Fracture Database in the UK has been associated with improvements in care and survival of older people with hip fracture [79]. As a further example, the Fracture Liaison Service Database (FLS-DB) is a UK continuous audit, initiated to measure performance against standards of management of secondary prevention of fragility fractures set primarily by the National Institute for Clinical Excellence (NICE) and the Royal Osteoporosis Society. In 2017 there were 65 fracture liaison services operational in the UK who contributed data to the FLS-DB (https://www.fffap.org.uk/). Whilst the 2020 report demonstrates improvement in most key performance indicators, the audit highlights further opportunities to advance effective and efficient services.

9.6.3.2 End-of-Life Care

Lifestyle interventions, supplements and education to improve/maintain bone health are imperative to reducing population incidence of frailty, falls and fragility fractures. However, for those with severe frailty (CFS > 7) or end-stage disease, priorities are likely to be different and may require a refocus towards managing symptoms and comfort rather than disease prevention or cure (Chap. 21).

9.7 Summary

For all those working with older adults, it is important to have some insight into the complex interrelationship between bone health, fragility and fractures. Nutrition plays a key role in the promotion of bone health in the older population. The role of calcium and vitamin D is well established and dietary supplementation may be required. Less is known about the effects of dietary protein, acid-base balance and micronutrients.

Prevention of musculoskeletal frailty through a life-course approach focusing on a healthy diet, regular exercise and multi-component management of osteoporosis is recommended. Older adult and healthcare provider education is key to adherence to treatment strategies following fragility fractures; orthogeriatric services, fracture liaison services, fracture liaison nurses and feedback and audit processes should be considered a healthcare system priority.

Regardless of the age or stage of disease, individualised attention towards benefits versus burdens of potential interventions should be considered and where appropriate discussed with the older adult to guide patient-centred care. Actions to prevent initial disease onset and preventable complications must become the priority. Conversely, focus for management at the end of life is likely to be comfort, as at this stage it is unlikely that nutritional supplements, exercise or medication for bone health will be beneficial.

Take-Home Points

- Nutrition plays a key role in the promotion of bone health in the older population.
- There is a complex interrelationship between bone health, fragility and fractures.
- Orthogeriatric services, fracture liaison services, fracture liaison nurses and feedback and audit processes should be routinely embedded in practice.
- Engaging older adults, their carers, healthcare providers, organisations and professional bodies to prioritise a multi-component, life-course approach to preventing and managing bone health, fragility and fractures.

References

1. Barnsley J, Buckland G, Chan PE, Ong A, Ramos AS, Baxter M et al (2021) Pathophysiology and treatment of osteoporosis: challenges for clinical practice in older people. Aging Clin Exp Res 33:759
2. Maes HH, Neale MC, Eaves LJ (1997) Genetic and environmental factors in relative body weight and human adiposity. Behav Genet 27(4):325–351
3. Gordon CM, Zemel BS, Wren TA, Leonard MB, Bachrach LK, Rauch F et al (2017) The determinants of peak bone mass. J Pediatr 180:261–269
4. Lu J, Shin Y, Yen MS, Sun SS (2016) Peak bone mass and patterns of change in total bone mineral density and bone mineral contents from childhood into young adulthood. J Clin Densitom 19(2):180–191
5. Health NIo (2011) Dietary reference intakes for calcium and vitamin D. The national guidelines. Institute of Medicine (US), Washington, DC
6. Peterlik M, Cross HS (2009) Vitamin D and calcium insufficiency-related chronic diseases: molecular and cellular pathophysiology. Eur J Clin Nutr 63(12):1377–1386
7. Cribb VL, Northstone K, Hopkins D, Emmett PM (2015) Sources of vitamin D and calcium in the diets of preschool children in the UK and the theoretical effect of food fortification. J Hum Nutr Diet 28(6):583–592
8. Beverley Bates DC, Cox L, Nicholson S, Page P, Roberts C, Steer T, Swan G (2019) National diet and nutrition survey - years 1 to 9 of the rolling programme (2008/2009 – 2016/2017): time trend and income analyses. A survey carried out on behalf of Public Health England and the Food Standards Agency. Report No.: 2018756. Public Health England & Food Standards Agency, London
9. Derbyshire E (2018) Micronutrient intakes of British adults across mid-life: a secondary analysis of the UK National Diet and Nutrition Survey. Front Nutr 5:55
10. Winzenberg T, Shaw K, Fryer J, Jones G (2006) Effects of calcium supplementation on bone density in healthy children: meta-analysis of randomised controlled trials. BMJ 333(7572):775
11. Bolland MJ, Leung W, Tai V, Bastin S, Gamble GD, Grey A et al (2015) Calcium intake and risk of fracture: systematic review. BMJ 351:h4580
12. Sunyecz JA (2008) The use of calcium and vitamin D in the management of osteoporosis. Ther Clin Risk Manag 4(4):827–836
13. Dawson-Hughes B, Dallal GE, Krall EA, Sadowski L, Sahyoun N, Tannenbaum S (1990) A controlled trial of the effect of calcium supplementation on bone density in postmenopausal women. N Engl J Med 27;323(13):878–883
14. Lanham-New SA (2008) Importance of calcium, vitamin D and vitamin K for osteoporosis prevention and treatment: symposium on 'Diet and bone health'. Proc Nutr Soc 67(2):163–176
15. Jäpelt RB, Jakobsen J (2013) Vitamin D in plants: a review of occurrence, analysis, and biosynthesis. Front Plant Sci 4:136

16. Seamans KM, Cashman KD (2009) Existing and potentially novel functional markers of vitamin D status: a systematic review. Am J Clin Nutr 89(6):1997S–2008S
17. WHO (2003) Global strategy on diet, physical activity and health - diet, nutrition and the prevention of chronic diseases. Contract No.: 916 (TRS 916). Surveillance and Population-based Prevention Unit, Department of Chronic Diseases and Health Promotion, Geneva
18. Kimball SM, Holick MF (2020) Official recommendations for vitamin D through the life stages in developed countries. Eur J Clin Nutr 74(11):1514–1518
19. D SACoNSWGoV (2016) Vitamin D and health report. SACN advises on nutrition and related health matters. It advises Public Health England (PHE) and other UK government organisations
20. Ross AC, Manson JE, Abrams SA, Aloia JF, Brannon PM, Clinton SK et al (2011) The 2011 report on dietary reference intakes for calcium and vitamin D from the Institute of Medicine: what clinicians need to know. J Clin Endocrinol Metab 96(1):53–58
21. Aspray TJ, Bowring C, Fraser W, Gittoes N, Javaid MK, Macdonald H et al (2014) National osteoporosis society vitamin D guideline summary. Age Ageing 43(5):592–595
22. Spiro A, Buttriss JL (2014) Vitamin D: an overview of vitamin D status and intake in Europe. Nutr Bull 39(4):322–350
23. Holick MF, Binkley NC, Bischoff-Ferrari HA, Gordon CM, Hanley DA, Heaney RP et al (2011) Evaluation, treatment, and prevention of vitamin D deficiency: an Endocrine Society clinical practice guideline. J Clin Endocrinol Metab 96(7):1911–1930
24. Ward KA, Das G, Roberts SA, Berry JL, Adams JE, Rawer R et al (2010) A randomized, controlled trial of vitamin D supplementation upon musculoskeletal health in postmenarchal females. J Clin Endocrinol Metab 95(10):4643–4651
25. Tomlinson PB, Joseph C, Angioi M (2015) Effects of vitamin D supplementation on upper and lower body muscle strength levels in healthy individuals. A systematic review with meta-analysis. J Sci Med Sport 18(5):575–580
26. Chapuy MC, Arlot ME, Duboeuf F, Brun J, Crouzet B, Arnaud S et al (1992) Vitamin D3 and calcium to prevent hip fractures in elderly women. N Engl J Med 327(23):1637–1642
27. Dawson-Hughes B, Tosteson AN, Melton LJ III, Baim S, Favus MJ, Khosla S et al (2008) Implications of absolute fracture risk assessment for osteoporosis practice guidelines in the USA. Osteoporos Int 19(4):449–458
28. Stein MS, Wark JD, Scherer SC, Walton SL, Chick P, Di Carlantonio M et al (1999) Falls relate to vitamin D and parathyroid hormone in an Australian nursing home and hostel. J Am Geriatr Soc 47(10):1195–1201
29. Ooms ME, Lips P, Roos JC, van der Vijgh WJ, Popp-Snijders C, Bezemer PD et al (1995) Vitamin D status and sex hormone binding globulin: determinants of bone turnover and bone mineral density in elderly women. J Bone Miner Res 10(8):1177–1184
30. Reid IR, Bolland M, Grey A (2014) Effects of vitamin D supplements on bone mineral density: a systematic review and meta-analysis. Quality-assessed reviews. The University of York, 1995 - CfRaDU
31. Wacker M, Holick MF (2013) Sunlight and vitamin D: a global perspective for health. Dermatoendocrinology 5(1):51–108
32. Shampo MA, Kyle RA (1998) Henrik Dam-discoverer of vitamin K. Mayo Clin Proc 73:46
33. Gröber U, Reichrath J, Holick MF, Kisters K (2014) Vitamin K: an old vitamin in a new perspective. Dermatoendocrinology 6(1):e968490
34. Rodríguez-Olleros Rodríguez C, Díaz CM (2019) Vitamin K and bone health: a review on the effects of vitamin K deficiency and supplementation and the effect of non-vitamin K antagonist oral anticoagulants on different bone parameters. J Osteoporos 2019:2069176
35. Lewis R, Gómez Álvarez CB, Rayman M, Lanham-New S, Woolf A, Mobasheri A (2019) Strategies for optimising musculoskeletal health in the 21(st) century. BMC Musculoskelet Disord 20(1):164
36. Cooper C, Atkinson EJ, Hensrud DD, Wahner HW, O'Fallon WM, Riggs BL et al (1996) Dietary protein intake and bone mass in women. Calcif Tissue Int 58(5):320–325

37. Sahni S, Broe KE, Tucker KL, McLean RR, Kiel DP, Cupples LA et al (2014) Association of total protein intake with bone mineral density and bone loss in men and women from the Framingham Offspring Study. Public Health Nutr 17(11):2570–2576
38. Zhu K, Meng X, Kerr DA, Devine A, Solah V, Binns CW et al (2011) The effects of a two-year randomized, controlled trial of whey protein supplementation on bone structure, IGF-1, and urinary calcium excretion in older postmenopausal women. J Bone Miner Res 26(9):2298–2306
39. Darling AL, Manders RJF, Sahni S, Zhu K, Hewitt CE, Prince RL et al (2019) Dietary protein and bone health across the life-course: an updated systematic review and meta-analysis over 40 years. Osteoporos Int 30(4):741–761
40. Darling AL, Millward DJ, Torgerson DJ, Hewitt CE, Lanham-New SA (2009) Dietary protein and bone health: a systematic review and meta-analysis. Am J Clin Nutr 90(6):1674–1692
41. Palacios C (2006) The role of nutrients in bone health, from A to Z. Crit Rev Food Sci Nutr 46(8):621–628
42. Frost HM (1994) Wolff's Law and bone's structural adaptations to mechanical usage: an overview for clinicians. Angle Orthod 64(3):175–188
43. Wang L, You X, Lotinun S, Zhang L, Wu N, Zou W (2020) Mechanical sensing protein PIEZO1 regulates bone homeostasis via osteoblast-osteoclast crosstalk. Nat Commun 11(1):282
44. Blake GM, Fogelman I (2007) The role of DXA bone density scans in the diagnosis and treatment of osteoporosis. Postgrad Med J 83(982):509–517
45. Lorentzon M, Cummings SR (2015) Osteoporosis: the evolution of a diagnosis. J Intern Med 277(6):650–661
46. Unnanuntana A, Gladnick BP, Donnelly E, Lane JM (2010) The assessment of fracture risk. J Bone Joint Surg Am 92(3):743–753
47. Sözen T, Özışık L, Başaran NÇ (2017) An overview and management of osteoporosis. Eur J Rheumatol 4(1):46–56
48. Cauley JA (2011) Defining ethnic and racial differences in osteoporosis and fragility fractures. Clin Orthop Relat Res 469(7):1891–1899
49. Compston J, Cooper A, Cooper C, Gittoes N, Gregson C, Harvey N et al (2017) UK clinical guideline for the prevention and treatment of osteoporosis. Arch Osteoporos 12(1):43
50. Cosman F, de Beur SJ, LeBoff MS, Lewiecki EM, Tanner B, Randall S et al (2014) Clinician's guide to prevention and treatment of osteoporosis. Osteoporos Int 25(10):2359–2381
51. Mazziotti G, Canalis E, Giustina A (2010) Drug-induced osteoporosis: mechanisms and clinical implications. Am J Med 123(10):877–884
52. Oxford University (2010) Oxford dictionary of English, 3rd edn. Oxford University Press, Oxford
53. Berg KM, Kunins HV, Jackson JL, Nahvi S, Chaudhry A, Harris KA Jr et al (2008) Association between alcohol consumption and both osteoporotic fracture and bone density. Am J Med 121(5):406–418
54. Kanis JA, Johnell O (1999) The burden of osteoporosis. J Endocrinol Investig 22(8):583–588
55. Marsh D, Akesson K, Beaton DE, Bogoch ER, Boonen S, Brandi ML et al (2011) Coordinator-based systems for secondary prevention in fragility fracture patients. Osteoporos Int 22(7):2051–2065
56. Downey C, Kelly M, Quinlan JF (2019) Changing trends in the mortality rate at 1-year post hip fracture - a systematic review. World J Orthop 10(3):166–175
57. Chan S, Wong EKC, Ward SE, Kuan D, Wong CL (2019) The predictive value of the clinical frailty scale on discharge destination and complications in older hip fracture patients. J Orthop Trauma 33(10):497–502
58. Fried LP, Tangen CM, Walston J, Newman AB, Hirsch C, Gottdiener J et al (2001) Frailty in older adults: evidence for a phenotype. J Gerontol A Biol Sci Med Sci 56(3):M146–M156
59. Rockwood K (2005) Frailty and its definition: a worthy challenge. J Am Geriatr Soc 53(6):1069–1070
60. Cooper C, Arden NK (2011) Excess mortality in osteoarthritis. BMJ 342:d1407
61. Hanson MA, Cooper C, Aihie Sayer A, Eendebak RJ, Clough GF, Beard JR (2016) Developmental aspects of a life course approach to healthy ageing. J Physiol 594(8):2147–2160

62. Rockwood K, Theou O (2020) Using the clinical frailty scale in allocating scarce health care resources. Can Geriatr J 23(3):210–215
63. England PH (2020) Falls: applying all our health: gov.uk. Updated 31 January 2020. https://www.gov.uk/government/publications/falls-applying-all-our-health/falls-applying-all-our-health
64. Lackoff AS, Hickling D, Collins PF, Stevenson KJ, Nowicki TA, Bell JJ (2020) The association of malnutrition with falls and harm from falls in hospital inpatients: findings from a 5-year observational study. J Clin Nurs 29(3–4):429–436
65. (NICE) NIfHaCE (2013) Falls in older people: assessing risk and prevention
66. Registry AaNZHF (2020) Annual report of hip fracture care. Annual report. Australian and New Zealand hip fracture registry, Registry AaNZHF, Sidney
67. Cheraghi Z, Doosti-Irani A, Almasi-Hashiani A, Baigi V, Mansournia N, Etminan M et al (2019) The effect of alcohol on osteoporosis: a systematic review and meta-analysis. Drug Alcohol Depend 197:197–202
68. Movassagh EZ, Vatanparast H (2017) Current evidence on the Association of Dietary Patterns and Bone Health: a scoping review. Adv Nutr 8(1):1–16
69. Royal Osteoporosis Society (2019) Strong, steady and straight: physical activity and exercise for osteoporosis quick guide: summary. https://theros.org.uk/media/0o5h1l53/ros-strong-steady-straight-quick-guide-february-2019.pdf
70. Fatoye F, Smith P, Gebrye T, Yeowell G (2019) Real-world persistence and adherence with oral bisphosphonates for osteoporosis: a systematic review. BMJ Open 9(4):e027049
71. Rampakakis E, Sampalis JS (2012) What can be done to maximize adherence of bisphosphonates in patients with osteoporosis? Int J Clin Rheumatol 7(4):361–364
72. Parsons CM, Harvey N, Shepstone L, Kanis JA, Lenaghan E, Clarke S et al (2020) Systematic screening using FRAX(®) leads to increased use of, and adherence to, anti-osteoporosis medications: an analysis of the UK SCOOP trial. Osteoporos Int 31(1):67–75
73. Yardley L, Donovan-Hall M, Francis K, Todd C (2006) Older people's views of advice about falls prevention: a qualitative study. Health Educ Res 21(4):508–517
74. Marsh D, Mitchell P, Falaschi P, Beaupre L, Magaziner J, Seymour H et al (2021) The multidisciplinary approach to fragility fractures around the world: an overview. In: Falaschi P, Marsh D (eds) Orthogeriatrics: the management of older patients with fragility fractures. Springer International Publishing, Cham, pp 3–18
75. Dreinhöfer KE, Mitchell PJ, Bégué T, Cooper C, Costa ML, Falaschi P et al (2018) A global call to action to improve the care of people with fragility fractures. Injury 49(8):1393–1397
76. Riemen AHK, Hutchison JD (2016) The multidisciplinary management of hip fractures in older patients. Orthop Traumatol 30(2):117–122
77. Huntjens KM, van Geel TA, van den Bergh JP, van Helden S, Willems P, Winkens B et al (2014) Fracture liaison service: impact on subsequent nonvertebral fracture incidence and mortality. J Bone Joint Surg Am 96(4):e29
78. Jmmjyl J (1991) The illness experience: dimensions of suffering. Sage publications Inc., Thousand Oaks, CA
79. Neuburger J, Currie C, Wakeman R, Tsang C, Plant F, De Stavola B et al (2015) The impact of a national clinician-led audit initiative on care and mortality after hip fracture in England: an external evaluation using time trends in non-audit data. Med Care 53(8):686–691

10

Psychological Barriers and Nutritional Care

Maria Eduarda Batista de Lima and Stefano Eleuteri

Abstract

Eating habits are inseparably linked with people's physical and psychological health and well-being. Many factors impact on eating behavior and nutritional status in older adults. Motivational and multidisciplinary interventions have been shown to be highly effective in promoting healthy eating, especially in hospitalized patients, but are often overlooked or not considered. The aim of this chapter is to discuss how to overcome the psychological barriers that lead older patients away from an appropriate nutritional intake and the importance of motivational interventions for adherence to nutritional care, providing useful evidence and direction for further research.

Keywords

Motivational interventions · Nutritional care adherence · Older adults · Motivation · Nutritional therapy

This chapter is a component of Part I: Nutritional Care in Old Age.
For an explanation of the grouping of chapters in this book, please see Chap. 1: "Geriatrics and Orthogeriatrics: Providing Nutrition Care."

M. E. Batista de Lima (✉)
Education Committee, Fragility Fracture Network, NHS South East Tuscany, Siena, Italy

S. Eleuteri
Education Committee, Fragility Fracture Network, Sapienza University of Rome, Rome, Italy
e-mail: stefano.eleuteri@uniroma1.it

Learning Outcomes
By the end of this chapter, you will be able to:

- Recognize the complexities of diverse psychological barriers and enablers to nutritional care in older adults.
- Share understanding regarding older adults' perspectives regarding the relationship between food and nutritional care.
- Describe opportunities to improve the role of caregivers and the community in supporting patient motivation and adherence to nutritional care.
- Explain the rationale and benefit of interdisciplinary teams in supporting positive nutrition-related behavior change in older adults.

10.1 Introduction

The nutritional status of older frail and hospitalized patients has been shown to be of high importance for general well-being and for their recovery. Patients at risk of malnutrition are known to have increased rates of infections and mortality. Nutritional risk also seems important for the degree of health and strength that patients recover after hospitalization [1, 2].

During the last years, guidelines have been developed to ensure the right care for patients at nutritional risk during hospitalization [3]. These guidelines consider screening for nutritional risk, nutrition plan, and monitoring as well as communication to other healthcare providers, when the patient still needs nutritional assistance at transferal between hospital departments or at discharge. A concrete division of tasks within the nutrition process has been shown important for good nutritional practice. Nurses play a significant role in nutritional care [4, 5].

Evidence suggests that approximately 30% of patients with nutritional risk are in hospitals, although estimates vary with differences in populations. More than half of these patients have a daily energy and protein intake of less than 75% of their needs, and up to 40% lose weight during hospitalization [6, 7]. The reasons for this insufficient food intake are multiple and complex. Insufficient knowledge of hospital staff about nutritional needs and a lack of attention to nutritional problems, especially among nurses, has been described [2, 7–10].

Some clinical controlled trials between specific patient groups have shown that active patient involvement in their own nutritional care and mentoring of patients could increase the patient's energy intake [8, 10]. This is underlined by surveys which point out that patients have quite concrete expectations about their nutritional care, but do not seem to express them to staff [7, 8].

Of all older adults admitted to the acute setting, orthopedic patients have been shown to be among those most severely undernourished. The attention to nutritional aspects as part of patient care is undervalued and underdeveloped [11]. Creating strategies within which effective nutritional treatment can be achieved is vital. Effective management of nutrition for those at risk will speed recovery and reduce the incidence of secondary complications and mortality, reducing nursing workload in both hospitals and community settings [12].

Traditionally, nutrition has been a nursing responsibility, as caring for the patients' basic needs [13]. Today, nutrition is an interdisciplinary field shared across several professions. Interdisciplinary and multimodal nutritional assistance facilitates the exploration of the barriers presented by the patient that prevent receipt of quality nutrition. The involvement of healthcare providers helps to identify these barriers and implement targeted practical and motivational solutions, offering a greater proportional increase in protein and energy intake and improved patient-reported experience measures [12, 14–16].

10.2 The Relationship Between Older Adults and Food as a First Step Toward Overcoming Psychological Barriers

Many studies demonstrate that food preferences in older adults take into consideration how people's experiences change with aging: changes in taste, diet, and food choice. Primarily, this occurs when most people approach the age of 70 or older. Influencing variables can include social and cultural environment, gender, and personal habits as well as physical and mental health. Scientific studies attempting to explain why people like or dislike certain foods have been performed to deepen understanding of these issues [17–19].

Research is continuously examining the variables that cause older adults to change food preferences, one example being the Elderly Nutrition Program (ENP). To improve the quality of meal programs, the ENP explored how food preferences varied depending on biological sex and ethnic groups. A total of 2024 participants aged 60 years or older were interviewed. Most of the participants were female, served by congregate meal programs, or meals served in community settings such as senior centers, churches, or senior housing communities [20].

A general impression of the meals and preferences for 13 food groups (fresh fruit, chicken, soup, salad, vegetables, potatoes, meat, sandwiches, pasta, canned fruit, legumes, deli meats, and ethnic foods) was assessed. In addition, compared with African Americans, the study found that Caucasians demonstrated higher percentages of preference for 9 of 13 food groups, including pasta, meat, and fresh fruit, and recommended that to improve the quality of the ENP and to increase dietary compliance of the older adults to the programs, the nutritional services require a strategic meal plan that solicits and incorporates older adults' food preferences [20, 21].

There are multiple factors in an older adult's life that can affect food preferences. Aspects like the environment, mental and physical health medications, food access, and lifestyle choices can all contribute to the individual taste and/or habits. It has been long recognized that the nutritional status of older adults relates to their quality of life, ability to live independently, and their risk for developing costly chronic illnesses [22]. An aging adult's nutritional well-being can be affected by multiple socio-environmental factors, including access to healthy and affordable foods, congregate meal sites, and nutritious selections at restaurants. The Academy of Nutrition and Dietetics, the American Society for Parenteral and Enteral Nutrition (ASPEN), and the Society for Nutrition Education and Behavior have identified an older adult's access to a balanced diet to be critical for the prevention of disease and promotion of nutritional wellness so that quality of life and independence can be maintained throughout the aging process and excessive healthcare costs can be reduced [3, 23].

10.2.1 Age: Younger and Older Adults

As people age, their bodies change. This can include their taste buds, their needs of certain vitamins and nutrients, and their desire for different types of food. A study was performed with the participation of 50 young adults and 48 older adults [24]. "Young" subjects ranged from 18 to 35 years of age and "older" subjects were defined as 65 years of age or older. There were more females than males in the study, but there were approximately equal proportions of males and females in the two age groups. The study observed that younger females had stronger cravings for sweets than older females. Causation theories included accounting this difference in preference with the younger female test subject's menstrual cycles and the fact that older women no longer go through menopause. The study also postulated that 91% of the cycle-associated cravings were said to occur in the second half of the cycle (between ovulation and the start of menstruation). These physical changes can be considered when assessing why someone of an older age might not be getting the nutrition they need. As taste buds change with age, certain foods might not be seen as appetizing, for example, the suggestion that as we age, our sense for tasting salty foods goes away slowly [25].

10.2.2 Biological Sex: Older Male and Female

Food preferences also differ among biological sexes. A study demonstrated that older males were "significantly more likely to prefer deli meats, meat, legumes, canned fruit, and ethnic foods compared to females" [13, 14]. Another research concluded that females had significantly more cravings for sweets and for chocolate than males; and the study results suggested that males had more cravings or preferences for savory foods than sweets [24].

10.2.3 Personal Health

10.2.3.1 Physical Health

With age, some people tend to avoid food or are unwilling to modify their diets due to oral health problems. These issues, such as ill-fitting dentures (false teeth) or gum disease, are associated with significant differences in dietary quality, which is a measure of the quality of the diet using a total of eight recommendations regarding the consumption of foods and nutrients from the National Academy of Sciences

(NAS). Approaches to minimize food avoidance and promote changes to the diets of people that have eating difficulties due to oral health conditions are needed desperately because without being able to chew or take in food properly, their health is affected drastically, and their food preferences are limited greatly (to soft or liquids only) [26] (Chap. 18).

Due to varying factors of older adults' physical and mental well-being, eating choices can become more and more restricted. Many older adults are constrained into eating softer foods, foods that incorporate fiber and protein, drinking calcium-packed liquids, and so on. Six of the leading causes of death for older adults, including cardiovascular disease, cancer, chronic lower respiratory disease, stroke, Alzheimer's, and diabetes mellitus, have nutrition-related causes and/or respond favorably to nutritional interventions. These six illnesses can implement certain restrictions and heavily influence the diet [27].

Declining physical health (e.g., patients with arthritis) can also cause dietary deterioration due to difficulties in food purchasing, preparation, and consumption [26].

Some authors noted that old adults are less active and have lower metabolism with a consequent lower need to eat. In addition, they tend to have existing diseases and/or take medications that interfere with nutrient absorption. Based on their research dietary requirements, one study developed specific recommendations for adults over 70 [28].

10.2.3.2 Mental Health

The impact of certain diseases can also impact the quality of nutritional intake in the old population, especially those that are in care facilities. Certain risk factors include conditions that impair cognitive function, such as dementia [29].

As a result of certain mental health conditions and/or diseases—like Alzheimer's and Parkinson's disease—a person's food preferences might become affected. Since the experience of flavor is significantly altered, people with dementia can often change their eating habits and take on entirely new food preferences. In this study, the researchers found that these dementia patients had trouble identifying flavors and appeared to have lost the ability to remember tastes, therefore leading to a theory that dementia caused the patients to lose their knowledge of flavors [30].

Psychological conditions can also affect eating habits. For instance, length of widowhood may affect nutrition [31]. Depression in old people is also associated with a risk of malnutrition [29, 31].

10.2.4 Lifestyle Choices

Old adults have different lifestyle choices involved in their eating habits. Dietary choices are often a result of personal beliefs and preferences.

A survey based on self-reporting found that many rural communities adopted eating habits that provided inadequate levels of some key nutrients and most did not take supplements to correct the deficiencies. In contrast, a restaurant study found that the impact of a lifestyle of health and sustainability on healthy food choices is much stronger for senior diners than for non-senior diners [32].

Other research has found that adults, regardless of age, will tend to increase fruit and vegetable consumption following a diagnosis of breast, prostate, or colorectal cancer [33].

10.2.5 Social Environment and Conditioning

The environment can greatly impact food preferences of older adults. Those around 75 years old and older are more likely to suffer with limited mobility due to health conditions and often rely on others for food shopping and preparation [34].

In some areas, homebound seniors receive one meal per day (several fresh and frozen meals may be included in a single delivery) by communities that offer congregate meals, or meals served in community settings such as senior centers, churches, or senior housing communities. These congregate meal programs are encouraged to offer a meal at least five times per week [13, 17].

Impeded access to transportation may also be an issue for old adults, especially in rural areas where there is less public transportation. This can vary greatly due to geographic location [34].

The type of social network can also influence the food choices of individuals in our older adult population. For example, one study showed that a person that has a larger social network and lower economic status is more likely to have proper nutrition that someone who has a smaller social network and higher economic status [35]. Health and social aid can be instrumental into introducing positive change for those at risk.

10.3 The Older Adult Perspective and the Quality of Nutritional Care

Clinical controlled trials have shown that actively involving patients in their own nutritional care and mentoring patients could increase the patient's energy intake. A study [36] demonstrated that the patient perspective contributes to the quality of nutritional care. Studies still show that patients felt a connection between their lack of physical and psychological well-being and their inability to eat enough [13, 37]. Both men and women experienced decreased physical strength. Lack of appetite, pain, bad taste, nausea, and early satiety were presented as the main reasons for not eating, in some studies. Within these findings, the amount of medication, especially tablets, was mentioned as a barrier to appetite, causing altered taste of food [37, 38].

A recent qualitative study considering enteral tube feeding in hip fracture highlighted key patient perspectives influencing nutrition support; these highlighted the need to consider patient (and/or carer) knowledge and understanding, perceived consequences and necessity of the nutritional intervention (or alternatives) in addition to ability to cope, attitude toward life duration, and the relative importance of tube feeding. Interestingly, three key potentially modifiable drivers were identified that were considered to facilitate or negate acceptance of tube feeding: personal perception of the situation, the value of nutrition, and perceived quality of life [39].

Another important factor to consider according to some research [39] is the food neophobia, defined as the "reluctance to eat and/or avoidance of novel foods." This may act as a barrier to the consumption of novel foods and may act as a barrier to the consumption of novel fortified foods or foods that have been specially developed for older adults. The negative impacts of this association will also be exacerbated when older adults are already at increased risk of malnutrition. Oral nutritional supplements and fortified foods may be comparable to functional foods, and food neophobia scores have been related to a reluctance to try new functional foods in adults, including older adults.

The timing of meal delivery and the presentation of the dish were considered important in some research. Patients stated that they appreciated being taken care of, especially with individually served snacks. Patients had a clear opinion about the commitment of the healthcare providers to the management of food service and stated that their attention stimulated them to eat more [40].

10.3.1 The Role of Caregivers and Community

The role and involvement of relatives with various aspects of nutritional care are important to patients. However, the practical role of relatives especially at discharge or leave from hospital should be considered carefully. Today, it is common that relatives are taken into practical planning of nutritional care and are taught by dietitians and nursing staff how to make food more energy dense and how to serve small portions, snacks, and supplements. Not least, urging to eat from relatives was mentioned as problematic [38]. The patients in this study described that they understood and appreciated the concern from their relatives, but at the same time, they felt they were under substantial pressure from them and felt they had no understanding toward their situation. As seen in advanced patients with cancer [41], families were concerned that their encouragement to make patients eat might become nagging and worsen the situation. Some even found that relative surging the patients to eat made them decrease nutrition intake rather than increase it. This situation should maybe be discussed with patients and relatives at leave or discharge. Fellow patients had a significant role to the patients feeling of comfort during hospitalization. A fellow patient in a futile situation seemed to have negative impact on the weak and passive patients, whereas companionship, trust, and support between fellow patients in similar situations seemed to be important and give the patient's life courage [42].

Studies such as these show the utmost importance of considering the patient's perceptions of their own nutrition and their expectations regarding the nutritional regimen prescribed by the nutritional team. This would be the first step to personally motivate each patient at nutritional risk.

10.4 The Effectiveness of Multidisciplinary Nutritional Care to Increase Patient Motivation

Many studies have aimed to determine the effectiveness of a multidisciplinary intervention program on nutritional intake and of nutritional intake on nutritional status and quality of life in older patients treated for a hip fracture.

Among older adults with a hip fracture, a multidisciplinary postoperative approach of nutritional care has been associated with an increase of energy and protein intake during hospitalization, reduced malnutrition incidence, and improved home discharge rates [43]. Other works demonstrate that effective management of nutrition for those at risk will speed recovery and reduce the incidence of secondary complications and mortality, reducing nursing workload in both hospitals and community settings. Of particular interest for this chapter are studies demonstrating the positive effects of care models that combine interdisciplinary motivational care with nutrition consultation, depression management, and fall prevention in older patients with hip fracture [44]. While multidisciplinary nutrition support teams routinely include medical, nursing, dietetics, and pharmaceutical professionals, in order to consider all the important factors involved in managing nutritional care in older, multimorbid patients, these should also include psychologists and other healthcare professionals [45]. In view of the multiculturalism of patients and health professionals, the multi-professional team is recommended to have an anthropological view that will allow even more the personalization of the dietary plan and the patient's nutritional adherence.

Clearly defined responsibilities, education and training of hospital staff, cooperation between all staff groups, and the involvement of hospital management are essential measures to effectively prevent and treat malnutrition in the hospital setting [46]. In addition to consider the patient's psychological barriers that affect their nutrition, the multidisciplinary team should also consider the system's barriers and their expectations regarding the patient's nutrition plan. Some studies demonstrate that health professions' responsibilities and roles related to such care should be more formally defined. The lack of proper instructions and of assignment of responsibility means that nobody is clearly accountable for the patients' nutrition, and undernourishment is more likely to be left unrecognized and undertreated [11, 46]. Moreover, poor cooperation among all hospital staff groups has been defined as a common barrier to good nutritional practice [47] resulting in inadequate nutrition in the chain of care.

10.5 Summary

In conclusion, in order to increase adherence and motivation, nutritional care recommendations must take into consideration patients' lifestyles, preferences, and psychological aspects in the nutritional care assessment, planning, intervention, and evaluation phases. Older adults and caregivers must also have an awareness of nutritional care basics and adequate nutritional literacy to support making informed choices about nutritional care. The possibility to understand why certain foods and fluids are to be prioritized and to choose between different options helps in moving the responsibility from the healthcare providers to the older adults, giving them the opportunity to feel to be more involved (and so more adherent and motivated) in nutritional care. In concluding, personalization is the most important point: what works with a patient is not certain to work with another, and what matters to one older adult may not be the same as what matters to another; so planning and evaluation in the multidisciplinary team should serve to consider this aspect.

Take-Home Points

- There are diverse psychological barriers and enablers that should be considered when assessing, treating, and evaluating nutrition care processes for older adults with or at risk of malnutrition.
- Despite the barriers that staff experience in day-to-day work in hospital wards to ensure adequate nutritional care for undernourished seniors, interdisciplinary work among health workers is a key enabler to meeting the complex needs of older people and motivating nutritional behavior change.
- Increasing patient motivation and adherence to nutritional care demands considering the patient's perceptions of their own nutrition, engaging them in care planning, and evaluating their expectations and experiences regarding the nutritional prescriptions recommended and enacted.

References

1. Nieuwenhuizen WF, Weenen H, Rigby P, Hetherington MM (2010) Older adults and patients in need of nutritional support: review of current treatment options and factors influencing nutritional intake. Clin Nutr 29(2):160–169
2. Bauer J, Biolo G, Cederholm T, Cesari M, Cruz-Jentoft AJ, Morley JE et al (2013) Evidence-based recommendations for optimal dietary protein intake in older people: a position paper from the PROT-AGE Study Group. J Am Med Dir Assoc 14(8):542–559
3. Volkert D, Beck AM, Cederholm T, Cruz-Jentoft A, Goisser S, Hooper L et al (2019) ESPEN guideline on clinical nutrition and hydration in geriatrics. Clin Nutr 38(1):10–47
4. Tappenden KA, Quatrara B, Parkhurst ML, Malone AM, Fanjiang G, Ziegler TR (2013) Critical role of nutrition in improving quality of care: an interdisciplinary call to action to address adult hospital malnutrition. JPEN J Parenter Enteral Nutr 37(4):482–497
5. Ten Cate D, Ettema RGA, Huisman-de Waal G, Bell JJ, Verbrugge R, Schoonhoven L et al (2020) Interventions to prevent and treat malnutrition in older adults to be carried out by nurses: a systematic review. J Clin Nurs 29(11–12):1883–1902
6. Fávaro-Moreira NC, Krausch-Hofmann S, Matthys C, Vereecken C, Vanhauwaert E, Declercq A et al (2016) Risk factors for malnutrition in older adults: a systematic review of the literature based on longitudinal data. Adv Nutr 7(3):507–522
7. de Morais C, Oliveira B, Afonso C, Lumbers M, Raats M, de Almeida MD (2013) Nutritional risk of European elderly. Eur J Clin Nutr 67(11):1215–1219

8. van der Schueren MAEB, Lonterman-Monasch S, de Vries OJ, Danner SA, Kramer MH, Muller M (2013) Prevalence and determinants for malnutrition in geriatric outpatients. Clin Nutr 32(6):1007–1011
9. Zeanandin G, Molato O, Le Duff F, Guérin O, Hébuterne X, Schneider SM (2012) Impact of restrictive diets on the risk of undernutrition in a free-living elderly population. Clin Nutr 31(1):69–73
10. Furuta M, Komiya-Nonaka M, Akifusa S, Shimazaki Y, Adachi M, Kinoshita T et al (2013) Interrelationship of oral health status, swallowing function, nutritional status, and cognitive ability with activities of daily living in Japanese elderly people receiving home care services due to physical disabilities. Community Dent Oral Epidemiol 41(2):173–181
11. Bell J, Bauer J, Capra S, Pulle CR (2013) Barriers to nutritional intake in patients with acute hip fracture: time to treat malnutrition as a disease and food as a medicine? Can J Physiol Pharmacol 91(6):489–495
12. Bell JJ, Rossi T, Bauer JD, Capra S (2014) Developing and evaluating interventions that are applicable and relevant to inpatients and those who care for them; a multiphase, pragmatic action research approach. BMC Med Res Methodol 14:98
13. Reinders I, Wijnhoven HAH, Jyväkorpi SK, Suominen MH, Niskanen R, Bosmans JE et al (2020) Effectiveness and cost-effectiveness of personalised dietary advice aiming at increasing protein intake on physical functioning in community-dwelling older adults with lower habitual protein intake: rationale and design of the PROMISS randomised controlled trial. BMJ Open 10(11):e040637. https://doi.org/10.1136/bmjopen-2020-040637. http://europepmc.org/abstract/MED/33444206, https://europepmc.org/articles/PMC7682452, https://europepmc.org/articles/PMC7682452?pdf=render
14. Chang M, Geirsdottir OG, Launer LJ, Gudnasson V, Visser M, Gunnarsdottir I (2020) A poor appetite or ability to eat and its association with physical function amongst community-dwelling older adults: age, gene/environment susceptibility-Reykjavik study. Eur J Ageing
15. Bell JJ, Bauer JD, Capra S, Pulle RC (2014) Multidisciplinary, multi-modal nutritional care in acute hip fracture inpatients - results of a pragmatic intervention. Clin Nutr 33(6):1101–1107
16. Bell JJ, Young AM, Hill JM, Banks MD, Comans TA, Barnes R et al (2021) Systematised, Interdisciplinary Malnutrition Program for impLementation and Evaluation delivers improved hospital nutrition care processes and patient reported experiences - an implementation study. Nutr Diet. Early view: https://doi.org/10.1111/1747-0080.12663
17. Nematy M, Hickson M, Brynes AE, Ruxton CH, Frost GS (2006) Vulnerable patients with a fractured neck of femur: nutritional status and support in hospital. J Hum Nutr Diet 19(3):209–218
18. Sánchez López AM, Moreno-Torres Herrera R, Pérez de la Cruz, AJ, Orduña Espinosa R, Medina T, López Martínez C (2005) [Malnutrition prevalence in patients admitted to a rehabilitation and orthopedic surgery hospital]. Nutr Hosp 20(2):121–130
19. Gustafsson K, Sidenvall B (2002) Food-related health perceptions and food habits among older women. J Adv Nurs 39(2):164–173
20. Brewster PW, Melrose RJ, Marquine MJ, Johnson JK, Napoles A, MacKay-Brandt A et al (2014) Life experience and demographic influences on cognitive function in older adults. Neuropsychology 28(6):846–858
21. Mowe M, Bosaeus I, Rasmussen HH, Kondrup J, Unosson M, Irtun Ø (2006) Nutritional routines and attitudes among doctors and nurses in Scandinavia: a questionnaire based survey. Clin Nutr 25(3):524–532
22. Westergren A, Unosson M, Ohlsson O, Lorefält B, Hallberg IR (2002) Eating difficulties, assisted eating and nutritional status in elderly (> or = 65 years) patients in hospital rehabilitation. Int J Nurs Stud 39(3):341–351
23. Grzegorczyk PB, Jones SW, Mistretta CM (1979) Age-related differences in salt taste acuity. J Gerontol 34(6):834–840
24. Savoca MR, Arcury TA, Leng X, Chen H, Bell RA, Anderson AM et al (2010) Association between dietary quality of rural older adults and self-reported food avoidance and food modification due to oral health problems. J Am Geriatr Soc 58(7):1225–1232

25. Jung SE, Lawrence J, Hermann J, McMahon A (2020) Application of the theory of planned behavior to predict nutrition students' intention to work with older adults. J Nutr Gerontol Geriatr 39(1):44–55
26. Field K, Duizer LM (2016) Food sensory properties and the older adult. J Texture Stud 47(4):266–276
27. Lee RJ, Collins PF, Elmas K, Bell JJ (2021) Restrictive diets in older malnourished cardiac inpatients: a cross-sectional study. Nutr Diet 78:121
28. Lawrence AS (2021) The Australian Dietary Guidelines review: time to plan for wider dissemination via general practitioners. Aust J Gen Pract 50(4):252–253
29. Ghimire S, Baral BK, Pokhrel BR, Pokhrel A, Acharya A, Amatya D et al (2018) Depression, malnutrition, and health-related quality of life among Nepali older patients. BMC Geriatr 18(1):191
30. Quandt SA, McDonald J, Arcury TA, Bell RA, Vitolins MZ (2000) Nutritional self-management of elderly widows in rural communities. Gerontologist 40(1):86–96
31. Vafaei Z, Mokhtari H, Sadooghi Z, Meamar R, Chitsaz A, Moeini M (2013) Malnutrition is associated with depression in rural elderly population. J Res Med Sci 18(Suppl 1):S15–S19
32. Marshall TA, Stumbo PJ, Warren JJ, Xie XJ (2001) Inadequate nutrient intakes are common and are associated with low diet variety in rural, community-dwelling elderly. J Nutr 131(8):2192–2196
33. Kim MJ, Lee C-K, Kim W, Kim J-M (2013) Relationships between lifestyle of health and sustainability and healthy food choices for seniors. Int J Contemp Hosp Manag 25:558
34. Fitzpatrick K, Greenhalgh-Stanlcy N, Vcr PM (2016) The impact of food deserts on food insufficiency and SNAP participation among the elderly. Am J Agric Econ 98(1):19–40
35. Holst M, Rasmussen HH, Laursen BS (2011) Can the patient perspective contribute to quality of nutritional care? Scand J Caring Sci 25(1):176–184
36. Pedersen PU (2005) Nutritional care: the effectiveness of actively involving older patients. J Clin Nurs 14(2):247–255
37. Norman K, Kirchner H, Lochs H, Pirlich M (2006) Malnutrition affects quality of life in gastroenterology patients. World J Gastroenterol 12(21):3380–3385
38. Westergren A, Ohlsson O, Hallberg IR (2001) Eating difficulties, complications and nursing interventions during a period of three months after a stroke. J Adv Nurs 35(3):416–426
39. van den Heuvel E, Newbury A, Appleton KM (2019) The psychology of Nutrition with advancing age: focus on food neophobia. Nutrients 11(1):151
40. Almdal T, Viggers L, Beck AM, Jensen K (2003) Food production and wastage in relation to nutritional intake in a general district hospital--wastage is not reduced by training the staff. Clin Nutr 22(1):47–51
41. Nourissat A, Vasson MP, Merrouche Y, Bouteloup C, Goutte M, Mille D et al (2008) Relationship between nutritional status and quality of life in patients with cancer. Eur J Cancer 44(9):1238–1242
42. Hestevik CH, Molin M, Debesay J, Bergland A, Bye A (2020) Older patients' and their family caregivers' perceptions of food, meals and nutritional care in the transition between hospital and home care: a qualitative study. BMC Nutr 6:11
43. Odlund Olin A, Koochek A, Ljungqvist O, Cederholm T (2005) Nutritional status, well-being and functional ability in frail elderly service flat residents. Eur J Clin Nutr 59(2):263–270
44. Shyu YI, Liang J, Tseng MY, Li HJ, Wu CC, Cheng HS et al (2013) Comprehensive care improves health outcomes among elderly Taiwanese patients with hip fracture. J Gerontol A Biol Sci Med Sci 68(2):188–197
45. Nightingale J (2010) Nutrition support teams: how they work, are set up and maintained. Frontline Gastroenterol 1(3):171–177
46. Eide HD, Halvorsen K, Almendingen K (2015) Barriers to nutritional care for the undernourished hospitalised elderly: perspectives of nurses. J Clin Nurs 24(5–6):696–706

47. Ross LJ, Mudge AM, Young AM, Banks M (2011) Everyone's problem but nobody's job: staff perceptions and explanations for poor nutritional intake in older medical patients. Nutr Diet 68(1):41–46

11

Nutritional Improvements: Spread and Sustainability

Celia V. Laur and Jack J. Bell

Abstract

Previous chapters have described how to improve nutrition care with an emphasis on interdisciplinary approaches. The focus of this chapter is on keeping these improvements going (sustainability) and how to apply them to a new setting (spread).

Keywords

Sustainability · Spread · Quality of healthcare · Implementation · Nutrition · Evaluation · Equity

---

This chapter is a component of Part 1: Nutritional Care in Old Age.
For an explanation of the grouping of chapters in this book, please see Chap. 1: "Geriatrics and Orthogeriatrics: Providing Nutrition Care."

C. V. Laur (✉)
Women's College Hospital Institute for Health System Solutions and Virtual Care, and Women's College Research Institute, Women's College Hospital, Toronto, ON, Canada
e-mail: Celia.Laur@wchospital.ca

J. J. Bell
Allied Health, The Prince Charles Hospital, Chermside, Queensland, Australia

School of Human Movement and Nutrition Sciences, The University of Queensland, St Lucia, QLD, Australia
e-mail: jack.bell@health.qld.gov.au

Learning Outcomes
By the end of this chapter, you will be able to:

- Understand the key elements of sustainability and differentiate between spread and scale.
- Formulate strategies to include sustainability from the beginning of nutrition care improvements.
- Justify elements integral to building, sustaining, and spreading nutrition care improvements.
- Recognize common barriers and enablers to sustaining and spreading nutrition care improvements.
- Know some tools to use to help support sustainability planning.
- Recognize the importance of equity considerations in planning for sustainability and spread.

11.1 Getting Started

When you make a change that improves practice, you want to make sure that it continues to have the desired benefit. This is why it is important to think about sustainability of interventions or programs from the beginning of your work. There are ways to integrate sustainability plans from the beginning and strategies to use once the initiative is working to help make sure that the processes and benefits continue. Another way to have a longer-term impact is to have your work used in other locations by spreading the program or improvement. This chapter will go through definitions, strategies, barriers, and enablers to sustainability and spread, drawing on case examples from Canada and Australia.

11.1.1 Definitions

A major challenge when talking about sustainability is that there is no consistent definition or length of time used to determine if a program was "sustained" [1–5]. There are also many terms used to describe this concept, such as maintenance, normalization, institutionalization, and routinization [3, 6]. Moore et al.'s (2017) definition of sustainability is commonly used as it breaks sustainability into five main components regarding time, continued delivery of the intervention and/or behavior change, and recognition that the program may continue to adapt in order to produce benefits for individual/systems [3] (p. 6). As put by Scheirer and Dearing, sustainability is the "continued use of program components and activities for the continued achievement of desirable program and population outcomes" [7].

When planning for the use of a program or improvement in another setting, two common ways to explain this process are spread and scale. As with sustainability, there are no consistent definitions for spread and scale. This chapter focuses on spread, but it is important to understand the difference since these concepts are often used interchangeably. Differentiating between these concepts allows for more targeted strategies. Greenhalgh et al. (2019) define spread as "Replicating an initiative somewhere else (i.e. one site to another)" and scale as "Tackling the infrastructure problems that arise during full scale implementation (i.e. implementing provincial policy)" [8, 9]. Shaw et al. [10] further indicate that spread is for "complex" problems where following a specific formula may not work and you may need to extensively adapt the program to fix the context. Scale is for "complicated" problems where formulas are critical and a high level of expertise is needed, yet solutions do not need to be adapted [10, 11]. As an example, if a nutrition care program that was working well in one long-term facility was taken up in another and adapted to that setting, it would be called spread, while if a specific change were made across all facilities, this would be scale.

11.2 Case Example: Improving Nutrition Care in Hospital

To further understand the concepts of sustainability and spread, this case example, led by Prof Heather Keller from the University of Waterloo, demonstrates how hospitals across Canada were able to implement nutrition care activities including nutrition screening and assessment [12, 13], sustain those changes for several years [14], and spread to new hospitals with minimal researcher involvement [14]. This grassroot, or "bottom-up," approach focused on implementation, sustainability, and spread, while complemented by "top-down" effort from the Canadian Malnutrition Task Force, the Canadian Nutrition Society, and the Health Standards Organization to develop malnutrition standards which could be scaled across Canada.

11.2.1 Initial Implementation and Considering Sustainability from the Beginning

Five hospitals across Canada were tasked with implementing the Integrated Nutrition Pathway for Acute Care (INPAC), a consensus-based pathway for the prevention, detection, and treatment of hospital malnutrition [15, 16]. After 1 year, a multidisciplinary team of hospital staff and management had implemented nutrition screening and a standardized assessment [12], decreased barriers to food intake (i.e., when the meal tray is too far from the patient), and increased food intake monitoring [12, 17]. Another year later, those changes continued [14], and six new hospitals that had started INPAC implementation were able to reach similar levels with less support from a research team [14].

A summary of strategies for initial implementation of INPAC is provided in Fig. 11.1, and strategies for sustainability and spread are in Fig. 11.2. These figures are based on interviews and focus groups with those involved in the original five hospitals [13, 18]. An INPAC implementation toolkit has also been developed which walks through steps for implementation and sustainability (http://m2e.nutritioncareincanada.ca/).

To implement INPAC, a multidisciplinary implementation team worked together to build a reason to change practice. These reasons varied slightly depending on the

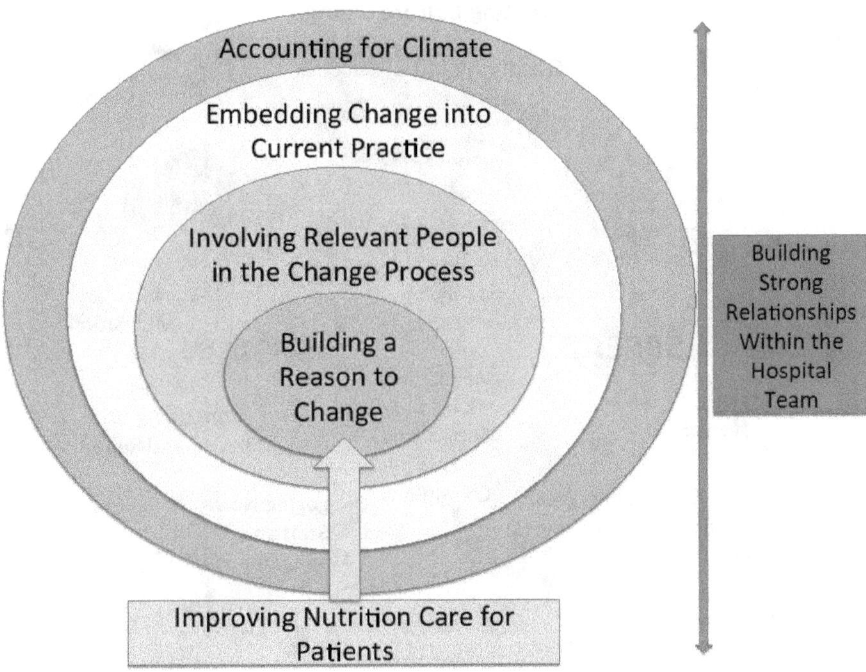

Fig. 11.1 A visual summary of how hospitals implemented nutrition care improvements and built the foundation for sustainable change [18]. (The figure is used with permission)

audience (management, nurses, and others), typically demonstrating the national and local prevalence (i.e., one in three patients are malnourished at admission) [19–22], the impact on length of stay (i.e., malnourished patients stay 2–3 days longer) [23], and the cost (i.e., approximately $2 billion CAN per year) [24]. These reasons for change were coupled with potential solutions, including ways that everyone can be involved in improving nutrition care.

This multidisciplinary approach led to the next main factor for change which was about involving the right people in the change process, including those most impacted (i.e., admission nurses who conduct nutrition screening). To be sustained, all changes had to be embedded into current practice, such as by adapting existing workflows and working with those impacted to see what made the most sense in that unit/hospital.

Context was key, so considering the external factors, such as hospital structure and overall climate, was needed. Climate focuses on the values of the organization, including the means, motivation, and opportunities for innovation [25]. For example, changes need to be within the regulations of the health region (context), while aligning with the hospital priorities (climate). Finally, strong relationships within the hospital teams were required throughout the change process, a factor that continues to apply through sustainability and spread.

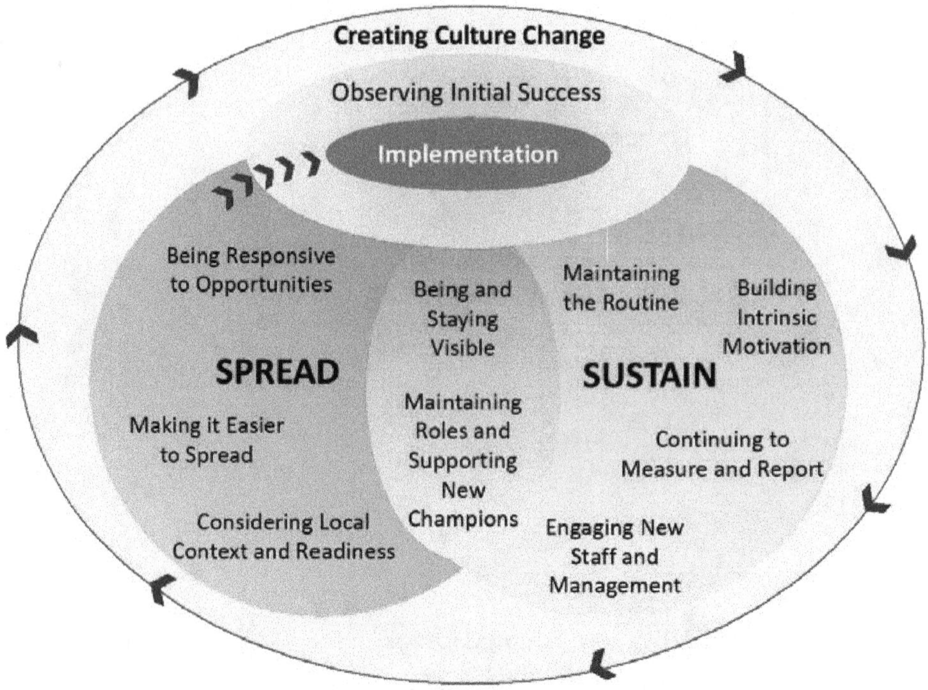

Fig. 11.2 The sustain and spread framework. This summary of strategies to support sustainability and spread begins once there is some initial implementation success.

11.2.2 Strategies for Sustainability and Spread

Nutrition care improvements, specifically nutrition screening and assessment, were sustained and spread [14]. Strategies for how these changes were sustained were explored with the original hospitals 1 year after initial implementation [13] and again 2 years later with six new hospitals [26]. A summary of these strategies is provided in Fig. 11.2.

Figure 11.1 could be placed in the "implementation" oval of Fig. 11.2. Strategies to encourage changes to be sustained or spread are included within each large circle, with the two overlapping strategies in the middle relevant to sustaining and spreading success. To spread to a new setting, it goes back to initial implementation (arrows from the spread circle back to implementation) in the new context. Working through several rounds of sustaining and spreading may potentially lead to culture change. The figure is used with permission [13].

To achieve sustainability, the multidisciplinary teams focused on maintaining the routine, building intrinsic motivation, continuing to measure and report, as well as engaging new staff and management. High staff turnover was common, making orientation sessions and quick introduction chats with new management key for continued success. Regular audits were also important, allowing teams to see their progress and to know when "booster" activities, such as reminders, were needed to maintain the momentum. Audits were less frequent than during initial implementation.

For spread, the teams mentioned the importance of being responsive to opportunities such as interest from other locations and finding ways to make it easier by learning from previous implementation experience. As with initial implementation, the new context needed to be considered, as well as how ready the new location was to start implementation. In the new location, the change needed to start again, thinking through each factor of implementation, ideally learning from what has come before.

Strategies important for both sustaining and spreading changes were about being and staying visible, such as having a member of the team regularly present where the change was taking place. Champions, those that bring the implementation efforts forward, were key to success. Champions for specific tasks or new locations were needed in order to decrease the burden on the original champion and facilitate sustainability. Attributes for effective champions have been suggested, such as influence, ownership, physical presence at the point of change, persuasiveness, grit, and a participative leadership style [27].

This case example was conducted in Canada, and the frameworks have not been validated in other settings. However, the Systematized, Interdisciplinary Malnutrition Pathway for impLementation and Evaluation (SIMPLE) in hospitals is based on INPAC and has used these strategies for improving nutrition care in Australia [28, 29].

11.3 Tools for Sustainability and Spread

There are many theories, models, frameworks, and tools that can be used as guides for implementation, sustainability, and spread [30, 31]. Although some tools may be more directed toward initial implementation and others toward sustainability, the most important factor is choosing what works for you and your team, and ideally, validated. A more detailed tool may provide useful ideas about factors to consider yet may not be practical for everyday use. Others may be too simplistic, focusing on key questions without providing direction on what to do with the information. Training courses have been developed, such as those from the Center for Implementation (https://thecenterforimplementation.com/courses), which can introduce you to several options and help you decide what makes sense for your work.

11.3.1 Sustainability Tools

While implementation tools can be used to plan for implementation and sustainability, it is recommended that sustainability be considered from the beginning, rather than only at the end, where it is typically placed. There are also tools focused on sustainability:

- **Program Sustainability Assessment Tool (PSAT)**: This is designed to support the implementation of an evidence-based program, typically in the community. The tool has several resources that help you understand, assess, review, and plan for sustainability [32]. The Clinical Sustainability Assessment Tool is also available (https://www.sustaintool.org/).
- **The NHS Sustainability Model and Guide**: This model focuses on staff, process, and organization and is designed to be used at several points throughout your implementation. This model allows you to work through a checklist and provides a quantitative score to inform your next steps [33].

11.4 Monitoring and Evaluation

It is difficult to know if the intended benefit or process is continuing without measuring it. Monitoring and evaluation are essential factors for initial implementation, and continued monitoring will allow you to know if your processes and outcomes are sustained [34]. The frequency of this monitoring may not need to be the same as during the earlier stages of implementation; however, an occasional check on progress will let you know if further effort or "boosters" are needed.

11.5 Barriers and Facilitators

There are many barriers and facilitators to implementation, sustainability, and spread [35–38]. Examples of facilitators include the continued role of the champion, ongoing organizational leadership and support, adequate funding and resources, continued effectiveness of the program, setting characteristics and policies, and fit of the program/intervention within the context. Examples of barriers include lack of funding, high staff turnover, or changes in policy. Using pre-established lists of barriers and facilitators [35–37] can help you think through possible factors; however, it is important to understand which factors are impacting your specific work before trying to overcome barriers that may not exist in your setting. Monitoring and evaluation, including discussions with those involved, can facilitate this understanding.

11.6 Considering Equity

When planning for a nutrition improvement to be sustained, spread, or scaled, it is important to take an equity lens to ensure the improvement is equitable, and not perpetuating or exacerbating existing inequities. Improvements also need to acknowledge the diverse experiences that impact implementation efforts and account for social influence, such as sociopolitical forces, physical structures, and economics [39]. A key goal in this work is to improve the quality and outcomes of services and make treatments and services available to multiple communities and settings [40, 41]. To achieve this goal, Baumann and Cabassa (2020) have listed five strategies [41]:

1. Focus on reach from the very beginning.
2. Design and select interventions for vulnerable populations and low-resource communities with implementation in mind.
3. Implement what works and develop implementation strategies that can help reduce inequities in care.
4. Develop the science of adaptations.
5. Use an equity lens for implementation outcomes.

11.7 Summary

When making nutrition care improvements in any setting, changes should be planned with the potential for sustainability and spread considered from the beginning. Focusing on improvements that are unlikely to be sustained can lead to wasted time and resources, which can be discouraging when trying to involve and motivate others for the next change. Not everything needs to be sustained and spread; evaluation and equity are key to this decision. Healthcare is constantly changing, making adaptability and flexibility key, and considering how to sustain or spread your improvement from the beginning will be beneficial for success.

Take-Home Points

- Sustainability and spread should be considered and planned for, if relevant, from the beginning of any change process.
- Sustainability is difficult to define; definitions typically focus on the continuation of program components which lead to the continuation of the desired outcomes.
- Distinguishing between spread and scale allows for more strategic approaches to have your nutrition care improvement used in other settings.
- Regular monitoring and evaluation allow for understanding of how a change is progressing and if "boosters" or reminders are needed.
- An equity lens is needed so that by sustaining and spreading nutrition care improvements you are not also sustaining and spreading inequities.

References

1. Ilott I et al (2013) Exploring scale-up, spread, and sustainability: an instrumental case study tracing an innovation to enhance dysphagia care. Implement Sci 8(1):128
2. Fleiszer AR et al (2015) The sustainability of healthcare innovations: a concept analysis. J Adv Nurs 71(7):1484–1498
3. Moore JE et al (2017) Developing a comprehensive definition of sustainability. Implement Sci 12(1):110

4. Proctor E et al (2015) Sustainability of evidence-based healthcare: research agenda, methodological advances, and infrastructure support. Implement Sci 10(1):88
5. Schell SF et al (2013) Public health program capacity for sustainability: a new framework. Implement Sci 8(1):15
6. Shelton RC, Cooper BR, Stirman SW (2018) The sustainability of evidence-based interventions and practices in public health and health care. Annu Rev Public Health 39:55–76
7. Scheirer MA, Dearing JW (2011) An agenda for research on the sustainability of public health programs. Am J Public Health 101(11):2059–2067
8. Greenhalgh T, Papoutsi C (2019) Spreading and scaling up innovation and improvement. BMJ 365:l2068
9. Barker PM, Reid A, Schall MW (2016) A framework for scaling up health interventions: lessons from large-scale improvement initiatives in Africa. Implement Sci 11:12. https://doi.org/10.1186/s13012-016-0374-x
10. Shaw J, Tepper J, Martin D (2018) From pilot project to system solution: innovation, spread and scale for health system leaders. BMJ Leader2: 87-90
11. Sholom Glouberman BZ (2013) Complicated and complex systems: what would successful reform of medicare look like? In: C.P.C. Office (ed) Discussion paper 8. Government of Canada
12. Keller HH et al (2019) Multi-site implementation of nutrition screening and diagnosis in medical care units: success of the More-2-Eat project. Clin Nutr 38(2):897–905
13. Laur C et al (2018) The Sustain and Spread Framework: strategies for sustaining and spreading nutrition care improvements in acute care based on thematic analysis from the More-2-Eat study. BMC Health Serv Res 18(1):930
14. Keller H et al (2020) More-2-Eat implementation demonstrates that screening, assessment and treatment of malnourished patients can be spread and sustained in acute care; a multi-site, pretest post-test time series study. Clin Nutr 40(4):2100–2108
15. Keller HH et al (2015) The Integrated Nutrition Pathway for Acute Care (INPAC): building consensus with a modified Delphi. Nutr J 14:63
16. Keller H et al (2018) Update on the Integrated Nutrition Pathway for Acute Care (INPAC): post implementation tailoring and toolkit to support practice improvements. Nutr J 17(1):2
17. Laur C et al (2019) Impact of facilitated behavior change strategies on food intake monitoring and body weight measurements in acute care: case examples from the More-2-Eat Study. Nutr Clin Pract 34(3):459–474
18. Laur C et al (2017) Changing nutrition care practices in hospital: a thematic analysis of hospital staff perspectives. BMC Health Serv Res 17(1):498
19. Ramage-Morin PL, Gilmour H, Rotermann M (2017) Nutritional risk, hospitalization and mortality among community-dwelling Canadians aged 65 or older. Health Rep 28(9):17–27
20. Correia M, Perman MI, Waitzberg DL (2017) Hospital malnutrition in Latin America: a systematic review. Clin Nutr 36(4):958–967
21. Schindler K et al (2017) nutritionDay: 10 years of growth. Clin Nutr 36(5):1207–1214
22. Leij-Halfwerk S et al (2019) Prevalence of protein-energy malnutrition risk in European older adults in community, residential and hospital settings, according to 22 malnutrition screening tools validated for use in adults ≥65 years: a systematic review and meta-analysis. Maturitas 126:80–89
23. Allard JP et al (2016) Malnutrition at hospital admission-contributors and effect on length of stay: a prospective cohort study from the Canadian Malnutrition Task Force. JPEN J Parenter Enteral Nutr 40(4):487–497
24. Curtis LJ et al (2017) Costs of hospital malnutrition. Clin Nutr 36(5):1391–1396
25. Weiner BJ et al (2011) The meaning and measurement of implementation climate. Implement Sci 6(1):78
26. Keller H et al (2021) More-2-Eat implementation demonstrates that screening, assessment and treatment of malnourished patients can be spread and sustained in acute care; a multi-site, pretest post-test time series study. Clin Nutr 40(4):2100–2108

27. Bonawitz K et al (2020) Champions in context: which attributes matter for change efforts in healthcare? Implement Sci 15(1):62
28. Bell JJ et al (2018) Rationale and developmental methodology for the SIMPLE approach: a systematised, interdisciplinary malnutrition pathway for implementation and evaluation in hospitals. Nutr Diet 75(2):226–234
29. Bell, JJ, Young, AM, Hill, JM, et al (2021) Systematised, Interdisciplinary Malnutrition Program for impLementation and Evaluation delivers improved hospital nutrition care processes and patient reported experiences – An implementation study. Nutr Diet 1–10. https://doi.org/10.1111/1747-0080.12663
30. Nilsen P (2015) Making sense of implementation theories, models and frameworks. Implement Sci 10(1):53
31. Moullin JC et al (2015) A systematic review of implementation frameworks of innovations in healthcare and resulting generic implementation framework. Health Res Policy Syst 13:16
32. Luke DA et al (2014) The program sustainability assessment tool: a new instrument for public health programs. Prev Chronic Dis 11:E12
33. Doyle C et al (2013) Making change last: applying the NHS institute for innovation and improvement sustainability model to healthcare improvement. Implement Sci 8:127
34. Graham ID et al (2006) Lost in knowledge translation: time for a map? J Contin Educ Heal Prof 26(1):13–24
35. Hailemariam M et al (2019) Evidence-based intervention sustainability strategies: a systematic review. Implement Sci 14(1):57
36. Milat AJ, Bauman A, Redman S (2015) Narrative review of models and success factors for scaling up public health interventions. Implement Sci 10(1):113
37. Geerligs L et al (2018) Hospital-based interventions: a systematic review of staff-reported barriers and facilitators to implementation processes. Implement Sci 13(1):36
38. Birken SA et al (2020) Advancing understanding and identifying strategies for sustaining evidence-based practices: a review of reviews. Implement Sci 15(1):88
39. Woodward EN et al (2019) The health equity implementation framework: proposal and preliminary study of hepatitis C virus treatment. Implement Sci 14(1):26
40. Chinman M, et al (2017) Harnessing implementation science to increase the impact of health equity research. Med Care 55 Suppl 9 Suppl 2(Suppl 9 2):S16–S23.
41. Baumann AA, Cabassa LJ (2020) Reframing implementation science to address inequities in healthcare delivery. BMC Health Serv Res 20(1):190

12

Nutritional Care: Role of Interprofessional Education for Interdisciplinary Cooperation

Julie Santy-Tomlinson, Celia V. Laur and Sumantra Ray

Abstract

Previous and forthcoming chapters describe how to improve nutrition care with an emphasis on interdisciplinary approaches. Developing and improving the skills and knowledge of the interdisciplinary team through interprofessional education are essential for embedding evidence-based, collaborative, nutritional care. This capacity building in turn supports delivery of effective nutritional care for older adults.

Keywords

Interdisciplinary teams · Interprofessional education · Nutritional care

This chapter is a component of Part I: Nutritional Care in Old Age.
For an explanation of the grouping of chapters in this book, please see Chap. 1: 'Geriatrics and Orthogeriatrics: Providing Nutrition Care'.

J. Santy-Tomlinson (✉)
Orthopaedic Nursing, Odense University Hospitals/University of Southern Denmark, Odense, Denmark
e-mail: juliesanty@tomlinson15.karoo.co.uk

C. V. Laur
Women's College Hospital Institute for Health System Solutions and Virtual Care, and Women's College Research Institute, Women's College Hospital, Toronto, ON, Canada

NNEdPro Global Centre for Nutrition and Health, Cambridge, UK
e-mail: Celia.Laur@wchospital.ca; cvlaur@uwaterloo.ca

S. Ray
NNEdPro Global Centre for Nutrition and Health, Cambridge, UK

School of Biomedical Sciences, Ulster University at Coleraine, Coleraine, UK

School of Humanities and Social Sciences, University of Cambridge, Cambridge, UK
e-mail: S.Ray@nnedpro.org.uk

Learning Outcomes
By the end of this chapter, you will be able to:

- Describe the importance of education in developing effective evidence-based interdisciplinary nutritional care.
- Discuss the benefits of interprofessional education in improving teamworking and collaboration in nutritional care.
- Summarise approaches to interprofessional education for nutritional care.
- Outline the value of education in practice improvement initiatives for nutrition care.

12.1 Introduction

Best practice in nutritional care needs to be evidence-based and delivered using a team approach. Even though nutrition specialists such as dietitians are the experts in the management of disease-related malnutrition, it is essential that effective evidence-based nutritional care is delivered by all members of the healthcare team. This need requires a collaborative culture where every practitioner has a fundamental understanding of their own role and the role of others in meeting the nutritional needs of their patients and the public [1]. This collaborative approach will not only improve care for all older adults but will also allow nutrition specialists to direct their expertise and specialist resources where they are most needed, including supporting high-risk individuals.

Healthcare practitioners rarely practise in isolation, working collaboratively with other health and social care professionals to achieve patient-centred goals using the collective skills of the team [2, 3]. The importance of interdisciplinary team approaches in the prevention and management of malnutrition in hospitalised older people has been discussed frequently throughout this book (Chaps. 1, 6, and 13). This chapter introduces the education perspectives of developing interdisciplinary teams. For clarity, working definitions of common terms used when referring to interdisciplinary collaboration and interprofessional education are provided in Table 12.1.

12.2 The Role of Interdisciplinary Teams

The complexity of human health, combined with the cross-cutting nature of nutrition, means that individuals and communities need all the skills of the healthcare team [5] in all aspects of nutritional care. An example of interdisciplinary nutrition care is monitoring food intake in hospital, where staff involved in supervising and supporting eating and drinking may record food intake, the

Table 12.1 Working definitions of common terms relating to interdisciplinary/interprofessional collaboration in education

Silo (professional silo)	A culture in which healthcare professionals operate solely within their own profession and avoid sharing information or collaborating, which may cause inadvertent duplication of efforts and resources.
Multidisciplinary	Professionals from several different disciplines collaborating, with each drawing on their own professional knowledge and skills applied to a common focal point.
Interdisciplinary	Professionals from several different disciplines collaborating by integrating and synthesising knowledge and skills from their different disciplines. Multiple angles on solving shared problems can offer innovative solutions that cannot be generated by a single discipline alone.
Transdisciplinary	Professional collaboration through creating a new discipline that transcends the boundaries of disciplinary roles with a polymathic approach that does not sit neatly in any one discipline. Nutrition can be considered transdisciplinary in relation to the natural, biomedical and social sciences as well as the humanities.
Collaboration	Cooperatively working together, sharing responsibility for problem-solving, making decisions and providing patient care in a culture of mutual trust, respect and collaboration. Requires a clear recognition of boundaries, areas of overlap and thresholds for seamless referral and transfer of care.
Interprofessional education (IPE)	IPE occurs when two or more professions learn with, from and about each other to improve collaboration and the quality of care [4].

specialist nutrition practitioner can follow up if intake is low, and a physician can consider low intake as part of their assessment. Each team member has an important role in ensuring that the food intake of a patient is documented and that appropriate action is taken if intake is inadequate, thus positively impacting on patient recovery and care outcomes.

If nutrition care practices are to be improved so that every malnourished or at-risk patient is identified and treated effectively, it is important to identify the barriers impacting the provision of nutrition care [6]. Two of these barriers are; (1) failures in multidisciplinary team collaboration and, (2) gaps in the interdisciplinary education of healthcare professionals.

Effective interdisciplinary teamworking requires team collaboration and involves open communication and information sharing within the team, ensuring that all team members are working towards the same goals. Successful teams work in an environment in which every member of the team is valued and respected and each has a clear role and understanding of the tasks which are their responsibility. These teams are also well-led, well-managed and effectively resourced in an environment in which performance is constantly reviewed and improved with a focus on patient outcomes [7]. An example of a successful practical strategy for the improvement of teamwork and communication can be found in Box 12.1.

Box 12.1 An example of a successful strategy for improving teamwork

Communication failures in healthcare teams are associated with medical errors and negative health outcomes. For this reason, team-based communication strategies have increased in the training of future health professionals. For example, in 2018, Brock et al., [8] explored the impact of a simulation-based interprofessional TeamSTEPPS (Team Strategies and Tools to Enhance Performance and Patient Safety, https://www.ahrq.gov/teamstepps/index.html) training programme on student attitudes, knowledge and skills around interprofessional communication. In this study, medical, nursing, pharmacy and physician assistant students (n = 306) took part in a 4-h training that included a 1-h TeamSTEPPS didactic session and three 1-h team simulation and feedback sessions. Students worked in groups balanced by a professional programme in a self-selected focal area. Pre- and post-assessments found differences in attitudes towards team communication ($p < 0.001$), motivation ($p < 0.001$), utility of training ($p < 0.001$) and self-efficacy ($p = 0.005$). Attitudinal shifts for TeamSTEPPS skills included team structure ($p = 0.002$), situation monitoring ($p < 0.001$), mutual support ($p = 0.003$) and communication ($p = 0.002$). Shifts were reported for knowledge of TeamSTEPPS ($p < 0.001$), advocating for patients ($p < 0.001$) and communicating in interprofessional teams ($p < 0.001$). This is just one example of a training programme used to support team communication strategies for trainees.

How teams 'work together' may be considered as a continuum progressing from independently working in silos through multidisciplinary, interdisciplinary and then transdisciplinary approaches (Table 12.1; Chap. 1, Fig. 1.1). Progression along this continuum is contingent on collaboration, mutual respect, trust and shared responsibilities and decision-making. However, these qualities alone are inadequate to support models and teams that embrace multi-, inter- or transdisciplinary approaches. Sharing of knowledge and skills should be considered a cornerstone of advancing teams working together towards realising transdisciplinary care.

12.3 Nutrition Education and Interdisciplinary Team Collaboration

The education of health professionals aims to ensure that all clinical decisions are supported by accurate and current information that reflects the best available evidence to achieve the best patient outcomes [9]. Unfortunately, health professionals are often not well informed about best practice in nutritional support, and their education is central to successfully implementing team approaches to nutritional assessment and interventions [10, 11]. The specific aim of interprofessional nutrition education for health professionals is to ensure that clinicians delivering healthcare to older people who are, for example, malnourished or at risk of malnutrition, have the right skills, knowledge and attitudes to deliver evidence-based interdisciplinary care. This approach must extend not only across disciplines but also across settings and the care continuum to effectively manage and prevent malnutrition across communities and healthcare settings. To achieve this, nutrition education is such an important foundation for fundamental healthcare practice that it needs to be embedded in the curricula of undergraduate, postgraduate and continuing education for all healthcare professionals, no matter which discipline [12, 13]. Interprofessional nutritional education has significant potential to be both a facilitator of evidence-based nutritional care through skills enhancement and a driver of better interdisciplinary team collaboration, which then leads to beneficial skill sharing.

It has been recognised for many years that health professionals need education and training to support best practice in nutritional care, but the literature suggests that this goal has not been achieved [14, 15]. The evidence for a lack of nutritional education for medical students is particularly strong [12]. However, even though much of the literature in this area considers medical education, this is also true of most other health professional disciplines, creating a professional culture in which nutritional care is sometimes seen as 'someone else's job'.

Considering the transdisciplinarity of nutritional care and the benefits of interdisciplinary team collaboration, it is clear these need to be considered together. However, effective collaboration remains relatively rare in most healthcare settings [16]. One explanation for this is that practitioners from different professions tend to work in 'silos', groups in which one health professional group is educated and practises together but in isolation from others [17, 18]. For these barriers to be overcome, it is widely proposed that education for all healthcare professionals needs to be interprofessional [19, 20] focusing on knowledge, skills and attitudes, along with the critical appraisal skills to identify appropriate evidence [21, 22]. This could be as simple as, for example, having dietitians teach medical students or support development of course material to integrate nutrition throughout the curriculum.

Cultural reform that enables students to develop at least some of the skills of other professions, as well as their own, is recommended for collaboration to be realised [23]. While most health professionals receive fundamental education and training about nutritional aspects, this is rarely sufficient for them to be confident and competent in providing effective nutritional care, especially in settings where nutritionists and dietitians are scarce or not available [1]. Interprofessional education is proposed as one of the ways of bridging skills gaps across the interdisciplinary team. In the case of nutritional care, it is one way that other healthcare professionals can learn about and operationalise the role of the nutritionist and their own and each other's roles in preventing and managing malnutrition.

Interdisciplinary healthcare is essential for the person-centred and effectively coordinated complex care required for frail older people. When healthcare is not person centred and/or not coordinated across the continuum, it is less effective and more likely to have a detrimental effect on outcomes. Considering this context within the aim of IPE, care for older adults can be improved through an interactive learning process that includes collaboration in itself. In this way, healthcare professionals learn, both individually and in teams, how to collaborate and communicate

Box 12.2 Case example of improvement in collaborative nutrition care through applied education and practice

In 2014, junior doctors from three hospitals across England were provided training in the basics of nutrition care along with an introduction to change management and leadership. These skills set them up to be nutrition champions, and when the trainees returned to their hospital, they put those skills into practice by running nutrition awareness weeks. To run these weeks, the champions worked with clinicians, administrators, staff and leaders across the hospital (transdisciplinary team building) to highlight the importance of nutrition (nutrition knowledge) and champion an event in their hospital (leadership) [26]. More recently, this model has been expanded on in nutrition education training across the UK.

within an interdisciplinary context so that such learning can then be transferred to day-to-day practice [24].

There is limited research that demonstrates the long-term outcomes of IPE on aspects of practice such as performance and care quality, but there are some examples of good practice, and studies that evaluate the impact of education on professional behaviour are challenging to conduct [25]. Even so, health professional educators agree that interprofessional education has significant potential to improve collaborative practice between each of the healthcare disciplines and, hence, have a positive impact on the quality of care [17]. Nutrition education is proposed as an approach to enabling practitioners to understand each other's roles and collaborate more effectively since nutrition is an aspect of practice where there is an important role for every member of the team. An example of such an approach is described in Box 12.2.

12.4 Approaches to Interprofessional Education for Nutritional Care

In recognition that education programmes for healthcare professionals inadequately prepare clinicians for a collaborative approach to nutritional care, a coordinated approach to interprofessional education aimed at improving nutrition practice across the entire team is needed. This means that each profession needs to review its current nutrition-related competence and use this to redevelop education curricula and delivery to ensure they facilitate collaborative nutritional practice rather than the current profession-specific programmes [11]. This requires nationwide, possibly global, overhaul of health professional curricula.

12.4.1 Curriculum

Curricula are blueprints for the content and delivery of education programmes that describe how learning needs are to be met, how content is to be learned and delivered, how the resources and assessment methods are to be and how effectiveness of programmes is to be evaluated [27]. The development of curricula needs to be driven by the competencies needed by the whole multidisciplinary team to deliver effective nutritional care led by dietetic practitioners [28]. For this to happen, those designing IPE programmes need to define common learning outcomes for all leaners who will be involved in the IPE programme [17]. These learning outcomes need to reflect the core collective nutrition learning needs [15] as well as the individual learning programmes in which students are individually engaged and require development through collaborative approaches that involve faculty from all the health professions involved. Such coordination is not a simple undertaking and constitutes a common barrier to the development of IPE outcomes that can only be overcome by collaborative working in education/academic institutions.

An essential aspect of curriculum is the design of assessment that will enable students to demonstrate learning that reflects the learning outcomes of the programme. The strategy for assessment will need to ensure that students can demonstrate the skills, competencies, knowledge and attitudes needed for successful collaborative nutritional care.

12.4.2 Delivery

It is important to consider how healthcare students and practitioners learn to work together across disciplines [29]. The way in which curricula are delivered needs to meet the learning needs of all health professionals being educated at the same time as bringing them together to learn. This involves careful consideration of teaching and learning methods to be employed as these need not only to meet the learning outcomes but fit the different needs of all team members. As clinical experts, dietetic practitioners have a central role in educating other health professionals for best practice in nutrition care in such programmes [29]. At a time when the value of traditional learning methods such as face-to-face lectures and seminars is being questioned, innovative and imaginative methods such as team-based learning, inquiry-based learning, evidence-based learning, scenario-based learning and problem-based learning are increasingly being used to foster collaboration in interprofessional healthcare education. A common theme in all these options is that students from varied professional groups use clinical exemplars to work together to understand the needs of patients and collaborate in identifying priorities, plan and deliver care.

Team-based learning (TBL) has, for example, been used successfully in providing interprofessional education relating to nutrition and lifestyle interventions [30, 31] but is less tried and tested in the field of practice improvement in preventing and managing malnutrition. In other fields of healthcare, TBL has been shown to engage students in authentic experiences of working in teams to solve real-life clinical problems [29]. Students work in teams and follow a specific sequence of activities throughout a unit of learning involving three phases [32]: (1) a preparation assignment prior to the first session, (2) individual and group readiness assurance tests and, (3) group activity that requires students to apply the material from the preparation assignment to a 'real-world' scenario. Using modes of learning such a TBL that engage students collaboratively in important patient safety issues such as malnutrition has the potential to significantly influence practice in the future.

There has been much discussion, especially since the arrival of the COVID-19 pandemic, about the value of using online methods to support learning. Many education programmes have successfully used 'blended learning' approaches, using both online and small group face-to-face sessions. It has been suggested that this may be a way to overcome some of the traditional barriers to interprofessional education discussed earlier [33]. Blended learning is an approach to teaching and learning that combines aspects of face-to-face and online interactions using appropriate technology and the provision of learning materials and opportunities through online platforms. Fundamental elements of this flexible approach are that different learning styles are accommodated and learners actively participate in learning with a focus on peer-learning and self-reflection [34]. Both online and face-to-face sessions provide a more rounded learning experience and enable collaborative learning that supports future interprofessional practice.

Few IPE programmes/curricula have been fully described or evaluated using robust methods. It is essential that IPE programmes are fully evaluated to ascertain the success of programmes in delivering the aims of interprofessional collaboration in improving nutrition care. This should not only include learner reactions to the programme and its components but evaluate: (1) whether students' attitudes, perceptions, knowledge and skills have been modified, (2) whether changes in behaviour have occurred and, (3) whether there have been changes in practice across healthcare organisations that lead to benefit to patients [25].

Strategies are needed for the development of an evidence-base for interprofessional nutrition education. There is a need for studies that assess the effectiveness of IPE interventions compared to separate, profession-specific interventions, as well as those which examine the processes relating to the IPE and consequent nutrition practice changes as well as cost-benefit analyses [16].

12.5 Interdisciplinary Collaboration for Nutritional Care in Action

Education is an essential aspect of nutrition practice improvement, but it is not sufficient on its own to drive and sustain best practice. Practice improvement initiatives, which include education as part of the strategy, need to be planned, led and evaluated to reflect quality improvement principles.

One example of an organisation which incorporates nutrition education with an interdisciplinary approach to improve nutrition outcomes is the NNEdPro Global Centre for Nutrition and Health (https://www.nnedpro.org.uk/). The NNEdPro Global Centre for Nutrition and Health provides a strategic global approach to advance and implement interdisciplinary collaboration in nutrition knowledge and skills to improve health and well-being. As an international, interdisciplinary think tank, they bring together nutrition education, research, policy and innovation to develop adaptable and scalable educational models for nutrition capacity building in health systems (https://www.nnedpro.org.uk/about-us). Their mission is to develop a critical mass of self-sustaining knowledge, skills and capacity in nutrition and health within the global healthcare and public health workforce, resulting in significantly improved health practices and outcomes. Working with these types of global organisations not only encourages the integration of interdisciplinary nutrition education into medical curricula but also drives forward the importance of applying education to practice to support improved patient and public nutrition care outcomes, including for older adults.

12.6 Summary

Education of health professionals is central to developing effective evidence-based interdisciplinary nutritional care, and there are several examples of good practice. Interprofessional education is widely considered an effective approach to improving teamworking and collaboration and needs to be embedded in health professional education curricula using a variety of teaching and learning models and methods.

Take-Home Points

- To improve nutritional care several barriers need to be overcome including failures in multidisciplinary team collaboration and gaps in the interdisciplinary education of healthcare professionals.
- The aim of interprofessional nutritional education is to ensure that clinicians have the skills, knowledge and attitudes to deliver evidence-based interdisciplinary care to effectively manage and prevent malnutrition.
- Interprofessional nutrition education needs to be embedded in the curricula driven by the competencies needed by the whole multidisciplinary team and common learning outcomes for all leaners reflecting the core collective nutrition learning needs.
- Practice improvement initiatives are needed which include education as part of the strategy, and these need to be evaluated to ascertain the impact on practice.
- An organisational culture that is constructive and open to growth and development is key in enabling cross-disciplinary knowledge sharing from upstream domains considering food production, supply and sustainability through dietary choices, guided interventions and downstream impacts on nutritional status as well as health and disease outcomes in healthcare settings.

References

1. Bell JJ et al (2021) Nutritional care of the older patient with fragility fracture: opportunities for systematised, interdisciplinary approaches across acute care, rehabilitation and secondary prevention settings. In: Falaschi P, Marsh D (eds) Orthogeriatrics: the management of older patients with fragility fractures. Springer, Cham, pp 311–329

2. Dinh JV et al (2021) The study of teamwork processes within the dynamic domains of healthcare: a systematic and taxonomic review. Front Commun 6:3
3. Wei H et al (2020) A culture of caring: the essence of healthcare interprofessional collaboration. J Interprof Care 34(3):324–331
4. CAIPE (2002) Interprofessional education: today, yesterday and tomorrow. The Centre for the Advancement of Interprofessional Education 2002 [cited 2021 28.04.2021]. https://www.caipe.org/resources/publications/caipe-publications/caipe-2002-interprofessional-education-today-yesterday-tomorrow-barr-h
5. Thistlethwaite J, Jackson A, Moran M (2013) Interprofessional collaborative practice: a deconstruction. J Interprof Care 27(1):50–56
6. Tappenden KA et al (2013) Critical role of nutrition in improving quality of care: an interdisciplinary call to action to address adult hospital malnutrition. JPEN J Parenter Enteral Nutr 37(4):482–497
7. Margaret Slusser LG, Reed C-R, McGinnis PQ (2018) Foundations of interprofessional collaborative practice in health care, 1st edn. Mosby, Maryland Heights, p 280
8. Brock D et al (2013) Interprofessional education in team communication: working together to improve patient safety. BMJ Qual Saf 22(5):414–423
9. Lehane E et al (2019) Evidence-based practice education for healthcare professions: an expert view. BMJ Evid Based Med 24(3):103–108
10. Nightingale J (2010) Nutrition support teams: how they work, are set up and maintained. Frontline Gastroenterol 1(3):171–177
11. DiMaria-Ghalili RA et al (2014) Challenges and opportunities for nutrition education and training in the health care professions: intraprofessional and interprofessional call to action. Am J Clin Nutr 99(5 Suppl):1184s–1193s
12. Crowley J, Ball L, Hiddink GJ (2019) Nutrition in medical education: a systematic review. Lancet Planet Health 3(9):e379–e389
13. Ellis G, Sevdalis N (2019) Understanding and improving multidisciplinary team working in geriatric medicine. Age Ageing 48(4):498–505
14. Kohlmeier M et al (2015) Nutrition education for the health care professions. J Biomed Educ 2015:380917
15. Kris-Etherton PM et al (2014) The need to advance nutrition education in the training of health care professionals and recommended research to evaluate implementation and effectiveness. Am J Clin Nutr 99(5 Suppl):1153s–1166s
16. Reeves S et al (2017) Interprofessional collaboration to improve professional practice and healthcare outcomes. Cochrane Database Syst Rev 6(6):CD000072
17. Thistlethwaite JE (2015) Interprofessional education: implications and development for medical education. Educ Med 16(1):68–73
18. Abu-Rish E et al (2012) Current trends in interprofessional education of health sciences students: a literature review. J Interprof Care 26(6):444–451
19. Mladenovic J (2017) Strategies for overcoming barriers to IPE at a health sciences university. J Interprofessional Educ Pract 8:10–13
20. Homeyer S et al (2018) Effects of interprofessional education for medical and nursing students: enablers, barriers and expectations for optimizing future interprofessional collaboration—a qualitative study. BMC Nurs 17:13
21. Green BN, Johnson CD (2015) Interprofessional collaboration in research, education, and clinical practice: working together for a better future. J Chiropr Educ 29(1):1–10
22. Bridges DR et al (2011) Interprofessional collaboration: three best practice models of interprofessional education. Med Educ Online 16
23. Grace S (2020) Models of interprofessional education for healthcare students: a scoping review. J Interprof Care:1–13
24. Buring SM et al (2009) Interprofessional education: definitions, student competencies, and guidelines for implementation. Am J Pharm Educ 73(4):59
25. Anderson E, Smith R, Hammick M (2016) Evaluating an interprofessional education curriculum: a theory-informed approach. Med Teach 38(4):385–394

26. Ray S et al (2014) Nutrition education and leadership for improved clinical outcomes: training and supporting junior doctors to run 'Nutrition Awareness Weeks' in three NHS hospitals across England. BMC Med Educ 14:109
27. Lee A, Steketee C, Rogers G, Moran M (2013) Towards a theoretical framework for curriculum development in health professional education. Focus Health Profess Educ 14(3):64–77
28. Hark LA, Deen D (2017) Position of the Academy of Nutrition and Dietetics: interprofessional education in nutrition as an essential component of medical education. J Acad Nutr Diet 117(7):1104–1113
29. Burgess A et al (2020) Interprofessional team-based learning (TBL): how do students engage? BMC Med Educ 20(1):118
30. Pogge E (2013) A team-based learning course on nutrition and lifestyle modification. Am J Pharm Educ 77(5):103
31. Khalafalla FG et al (2020) Enhancing nutrition and lifestyle education for healthcare professional students through an interprofessional, team-based training program. Curr Pharm Teach Learn 12(12):1484–1490
32. Reimschisel T et al (2017) A systematic review of the published literature on team-based learning in health professions education. Med Teach 39(12):1227–1237
33. Chen AK et al (2017) Teaching interprofessional collaborative care skills using a blended learning approach. J Interprofess Educ Pract 8:86–90
34. Swaminathan N et al (2020) Blended learning and health professional education: Protocol for a mixed-method systematic review. J Educ Health Promot 9:46

Part 2

Geriatric Nutritional Care: Distinctive Topics

13

Geriatric Malnutrition: A Multidisciplinary Approach

Heather Keller, Susan Slaughter, Leah Gramlich, Ashwini Namasivayam-MacDonald and Jack J. Bell

Abstract

Geriatric malnutrition prevention, detection, and treatment benefit from a multidisciplinary approach, regardless of the care setting. Nutrition care pathways have been created to support multidisciplinary care for hospitals and for transitions and primary care. Conceptual models for supporting nutrition in long-term care emphasize a multidisciplinary approach.

This chapter is a component of Part II: Special Topic in Geriatric Nutrition.
For an explanation of the grouping of chapters in this book, please see Chap. 1: "Geriatrics and Orthogeriatrics: Providing Nutrition Care."

H. Keller (✉)
Schlegel-University of Waterloo Research Institute for Aging, University of Waterloo, Waterloo, ON, Canada
e-mail: hkeller@uwaterloo.ca

S. Slaughter
Faculty of Nursing, University of Alberta, Edmonton, AB, Canada
e-mail: sslaught@ualberta.ca

L. Gramlich
Department of Medicine, Faculty of Medicine and Dentistry, University of Alberta, Edmonton, AB, Canada
e-mail: lg3@ualberta.ca

A. Namasivayam-MacDonald
School of Rehabilitation Science, McMaster University, Hamilton, ON, Canada
e-mail: namasia@mcmaster.ca

J. J. Bell
Allied Health, The Prince Charles Hospital, Chermside, Queensland, Australia

School of Human Movement and Nutrition Sciences, The University of Queensland, St Lucia, QLD, Australia
e-mail: jack.bell@health.qld.gov.au

Keywords
Acute care · Long-term care · Malnutrition · Multidisciplinary care · Nutrition assessment · Nutrition therapy · Nutritional support

Learning Outcomes
By the end of this chapter, you will be able to:

- Explain the difference between screening and assessment and how different healthcare professionals can take part in detection of geriatric malnutrition.
- Describe the various roles the multidisciplinary team contributes to the prevention, detection, and treatment of malnutrition.
- Formulate a plan for multidisciplinary geriatric malnutrition care using existing nutrition care pathways and conceptual frameworks designed for specific sectors.

13.1 Malnutrition, Assessment, and Screening

Malnutrition is defined as the inadequate intake or use of energy and nutrients resulting in changes in body composition that impact mental and cognitive function and impair clinical outcomes from acute disease [1]. Malnutrition is extremely common in older adults [2, 3]. Prevalence varies based on how malnutrition is assessed [4], as well as disease subpopulations, but is approximated at a third of acute care patients [5] and up to half of residents in long-term care [6]. Prevalence of malnutrition in community living older adults is more elusive [7]. Nutrition risk precedes malnutrition and is an indication that the individual has risk factors that impair food intake or has increased requirements which could lead to malnutrition: prevalence is approximated at one-third of community-living older adults [8]. This prevalence necessitates a multidisciplinary approach, as access to dietitians, whose scope of practice includes malnutrition assessment and treatment, is limited across all sectors.

Nutrition screening is a quick and easy-to-complete process of identifying nutrition risk using a validated screening tool [1]. Malnutrition screening can be completed by any healthcare professional with minimal training. Electronically captured data can also be used to screen for malnutrition, and in some settings, patient-administered tools are available [9, 10]. As these tools vary, the training requirements will also vary. For example, screening tools that require the measurement of body mass index or calf circumference (e.g., Mini Nutritional Assessment—Short Form [11]) will require more training than tools that are based on questions (e.g., Canadian Nutrition Screening Tool [12]). Screening tools may be specific to the population and sector for which they are created. For example, the Canadian Nutrition Screening Tool [12] is recommended for acute care, and the SCREEN-14 for community-living seniors [13]. Other tools can be used across sectors, such as the MNA-SF [11].

A comprehensive nutrition assessment includes anthropometry and body composition measures; nutrition-focused biochemistry; a history of dietary intake and adequacy of this intake; food security; assessment of functional capacity; a physical exam for muscle and fat wasting and physical signs of micronutrient deficiency; clinical history of disease states, medications and surgeries, and substance abuse issues; and social history (e.g., living situation, food-related activities of daily living, such as grocery shopping, cooking, and eating ability) [1]. The clinician completing a nutritional assessment tailors these components dependent on the age, disease, and other contexts of the patient (e.g., living in the community vs. long-term care).

13.2 Multidisciplinary Roles in Malnutrition Care

13.2.1 Dietitian Role

Dietitians in many countries of the world have been trained to complete a comprehensive, individualized nutrition assessment to detect malnutrition and counsel patients [14] on nutritional means for mitigating malnutrition (e.g., low-dose vitamin pills, oral nutritional supplements (ONS), diet enhancements, diet modifications, etc.), as well as other strategies to support nutritional status (e.g., the use of adapted utensils, grocery delivery, etc.). Dietitians have specialized knowledge on nutrient requirements for age, sex, and disease groups, as well as a comprehensive understanding of the nutritional value of food and supplements [15], and as such can tailor a therapeutic diet to support nutritional status and health goals. As malnutrition assessment and treatment are a core area of practice, dietitians are readily able to detect and treat malnutrition. However, not all dietitians have the specialized knowledge for malnutrition care in geriatrics, especially considering the complexity of comorbid conditions, frailty [16], and dementia [17] in this subgroup. Further, dietitians are a limited resource in all sectors of healthcare [18, 19], and it is not realistic that all at-risk patients will see a dietitian for treatment [20]. The greater healthcare team is needed to support malnutrition care.

13.2.2 Physician Role

Another important member of the multidisciplinary team is the physician. Physicians can play a central role in identifying malnutrition. Some physicians are nutrition specialists and have been trained to complete a comprehensive nutritional assessment. However, a majority of physicians, with training, are able to identify risk and diagnose malnutrition using standardized tools such as the subjective global assessment [21]. Where dietitians are involved in assessing patients, the dietitian can communicate the diagnosis of malnutrition to the physician, allowing prioritization of appropriate nutrition care. Physicians are also central to identifying, diagnosing, and treating symptoms which preclude oral intake. In addition, they are well positioned to anticipate the patients' trajectory and how medical care and intercurrent illness will impact nutrition care in a given patient. In addition to identifying risk and/or diagnosing malnutrition, physicians are integral to communicating and emphasizing the importance of a malnutrition diagnosis to older patients and how this malnutrition may be linked to their other health conditions or geriatric syndromes, including frailty as discussed in Chap. 7. The physician is well poised to support nutritional treatment by prescribing oral nutritional supplements [22], higher-dose micronutrients, as well medications to mitigate potential causes of poor food intake. A critical function of the physician is working with dietitians and other health professionals to implement complex nutrition care processes, such as artificial feeding or how to address continuing weight loss.

13.2.3 Role of the Speech-Language Pathologist

Speech-language pathologists (SLPs) are integral to the multidisciplinary team as some, and specifically those with a geriatric practice, are specialists in swallowing and swallowing impairments (dysphagia). SLPs, however, are not readily available in all care settings, especially in under-resourced areas. Dysphagia is independently associated with malnutrition and dehydration in older adults [23]. Food and fluid intake may be reduced or eliminated for many older adults with both acute and chronic conditions, such as a post-stroke, post brain injury, dementia, Parkinson disease, head and neck cancer, etc., due to risk for aspiration (i.e., food or liquid entering the airway, increasing risk for pneumonia). Food and fluid may also be modified in texture, which is unpalatable for many patients, leading to reduced intake. Finally, modified texture food itself may lead to malnutrition if it is not sufficient in energy and micronutrients [24]. Dysphagia is prevalent among older adults. Similar to malnutrition, prevalence is dependent on the assessment method (bedside or instrumental), patient population, and setting. Poststroke, acute dysphagia is estimated to be present in up to 80% of patients [25], while dysphagia risk due to a variety of geriatric-related diseases, including dementia, could be as high as 60% in long-term care [26]. It is also present in up to 29% of community-dwelling older adults [27]. SLPs have the requisite skills to assess risk of aspiration and the swallowing physiology and function of patients. Working with the team, they recommend and train the team and patient on compensatory strategies (e.g., chin tucks, clearing swallows), provide rehabilitative treatment (e.g., tongue-strengthening exercises and other exercises to improve physiology), and recommend any necessary diet modifications. As dysphagia can resolve or worsen depending on the primary medical diagnosis and other complicating factors, it is ideal that the SLP be involved in the ongoing reassessment of swallowing capacity for patients with dysphagia, to further limit malnutrition and dehydration. Dietitians, physicians, and nurses often include dysphagia risk screening for select geriatric groups (e.g., post-stroke, Parkinson disease, dementia) referring those with potential risk to SLP for assessment, when this resource is available. Commonly used screening tools include the Toronto Bedside Swallowing Screening Test [28], the 3-ounce water swallow test [29], and the Eating Assessment Tool-10 [30]. Best practice entails a formal screening for all patients/residents considered to be in at-risk populations (i.e., any neurological condition or head and neck cancer survivor) upon admission if a dysphagia diagnosis has not previously been given, to reduce risk of pneumonia [31] and malnutrition [23] (Chap. 18).

13.2.4 Other Health Professionals

In addition to dietitians, physicians, and SLPs, other health professions may be involved in malnutrition prevention and detection. Specifically, occupational therapists may be consulted in acute care to provide strategies and specialized equipment for self-feeding post-paresis or amputation. Together with physical therapists, they may be involved in the assessment of sarcopenia, a condition often comorbid with malnutrition, which also responds to nutritional therapy, as well as physical therapy and exercise (Chaps. 8 and 14). Pharmacists can support optimization of medications, minimizing side effects that impact appetite or food intake (Chap. 20). Social workers support patients with identification of community services such as grocery shopping or help with cooking allowing older adults to leave hospital sooner and remain at home for as long as possible. In acute and long-term care, dietary service aides/nutrition aides provide food to residents and patients and see them on a meal-to-meal basis and thus can help to identify preferred foods, especially when intake is poor. All members of the team are essential in encouraging the person to eat, emphasizing the importance of food to their recovery and health, and identifying potential risks with eating that need to be discussed with other specialized members of the team. Allied health providers can also support residents with getting to the dining room and using this time for mobilization.

13.2.5 The Nursing Role in Malnutrition

The nursing team links the entire multidisciplinary team together. Consisting of registered nurses, registered or licensed practical nurses, and care aides, nursing staff are essential for all core activities that involve prevention, detection, and treatment of malnutrition (Chaps. 1–6). For example, during their assessment, nurses identify potential challenges that impact food access and consumption. They also complete ongoing monitoring of patients and residents during meals, such as how much is consumed and if eating challenges occur, to not only prevent malnutrition but also determine the effectiveness of treatments. They measure body weight and are commonly the team member that completes nutrition screening and dysphagia screening [12, 32]. They are integral in identifying potential risk of malnutrition, dysphagia, and/or issues with self-feeding given their consistent interactions with patients and residents. Nurses often initiate referrals to other members of the multidisciplinary team and community services. They can be involved in delivering oral nutritional supplements during medication passes [32], as well as micronutrient pills. Where dietitians are unavailable in the community setting, nurses are vital to preventing, detecting, and treating malnutrition of vulnerable older adults and may be involved in providing basic nutrition counseling [33]. As the nursing team is most involved with the patient on a day-to-day basis, it is important that they are well educated on malnutrition (Chap. 12).

13.2.6 Management and Healthcare Leaders

Directors of care, managers, and practice and other healthcare leaders also have responsibility for promoting quality nutrition care and prevention of malnutrition in older adults [18]. Specifically, leaders can support a care culture that supports the use of appropriate screening tools, protocols, and standards that are based on best available evidence, quality food; systems that support food delivery, removal of barriers to food intake, and identification and treatment of those who are malnourished; and clarifying roles and training staff on these roles [34].

13.3 Multidisciplinary Models of Malnutrition Care

The Making the Most of Mealtimes conceptual model [35] provides a basis for considering the multidisciplinary team approach to promoting food and fluid intake and preventing malnutrition in long-term care. Resident, staff, and home determinants impact food intake, but central to this model is that meal access, meal quality, and mealtime experience directly impact food intake and can be modified by team actions. This conceptual model was confirmed in the Making the Most of Mealtimes prevalence study, identifying that eating assistance, food quality, and mealtime experience were all important for promoting food intake in over 600 residents across 32 long-term care homes [26]. Thus, multidisciplinary care is needed to prevent malnutrition in the residential setting.

Best practice pathways for acute care, transitions, and primary care provide guidance on multidisciplinary care of malnourished patients. Several pathways have been created for specific patient groups. An example is the Integrated Nutrition Pathway for Acute Care [36] designed to provide direction on the prevention, detection, and treatment of malnutrition. Screening is completed on admission by admitting personnel, including nurses and admitting clerks, or potentially by electronic assembly and alerting based on admission data. Those identified to be at risk are assessed, usually by dietitians, using the subjective global assessment [21] to diagnose malnutrition. Standard care practices to promote food intake are commonly identified and implemented by nursing staff, such as reducing barriers to food intake (e.g., the need for eyeglasses and dentures, positioning patients for meals) or determining if the patient is at risk for dysphagia. Monitoring food intake is commonly completed by nursing staff members, such as care aides or dietary aides, to identify improvements and determine if a patient needs intervention before there are significant weight changes [37]. Weight monitoring is also completed. Nurses deliver medications and pass out oral nutritional supplements as an advanced care strategy. Dietitians are involved in identifying specialized diet prescriptions for malnourished patients and work with physicians to prescribe enteral or parenteral nutrition as necessary. Discharge planning involves the entire multidisciplinary team to plan for a successful transition home, including referral to the primary care team, continuing dietitian treatment post discharge, and referral to community services. The Primary Care Nutrition Pathway for Hospital to Community Transitions [38] outlines the multidisciplinary roles involved to continue the nutrition care. The primary responsible healthcare provider (e.g., nurse practitioner, family physician) is central to this care, linking malnourished patients to community dietitians and services to support food access and monitoring the nutritional status of patients. When a dietitian is not available, the primary care provider can follow a basic nutrition plan to meet the needs of malnourished patients (https://nutritioncareincanada.ca/resources-and-tools/primary-community-care/nutrition-care-pathways). The companion Primary Care Nutrition Pathway for Older Adults (65+) provides specific guidance for older adults living in the community and is focused on early detection and prevention. In this pathway, the primary care provider initiates nutrition screening and provides educational resources and a basic nutrition care plan, referring high-risk patients to the dietitian for further assessment and treatment.

13.4 Standards and Policy Promote Multidisciplinary Malnutrition Care

In addition to bottom-up approaches by individual healthcare professionals and care institutions to provide quality nutrition care to prevent or treat malnutrition, top-down approaches also improve care. For example, accreditation has been demonstrated to lead to malnutrition screening at a national level [39]. Best practice pathway implementation is supported with policies or standards, as spread and scale are facilitated with the mandate of practices. An example is the Malnutrition Prevention, Detection and Treatment standard from the Health Standards Organization (https://healthstandards.org/), which describes an inclusive and comprehensive approach to multidisciplinary malnutrition care.

13.5 Examples of Multidisciplinary Malnutrition Care

The More-2-Eat study [5] is an example of the successful implementation of the multidisciplinary Integrated Nutrition Pathway for Acute Care [36]. Phase 1 demonstrated the feasibility of implementing the pathway in five hospitals and the vital role of the multidisciplinary team. Each hospital was led by a champion who was a nutrition manager, lead dietitian, or nurse. With the support of multidisciplinary site implementation team (nurse, physician, SLP, physiotherapist, food services manager, pharmacist, etc.), the pathway was tailored to the context of each hospital. For example, in one site, physical therapists supported nutrition monitoring by walking patients to weigh scales for their biweekly weights [37]. In another site, dietary team members completed admission screening while providing patients with menus and determining their preferences. Food intake monitoring was completed in some sites by the nursing staff, while in one site this was the domain of dietary staff who delivered and picked up trays [37]. Regardless of how the pathway was tailored, success in implementation was demonstrated, including improved practices and patient-reported outcomes and, in four of the five sites, decreased length of stay [32, 40]. Phase 2 demonstrated that implementation could be replicated in more sites and with only the resources available to the hospital [5, 41].

This example highlights the necessity of multidisciplinary nutrition care. There is a role for all members of the healthcare team to prevent, detect, and treat malnutrition with basic care interventions, especially when a dietitian is unavailable [42].

13.6 Summary

This chapter has provided an overview of malnutrition, how it is screened and diagnosed, and the role of the multidisciplinary team, across all healthcare sectors, in the prevention, detection, and treatment of malnutrition. Each discipline has a role to play [42, 43]. Nurses are an integral member of the team, preventing and detecting malnutrition and providing basic nutrition treatment, while linking other team members and community service providers together to ensure that older adults receive the care they need. Conceptual models and best practice pathways for malnutrition guide the process of multidisciplinary care for older adults.

Take-Home Points

- Malnutrition prevention, detection, and treatment benefit from a multidisciplinary model.
- Pathways of care have been developed to support a multidisciplinary process in malnutrition care for geriatric patients in acute care, transitions, and primary care.
- All health professionals have a role to play, due to the complexity of causes and treatment of geriatric malnutrition.
- Nurses play a central role in coordination of geriatric nutrition care.

References

1. Cederholm T, Barazzoni R, Austin P, Ballmer P, Biolo G, Compher C et al (2017) ESPEN guidelines on definition and terminology of clinical nutrition. Clin Nutr 36(1):49–64
2. Wolters M, Volkert C, Streicher M, Kiesswetter E, Torbahn G, O'Connor EM et al (2019) Prevalence of malnutrition using harmonized definitions in older adults from different settings—a MaNuEL study. Clin Nutr 38:2389–2398
3. Creda E, Pedrolli C, Klersy C, Bonardi C, Quarleri L, Cappello S et al (2016) Nutritional status in older persons according to healthcare setting: a systematic review and meta-analysis of prevalence data using MNA. Clin Nutr 35:1282–1290

4. Dent E, Hoogendijk EO, Visvanathan R, Wright ORL (2019) Malnutrition screening and assessment in hospitalised older people: a review. J Nutr Health Aging 23:431–441
5. Keller H, Morrison Koechl J, Laur C, Chen H, Curtis L, Dubin JA et al (2020) More-2-Eat implementation demonstrates that screening, assessment and treatment of malnourished patients can be spread and sustained in acute care; a multi-site, pretest post-test time series study. Clin Nutr 40(4):2100–2108. https://doi.org/10.1016/j.clnu.2020.09.034; S0261–5614(20)30506–9
6. Keller H, Vucea V, Slaughter SE, Jäger-Wittenaar H, Lengyel C, Ottery FD, Carrier N (2019) Prevalence of malnutrition or risk in residents in long term care: comparison of four tools. J Nutr Gerontol Geriatrics 38(4):329–344. https://doi.org/10.1080/21551197.2019.1640165
7. Marshall S, Craven D, Kelly J, Isenring E (2018) A systematic review and meta-analysis of the criterion validity of nutritional assessment tools for diagnosing protein-energy malnutrition in the older community setting (the MACRo study). Clin Nutr 37:1902–1912
8. Ramage-Morin PL, Garriguet D (2013) Nutritional risk among older Canadians. Health Rep 24(3):3–13
9. Power L, Mullally D, Gibney ER, Clarke M, Visser M, Volkert D et al (2018) A review of the validity of malnutrition screening tools used in older adults in the community and healthcare settings—a MaNuEL study. Clin Nutr 24:1–13
10. Keller HH (2016) Nutri-eSCREEN®: descriptive analysis of a self-management site for older adults (50+ years). BMC Nutr 2:1. https://doi.org/10.1186/s40795-015-0041-7
11. Kaiser MJ, Bauer JM, Ramsch C, Uter W, Guigoz Y, Cederholm T et al (2009) Validation of the Mini Nutritional Assessment short-from (MNA-SF): a practical tool for identification of nutritional status. J Nutr Health Aging 13(9):782–788
12. Laporte M, Keller H, Payette H, Allard JP, Duerksen DR, Bernier P, Jeejeebhoy K, Gramlich L, Vesnaver E, Teterina A (2015) Validity and reliability of the new Canadian Nutrition Screening tool in the 'real-world' hospital setting. Eur J Clin 69(5):558–564. https://doi.org/10.1038/ejcn.2014.270
13. Keller HH, Goy R, Kane S-L (2005) Validity and reliability of SCREEN II (seniors in the community: risk evaluation for eating and nutrition-version II). Eur J Clin Nutr 59(10):1149–1157
14. Andersen D, Baird S, Bates T, Chapel DL, Cline AD, Ganesh SN et al (2018) Academy of Nutrition and Dietetics: revised 2017 standards of practice in nutrition care and standards of professional performance for registered dietitian nutritionists. J Acad Nutr Diet 118(1):132–140.e15
15. Dorner B, Friedrich EK (2018) Position of the Academy of Nutrition and Dietetics: individualized nutrition approaches for older adults: long-term care, post-acute care and other settings. J Acad Nutr Diet 118:724–735
16. Verlaan S, Ligthart-Melis GC, Wijers SLJ, Cederholm T, Maier AB, de van der Schueren MAE (2017) High prevalence of physical frailty among community-dwelling malnourished older adults—a systematic review and meta-analysis. JAMDA 18:374–382
17. Livingston G, Sommerlad A, Orgeta V, Costafreda SG, Huntley J, Ames D et al (2017) Dementia prevention, intervention, and care. Lancet 390:2673–2734
18. Tappenden KA, Quatrara B, Parkhurst ML, Malone AM, Fanjiang G, Ziegler TR (2013) Critical role of nutrition in improving quality of care: an interdisciplinary call to action to address adult hospital malnutrition. J Acad Nutr Diet 113:1219–1237
19. Fleurke M, Voskuil DW, Beneken Genaamd Kolmer DM (2020) The role of the dietitian in the management of malnutrition in the elderly: a systematic review of current practices. Nutr Diet 77(1):60–75. https://doi.org/10.1111/1747-0080.12546
20. Bell J, Young A, Hill J, Banks M, Comans T, Barnes R, Keller H (2018) Rationale and developmental methodology for The SIMPLE Approach: a Systematized, Interdisciplinary Malnutrition Pathway for implementation and evaluation in hospitals. Nutr Diet 75(2):226–234. https://doi.org/10.1111/1747-0080.12406
21. Detsky AS, McLaughlin JR, Baker JP, Johnston N, Whittaker S, Mendelson RA, Jeejeebhoy KN (1987) What is subjective global assessment of nutritional status? J Parent Enteral Nutr 11(1):8–13

22. Van den Berg GH, Lindeboom R, van der Zwet WC (2015) The effects of the administration of oral nutritional supplementation with medication rounds on the achievement of nutritional goals: a randomized controlled trail. Clin Nutr 34(1):15–19
23. Namasivayam-MacDonald A, Morrison J, Steele CM, Keller H (2017) How swallow pressures and dysphagia affect malnutrition and mealtime outcomes in long-term care. Dysphagia 32(6):785–796. https://doi.org/10.1007/s00455-017-9925-z
24. Vucea V, Keller HH, Morrison JM, Duncan AM, Duizer LM, Carrier N, Lengyel CO, Slaugther SE (2017) Nutritional quality of regular and pureed menus in Canadian long term care homes: an analysis of the making the most of mealtimes (M3) project. BMC Nutr 3:80. https://doi.org/10.1186/s40795-017-0198-3
25. Takizawa C, Gemmell E, Kenworthy J, Speyer R (2016) A systematic review of the prevalence of oropharyngeal dysphagia in stroke, Parkinson's disease, Alzheimer's disease, head injury, and pneumonia. Dysphagia 31(3):434–441
26. Keller H, Carrier N, Slaughter S, Lengyel C, Steele CM, Duizer L, Morrison J, Brown KS, Chaudhury H, Yoon MN, Duncan AM, Boscart V, Heckman G, Villalon L (2017) Prevalence and determinants of poor food intake or residents living in long term care. J Am Med Dir Assoc 18(11):941–947. https://doi.org/10.1016/j.jamda.2017.05.003
27. Mulheren RW, Azola AM, Kwiatkowski S, Karagiorgos E, Humbert I, Palmer JB, González-Fernández M (2018) Swallowing changes in community-dwelling older adults. Dysphagia 33(6):848–856
28. Martino R, Silver F, Teasell R, Bayley M, Nicholson G, Streiner DL, Diamant NE (2009) The Toronto bedside swallowing screening test (TOR-BSST) development and validation of a dysphagia screening tool for patients with stroke. Stroke 40(2):555–561
29. Suiter DM, Leder SB (2008) Clinical utility of the 3-ounce water swallow test. Dysphagia 23(3):244–250
30. Belafsky PC, Mouadeb DA, Rees CJ, Pryor JC, Postma GN, Allen J, Leonard RJ (2008) Validity and reliability of the Eating Assessment Tool (EAT-10). Ann Otol Rhinol Laryngol 117(12):919–924
31. Hinchey JA, Shephard T, Furle K, Smith D, Wang D, Tonn S (2005) Formal dysphagia screening protocols prevent pneumonia. Stroke 36(9):1972–1976
32. Keller H, Valaitis R, Laur CV, McNicholl T, Xu Y, Dubin JA, Curtis L, Obiorah S, Ray S, Bernier P, Gramlich L, Stickles-White M, Laporte M, Bell J (2018) Multi-site implementation of nutrition screening and diagnosis in medical care units: success of the project More-2-Eat. Clin Nutr:1–9. https://doi.org/10.1016/j.clnu.2018.02.009
33. Vasiloglou MF, Fletcher J, Poulia KA (2019) Challenges and perspectives in nutritional counselling and nursing: a narrative review. J Clin Med 8:1489. https://doi.org/10.3390/jcm8091489
34. Keller HH, Vesnaver E, Davidson B, Allard J, Laporte M, Bernier P, Payette H, Jeejeebhoy K, Duerksen D, Gramlich L (2014) Providing quality nutrition care in acute care hospitals: perspectives of nutrition care personnel. J Hum Nutr Diet 27(2):192–202. https://doi.org/10.1111/jhn.12170
35. Keller H, Carrier N, Duizer L, Lengyel C, Slaughter S, Steele C (2014) Making the Most of Mealtimes (M3): grounding mealtime interventions with a conceptual model. J Am Med Dir Assoc 15(3):158–161. https://doi.org/10.1016/j.jamda.2013.12.001
36. Keller H, McCullough J, Davidson B, Vesnaver E, Laporte M, Gramlich L, Allard J, Bernier P, Duerksen D, Jeejeebhoy K (2015) Integrated nutrition pathway for acute care (INPAC): building consensus with a modified Delphi. Nutr J 14:63. https://doi.org/10.1186/s12937-015-0051-y
37. Laur C, Nasser R, Butterworth D, Valaitis R, Bell J, Marcell C, Murphy J, Ray S, Bernier P, Keller H (2019) Implementing food intake and body weight monitoring in acute care using behavior change techniques: case examples from the More-2-Eat study. Nutr Clin Pract 34(3):459–474. https://doi.org/10.1002/ncp.10207
38. Keller H, Donnelly R, Laur C, Goharian L, Nasser R (2021) Consensus-based nutrition care pathways for hospital-to-community transitions and older adults in primary and community care. J Paren Enter Nutr (online ahead of print). https://doi.org/10.1002/jpen.2068n

39. Leistra E, van Bokhorst-de van der Schueren M, Visser M, van der Hout A, Langius J, Kruizenga H (2014) Systematic screening for undernutrition in hospitals: predictive factors for success. Clin Nutr 33(3):495–501
40. Keller H, Xu Y, Dubin JA, Curtis L, Laur C, Bell J, for the More-2-Eat Team (2018) Improving the standard of nutrition care in hospital: mealtime barriers reduced with implementation of the Integrated Nutrition Pathway for Acute Care. Clin Nutr ESPEN 28:74–79
41. Keller H, Koechl JM, Laur C, Chen H, Curtis L, Dubin JA, Gramlich L, Ray S, Valaitis R, Yang Y, Bell J (2021) More-2-Eat implementation demonstrates that screening, assessment and treatment of malnourished patients can be spread and sustained in acute care; a multi-site, pretest post-test time series study. Clin Nutr 40(4):2100–2108. https://doi.org/10.1016/j.clnu.2020.09.034
42. Ten Cate D, Ettema RGA, Huisman-de Waal G, Bell JJ, Verbrugge R, Schoonhoven L et al (2020) Interventions to prevent and treat malnutrition in older adults to be carried out by nurses: a systematic review. J Clin Nurs 29(11–12):1883–1902
43. Laur C, Keller H (2015) Implementing best practice in multidisciplinary nutrition care: an example of using the Knowledge-to-Action Process for a research program. J Multidiscip Healthc 8:463–472. https://doi.org/10.2147/JMDH.S93103

14

Role of Physical Activity for Older Adults: Nutritional Aspects

Camila Astolphi Lima, Renato Barbosa dos Santos
and Monica Rodrigues Perracini

Abstract

Enhancing physical activity promotes positive health trajectories throughout the life course. Physical activity should be tailored and graded to suit older adults' capacities and needs and can be combined with rehabilitation interventions to manage geriatric syndromes and disability. This chapter provides a summary of current evidence about the role of physical activity for older adults, emphasizing nutritional aspects. We also present strategies to help health-care professionals to enhance physical activity participation.

Keywords

Physical activity · Exercise · Nutrition · Rehabilitation · Older adults

This chapter is a component of Part II: Special Topic in Geriatric Nutrition.
For an explanation of the grouping of chapters in this book, please see Chap. 1: "Geriatrics and Orthogeriatrics: Providing Nutrition Care."

C. A. Lima · R. B. dos Santos
Master's and Doctoral Programs in Physical Therapy, Universidade Cidade de São Paulo, São Paulo, SP, Brazil

M. R. Perracini (✉)
Master's and Doctoral Programs in Physical Therapy, Universidade Cidade de São Paulo, São Paulo, SP, Brazil

Master's and Doctoral Programs in Gerontology, Faculty of Medical Sciences, Universidade Estadual de Campinas, São Paulo, SP, Brazil
e-mail: monica.perracini@unicid.edu.br

Learning Outcomes
By the end of this chapter, you will be able to:

- Apply the updated recommendations of physical activity for older people.
- Justify health benefits of physical activity in older adults.
- Describe the rationale for combined exercise and nutritional interventions.
- Report strategies to enhance physical activity level.

14.1 Importance of Physical Activity in Older Adults

Healthy aging conceptualization is grounded in fostering the functional ability of older people, so they can be and do what they value [1]. Being physically active is a key factor to prevent and maintain intrinsic capacity and to optimize functional ability in old age. Physical activity (PA) is considered as any bodily movement produced by the contraction of muscles, increasing energy expenditure [2]. In a new and broader definition, PA involves people moving, acting, and performing within culturally specific spaces and contexts and is influenced by a unique array of interests, emotions, ideas, instructions, and relationships [3]. Exercise is defined as planned, structured, and repetitive movement to improve or maintain some component of physical fitness [2].

PA can be undertaken as part of recreation and work or as part of domestic tasks. While some PA activities can be more pleasant than others, with associated mental and social benefits, if older people undertake PA regularly and in a sufficient duration and intensity, they will have health benefits [4]. Reducing physical inactivity is part of World Health Organization (WHO) global strategy to manage noncommunicable diseases (NCDs). Implementing community-wide public education and awareness for PA and providing PA counseling and referral as part of routine primary health-care services are considered "best buys" interventions, particularly for low- and middle-income countries [5].

14.2 Recommendations for Physical Activity

Recommendations suggest 150–300 min of moderate-intensity aerobic physical activity or at least 75–150 min of vigorous-intensity aerobic physical activity or an equivalent combination of moderate- and vigorous-intensity activity throughout the week, for substantial health benefits [6]. Aerobic activity is recommended to be performed in bouts of at least 10 min each. There is high evidence of an inverse dose response relationship between volume of aerobic physical activity and risk of physical functional limitations in the general older adult population.

For older adults that are not able to complete the above recommendations, they should be physically active as their abilities and conditions allow [6]. As highlighted in the 2020 WHO recommendation, "Doing some physical activity is better than doing none."

Older adults should include multicomponent physical activity that combines aerobic, strengthening, and functional balance on 3 or more days a week; strength training for all major muscle groups should be considered 2 or more days a week [6]. For adults with chronic conditions, a frequency of 3 days a week is commonly recommended.

The types of PA most popular for older adults are light intensity, such as walking and gardening [2]. Older adults should gradually increase the duration and frequency of moderate-intensity activity rather than rapidly increasing to vigorous-intensity activity [6, 7]. Growing evidence supports that light-intensity activities, like a slow walking or housework (e.g., ironing and dusting), also offer a protective benefit against diseases and disability [8, 9]. Older adults should be as active as possible. Even when recommendations are not met, efforts to integrate more light-intensity activities into everyday life are beneficial.

14.3 Benefits of Physical Activity

Márcia has worked on a cattle ranch for most of her life. Although she was thin, she was a strong, hardworking, healthy, and happy woman who slept well at night. She did not take any medications and, although having annual checkups with the community nurse, had never needed to see the doctor or go to hospital.

Benefits of PA in middle age to older adult years include the maintenance of balance, strength, flexibility, and exercise capacity (Table 14.1). Whether achieved through prescribed multimodal or multicomponent exercises or mustering cattle and rural fencing, PA optimizes physical, mental, and musculoskeletal health, health-related quality of life, and functional independence and abilities and decreases the risk of falling.

Following a fall off her horse at the age of 76, Márcia spent most of her days in bed. She had poor dietary intake, ongoing falls, and urinary incontinence over the next 6 months. Márcia's son José eventually convinced her to receive a visit from the local community nurse. Shortly afterward, Márcia presented to hospital where multiple vertebral crush fractures, malnutrition, frailty, vitamin D deficiency, osteoporosis, and depression were diagnosed.

Older adults presenting with geriatric syndromes, such as falls and fragility fractures, malnutrition, frailty, depression, and urinary incontinence, may present with different levels of functional disability and deconditioning, resulting in low physical

Table 14.1 Benefits of physical activity in older adults

Potential benefit	Examples
Health conditions and mortality	• 22% ↓ all-cause mortality [10] • 12% ↓ risk of breast cancer [11] • Noncommunicable disease (e.g., coronary heart disease, type 2 diabetes) prevention/management [2, 12]
Cognitive function, mental health, and health-related quality of life	• 36% ↓ risk of cognitive decline [13, 14] • 24% ↓ all-cause dementia (moderate-intensity) • 28% ↓ all-cause dementia (high-intensity) [13, 14] • 40% ↓ Alzheimer's disease development [11] • 21% ↓ incident depression (high-intensity) [11] • Poor sleep quality and declining intrinsic capacity • Increased health-related quality of life
Musculoskeletal health	• 31% ↓ in relative risk of fracture (hip, wrist, and vertebral fractures) [15] • Improved lumbar spine bone mineral density,may improve hip (femoral neck) bone mineral density [15] • Probable positive impact on frailty and sarcopenia (resistance training, combination of resistance, balance, endurance, and function exercise) [16]
Physical function and disability	• Approximately 50% likely ↓ risk of functional limitations/ disability (moderate/high levels) [17] • Strongly recommended to ↓ loss of physical function and mobility (multimodal or multicomponent exercises including balance, strength, flexibility, and functional training) [17] • Delayed disability or functional limitation and prolonged disability-free life (high levels in middle age) [18]
Fall prevention	• 31% ↓ in falls (dance-based mind-motor activities [19] • 23% ↓ in falls (structured exercise) [20] • 42% estimated reduction in the rate of falls (exercise dose of more than 3 h/week of balance and functional exercises) [20] • Exercise as a single intervention did not reduce falls but was able to enhance mobility in frail older people recently discharged from hospital [21]

activity levels and the adoption of sedentary behavior over time. Appropriately prescribed exercise and PA are demonstrated to be safe and have a beneficial effect on functional ability; these benefits can be extended to older adults like Márcia, even in the presence of existing physical and functional limitations. Multimodal or multicomponent exercises including balance, strength, flexibility, and functional training are strongly recommended to manage significant loss of physical function and mobility [22].

Over the next 6 months, Márcia worked together with many different health-care providers in the hospital, rehabilitation center, and secondary prevention fracture clinic and achieved her goal of being back in the saddle within 1 year.

14.4 Nutrition Status and Physical, Functional, Exercise, and Rehabilitation Outcomes

Malnutrition can influence physical and functional activity, exercise, and rehabilitation processes of older adults [23], increasing the length of stay in the hospital and the rates of readmission [24]. Nutritional status has been correlated with poor basic activities of daily living (ADL) and instrumental activities of daily living (IADL) in community-dwelling [22], institutionalized [25], and hospitalized older adults [26]. Older people who report unintentional weight loss are at a higher risk of developing limitations in ADL such as bathing, dressing, and eating [27], as well as older people who report obesity [28]. Also, low body mass index (BMI) [29] and high BMI [28] have been shown as a risk factor for the onset of activities of daily living limitations. Particularly the combination of a high BMI and dynapenia, defined as dynapenic obesity, is associated with a poorer physical function when compared to obesity alone [30]. Malnutrition has also been associated with high risk of falling [31], harmful falls [32], hip fracture incidence, and reduced ability to recover pre-fracture functional capacity in patients after hip fracture [33].

Vitamin D and protein has an important function on muscle strength, so its deficits can lead to muscle weakness [34]. Administration of high-protein diets, with protein throughout the three meals associated with high doses of calcium and vitamin D, can improve muscle health and decrease the risk of fracture [34] (Chap. 9).

14.5 Combined Nutrition Physical Activity/ Exercise Interventions

Consequently, we make the case that in the absence of adequate nutrition, physical activity or exercise interventions are unlikely to lead to optimized health or health-related quality of life for older adults like Márcia. Although the evidence remains inconsistent, there is a growing body of evidence to support combined nutrition and exercise/PA interventions in older adults. Particularly the combination of protein intake and nutrition counseling with exercise has demonstrated reduced long-term mobility disability [17, 22], improved frailty scores [35], improved lower limb functionality [35], and increased independence in activities of daily living [35].

14.6 Physical Rehabilitation

Rehabilitation is a set of person-centered interventions across multiple disciplines with the key objective of optimizing functioning and reducing disability [36]. A person-centered care approach for older people includes the assessment and development of a care plan based on the assessment of vitality (including the nutritional care), visual, hearing, cognitive, locomotor, and psychological capacities; underlying diseases (and risk factors); caregiving needs; assessment, selection, and provision of assistive products (e.g., walking aids, therapeutic shoes, grab bars); physical environment modifications; and need for social care (Chaps. 1 and 13) [37].

A comprehensive care approach conducted by an interdisciplinary team allows tailoring older people and caregiver's needs and ensures interventions orientated toward relevant outcomes, avoiding unnecessary treatments, polypharmacy, and poor adherence to interventions. Particularly for older people with significant loss of mobility due to chronic conditions, the combination of rehabilitation interventions and the enhancement of PA level may amplify positive outcomes [6].

14.7 Enhancing Physical Activity Level Among Older People

Diverse health-care professionals can help older people to increase their PA levels by exploring, discussing, and intervening to reduce barriers and enhance facilitators for being more active (Table 14.2) [38]. These actions include establishing and negotiating individual realistic goals, taking into account specific needs, health conditions, and physical limitations, and creating a shared, tailored plan that addresses each recommended type of activity/exercise with specific goals, need of supervision, and safety procedures. Applying behavioral strategies of positive reinforcement using motivational interviewing strategies to stimulate participation in PA demonstrates successful long-term results. Goal setting and self-monitoring in combination with the use of digital technologies such as sensors (e.g., pedometers and accelerometers) have also proven beneficial [38, 39]. The use of smartphone, tablet apps, and mobile text messages is promising and appears to be acceptable and beneficial for the maintenance and improvement of PA in the short term [39]. E-health strategies are being increasingly used to promote and track physical activity among older people (e.g., mobile apps, wearable, digital PA coaching, online social support, video demonstrations, video games, etc.) with positive results in increasing the time spent on physical activity, the energy expenditure in physical activity, and the number of walking steps. These strategies should be used to enhance physical activity level among older adults [39].

14.8 Summary

Benefits of physical activity are substantial and contribute to healthy aging. Particularly, multicomponent exercises, nutritional interventions, and rehabilitation can improve physical functioning and prevent disability. Health-care professionals play a key role in implementing strategies to enhance physical activity participation.

Take-Home Points

- The recommendation is 150–300 min of moderate-intensity aerobic physical activity or at least 75–150 min of vigorous-intensity aerobic physical activity or

Table 14.2 Interdisciplinary opportunities for enhancing physical activity in older adults

Who	What	How
Medical doctor/ physician	Physical activity advice	Specific physical activity advice (type, frequency); plan of action and follow-up [40]; address individual motivators, facilitators, and barriers; refer to local physical activity opportunities or to a professional able to offer a specific physical activity or exercise plan
Physiotherapist	Promote physical activity [41] and provide tailored preventive interventions and/or rehabilitation program	Assess and prescribe appropriate program according to needs, preferences, abilities, and conditions; specific physical activity advice (type, frequency); plan of action and follow-up; encourage progress and participation [42]
Physical educator and fitness professionals	Provide tailored physical activity/ exercise program	Assess and prescribe appropriate program according to needs, preferences, abilities, and conditions; specific physical activity advice (type, frequency); plan of action and follow-up; encourage progress and participation
Nurse and other health-care professionals	Promote physical activity participation	Explore and discuss awareness of the benefits of being active; address individual motivators, facilitators, and barriers; refer to local physical activity opportunities or to a professional able to offer a specific physical activity or exercise plan [43, 44]
Volunteers and carers	Promote physical activity participation	Be a physical activity enthusiast; explore and discuss awareness of benefits of being active. Address motivators, facilitators, and barriers; refer to local physical activity opportunities or to a professional able to offer a specific physical activity or exercise plan [43]; provide support and/or company to those who need it [38]
Researchers	Promote and disseminate science	Generate and implement high-quality evidence for physical activity; investigate local barriers and facilitators for implementing successful strategies
Policy makers	Implement healthy aging policies, environments, and infrastructure	Provide free or low-cost exercise programs that are tailored to personal needs and preferences [4–6]; create safe environments, access to parks and other recreational facilities, and safe footpaths [45]

an equivalent combination of moderate- and vigorous-intensity activity throughout the week, for substantial health benefits.

- Older adults should combine aerobic, strengthening, and functional balance exercises.
- Exercise can be part of lots of things as recreation, work, or domestic activities.
- Doing some physical activity is better than doing none—it is important be physically active as their abilities and conditions allow.
- Nutritional treatment reduces the progression of functional decline, even further when associated with PA programs, reducing long-term mobility disability.
- The use of e-health strategies to enhance PA should be considered.

References

1. Global strategy and action plan on ageing and health (2017). World Health Organization, Geneva. Contract no.: CC BY-NC-SA3.0IGO
2. American College of Sports M, Chodzko-Zajko WJ, Proctor DN, Fiatarone Singh MA, Minson CT, Nigg CR et al (2009) American College of Sports Medicine position stand. Exercise and physical activity for older adults. Med Sci Sports Exerc 41(7):1510–1530
3. Piggin J (2020) What is physical activity? A holistic definition for teachers. Res Policy Makers Front Sports Act Living 2:72
4. WHO (2019) Global action plan on physical activity 2018–2030: more active people for a healthier world. World Health Organization, Geneva
5. Tackling NCDs: 'best buys' and other recommended interventions for the prevention and control of noncommunicable diseases (2017). World Health Organization, Geneva
6. WHO (2020) WHO guidelines on physical activity and sedentary behaviour: at a glance. World Health Organization, Geneva. Report no.: 9240014888
7. Piercy KL, Troiano RP, Ballard RM, Carlson SA, Fulton JE, Galuska DA et al (2018) The physical activity guidelines for Americans. JAMA 320(19):2020–2028
8. Sparling PB, Howard BJ, Dunstan DW, Owen N (2015) Recommendations for physical activity in older adults. BMJ 350:h100
9. Duvivier BM, Schaper NC, Bremers MA, van Crombrugge G, Menheere PP, Kars M et al (2013) Minimal intensity physical activity (standing and walking) of longer duration improves insulin action and plasma lipids more than shorter periods of moderate to vigorous exercise (cycling) in sedentary subjects when energy expenditure is comparable. PLoS One 8(2):e55542
10. Hupin D, Roche F, Gremeaux V, Chatard JC, Oriol M, Gaspoz JM et al (2015) Even a low-dose of moderate-to-vigorous physical activity reduces mortality by 22% in adults aged >/=60 years: a systematic review and meta-analysis. Br J Sports Med 49(19):1262–1267
11. Cunningham C, Sullivan RO, Caserotti P, Tully MA (2020) Consequences of physical inactivity in older adults: a systematic review of reviews and meta-analyses. Scand J Med Sci Sports 30(5):816–827
12. Lee IM, Shiroma EJ, Lobelo F, Puska P, Blair SN, Katzmarzyk PT et al (2012) Effect of physical inactivity on major non-communicable diseases worldwide: an analysis of burden of disease and life expectancy. Lancet 380(9838):219–229
13. Blondell SJ, Hammersley-Mather R, Veerman JL (2014) Does physical activity prevent cognitive decline and dementia? A systematic review and meta-analysis of longitudinal studies. BMC Public Health 14:510
14. Guure CB, Ibrahim NA, Adam MB, Said SM (2017) Impact of physical activity on cognitive decline, dementia, and its subtypes: meta-analysis of prospective studies. Biomed Res Int 2017:9016924
15. Qu X, Zhang X, Zhai Z, Li H, Liu X, Li H et al (2014) Association between physical activity and risk of fracture. J Bone Miner Res 29(1):202–211
16. Oliveira JS, Pinheiro MB, Fairhall N, Walsh S, Chesterfield Franks T, Kwok W et al (2020) Evidence on physical activity and the prevention of frailty and sarcopenia among older people: a systematic review to inform the World Health Organization physical activity guidelines. J Phys Act Health 17(12):1247–1258
17. Integrated care for older people: guidelines on community-level interventions to manage declines in intrinsic capacity (2017). World Health Organization, Geneva
18. Paterson DH, Warburton DE (2010) Physical activity and functional limitations in older adults: a systematic review related to Canada's Physical Activity Guidelines. Int J Behav Nutr Phys Act 7:38
19. Mattle M, Chocano-Bedoya PO, Fischbacher M, Meyer U, Abderhalden LA, Lang W et al (2020) Association of dance-based mind-motor activities with falls and physical function among healthy older adults: a systematic review and meta-analysis. JAMA Netw Open 3(9):e2017688

20. Sherrington C, Fairhall N, Kwok W, Wallbank G, Tiedemann A, Michaleff ZA et al (2020) Evidence on physical activity and falls prevention for people aged 65+ years: systematic review to inform the WHO guidelines on physical activity and sedentary behaviour. Int J Behav Nutr Phys Act 17(1):144
21. Sherrington C, Lord SR, Vogler CM, Close JC, Howard K, Dean CM et al (2014) A post-hospital home exercise program improved mobility but increased falls in older people: a randomised controlled trial. PLoS One 9(9):e104412
22. Ferdous T, Cederholm T, Razzaque A, Wahlin A, Nahar KZ (2009) Nutritional status and self-reported and performance-based evaluation of physical function of elderly persons in rural Bangladesh. Scand J Public Health 37(5):518–524
23. Diekmann R, Wojzischke J (2018) The role of nutrition in geriatric rehabilitation. Curr Opin Clin Nutr Metab Care 21(1):14–18
24. Kruizenga H, van Keeken S, Weijs P, Bastiaanse L, Beijer S, Huisman-de Waal G et al (2016) Undernutrition screening survey in 564,063 patients: patients with a positive undernutrition screening score stay in hospital 1.4 d longer. Am J Clin Nutr 103(4):1026–1032
25. Suominen M, Muurinen S, Routasalo P, Soini H, Suur-Uski I, Peiponen A et al (2005) Malnutrition and associated factors among aged residents in all nursing homes in Helsinki. Eur J Clin Nutr 59(4):578–583
26. Oliveira MR, Fogaca KC, Leandro-Merhi VA (2009) Nutritional status and functional capacity of hospitalized elderly. Nutr J 8:54
27. Arnold AM, Newman AB, Cushman M, Ding J, Kritchevsky S (2010) Body weight dynamics and their association with physical function and mortality in older adults: the Cardiovascular Health Study. J Gerontol A Biol Sci Med Sci 65(1):63–70
28. Kong HH, Won CW, Kim W (2020) Effect of sarcopenic obesity on deterioration of physical function in the elderly. Arch Gerontol Geriatr 89:104065
29. Beydoun MA, Popkin BM (2005) The impact of socio-economic factors on functional status decline among community-dwelling older adults in China. Soc Sci Med 60(9):2045–2057
30. Bouchard DR, Janssen I (2010) Dynapenic-obesity and physical function in older adults. J Gerontol A Biol Sci Med Sci 65(1):71–77
31. Adly NN, Abd-El-Gawad WM, Abou-Hashem RM (2020) Relationship between malnutrition and different fall risk assessment tools in a geriatric in-patient unit. Aging Clin Exp Res 32(7):1279–1287
32. Lackoff AS, Hickling D, Collins PF, Stevenson KJ, Nowicki TA, Bell JJ (2020) The association of malnutrition with falls and harm from falls in hospital inpatients: findings from a 5-year observational study. J Clin Nurs 29(3–4):429–436
33. Malafarina V, Reginster JY, Cabrerizo S, Bruyere O, Kanis JA, Martinez JA et al (2018) Nutritional status and nutritional treatment are related to outcomes and mortality in older adults with hip fracture. Nutrients 10(5):555
34. Artaza-Artabe I, Saez-Lopez P, Sanchez-Hernandez N, Fernandez-Gutierrez N, Malafarina V (2016) The relationship between nutrition and frailty: effects of protein intake, nutritional supplementation, vitamin D and exercise on muscle metabolism in the elderly. A systematic review. Maturitas 93:89–99
35. Han CY, Miller M, Yaxley A, Baldwin C, Woodman R, Sharma Y (2020) Effectiveness of combined exercise and nutrition interventions in prefrail or frail older hospitalised patients: a systematic review and meta-analysis. BMJ Open 10(12):e040146
36. Stucki G, Bickenbach J, Gutenbrunner C, Melvin J (2018) Rehabilitation: the health strategy of the 21st century. J Rehabil Med 50(4):309–316
37. Integrated care for older people (ICOPE): guidance for person-centred assessment and pathways in primary care (2019). World Health Organization, Geneva
38. Perracini MR, Franco MRC, Ricci NA, Blake C (2017) Physical activity in older people—case studies of how to make change happen. Best Pract Res Clin Rheumatol 31(2):260–274
39. Kwan RYC, Salihu D, Lee PH, Tse M, Cheung DSK, Roopsawang I et al (2020) The effect of e-health interventions promoting physical activity in older people: a systematic review and meta-analysis. Eur Rev Aging Phys Act 17:7

40. Hinrichs T, Brach M (2012) The general practitioner's role in promoting physical activity to older adults: a review based on program theory. Curr Aging Sci 5(1):41–50
41. Perracini MR, Freitas SMSF, Pires RS, Rico JMP, Alouche SR (2018) Promotion of physical activity for older people with neurological conditions. In: Nyman SR, Haines T, Musselwhite C, Victor CR (eds) The Palgrave handbook of ageing and physical activity promotion. Palgrave Macmillan, Basel, pp 145–163
42. Oliveira CB, Franco MR, Maher CG, Tiedemann A, Silva FG, Damato TM et al (2018) The efficacy of a multimodal physical activity intervention with supervised exercises, health coaching and an activity monitor on physical activity levels of patients with chronic, nonspecific low back pain (Physical Activity for Back Pain (PAyBACK) trial): study protocol for a randomised controlled trial. Trials 19(1):40
43. Palmer SJ (2020) Encouraging exercise in older adults: advice for nurses. Br J Community Nurs 25(2):95–97
44. Lee LL, Arthur A, Avis M (2008) Using self-efficacy theory to develop interventions that help older people overcome psychological barriers to physical activity: a discussion paper. Int J Nurs Stud 45(11):1690–1699
45. Peters M, Muellmann S, Christianson L, Stalling I, Bammann K, Drell C et al (2020) Measuring the association of objective and perceived neighborhood environment with physical activity in older adults: challenges and implications from a systematic review. Int J Health Geogr 19(1):47

15

Prevention and Management of Malnutrition and PIs

Donna Hickling, Tracy Nowicki and Julie Santy-Tomlinson

Abstract

Previous chapters have described how to implement and improve nutrition care with an emphasis on interdisciplinary approaches. The focus of this chapter is on the link between malnutrition and pressure injuries (PIs), focussing on nutritional screening, assessment and interdisciplinary interventions in preventing and managing PIs.

Keywords

Pressure injuries (PIs) · Pressure ulcers · Skin integrity · Screening · Malnutrition · Nutrition therapy

---

This chapter is a component of Part II: Specialist Versus Generalist Nutritional Care in Aging. For an explanation of the grouping of chapters in this book, please see Chap. 1: 'Geriatrics and Orthogeriatrics: Providing Nutrition Care'.

D. Hickling (✉)
Nutrition and Dietetics Department, The Prince Charles Hospital, Chermside, QLD, Australia
e-mail: Donna.Hickling@health.qld.gov.au

T. Nowicki
Quality Effective Support Team (QuEST), The Prince Charles Hospital, Chermside, QLD, Australia
e-mail: Tracy.Nowicki@health.qld.gov.au

J. Santy-Tomlinson
Orthopaedic Nursing, Odense University Hospitals/University of Southern Denmark, Odense, Denmark
e-mail: juliesanty@tomlinson15.karoo.co.uk

Learning Outcomes
By the end of this chapter, you will be able to:

- Outline the nutrition-related causes of PIs.
- Explain the importance of good nutrition in preventing and managing PIs.
- Explore nutrition care most likely to impact on the prevention and management of PIs as part of a holistic approach.

15.1 Pressure Injuries

Pressure injuries (PIs, also known as pressure ulcers) are localised areas of skin and underlying soft tissue damage [1] that are especially common in older people with impaired mobility and acute or chronic health problems and who are identified as frail [2]. PIs are mainly preventable, and, although there is abundant evidence-based guidance readily available, they remain common patient safety incidents attributed to missed care [3]. Multidisciplinary management of the extrinsic and intrinsic factors that contribute to the development of PIs is central to prevention and management.

PIs are classified by the severity and depth of tissue damage, ranging from intact skin with non-blanching erythema (stage I), partial skin loss with exposed dermis or blister (stage II) and full-thickness skin loss extending into the adipose layer (stage III) to full-thickness tissue loss with exposed underlying tissues (stage IV). Some PIs are unstageable because the base of the wound cannot be observed due to slough/eschar. Persistent non-blanchable, deep-red, maroon or purple discoloration with intact or non-intact skin indicates deep tissue injury [1]. It is essential to consider the significance of mucosal membrane pressure injuries: such damage to the mucosal lining of the respiratory, gastrointestinal and genitourinary tracts is usually caused by pressure from medical devices, such as ventilation or feeding tubes [4, 5]. Mucosal membrane PIs cannot be staged using the classification system described above.

15.2 The Aetiology of Pressure Injuries

PIs are caused by pressure exerted on the skin and soft tissue overlying a bony prominence or a combination of pressure and shear [1]. When these extrinsic forces are sustained, damage to the microcirculation of the skin leads to ischaemia, reduced nutrient supply to cells and accumulation of metabolites [6], resulting in tissue necrosis. Prolonged exposure of the skin surface to moisture (from urine, sweat, saliva, faeces and wound exudate) can also lead to inflammation and damage to the epidermis [7], increasing the risk of tissue injury. Medical devices (such as endotracheal and nasogastric tubes, oxygen tubing and masks, urinary catheters and casts) exert pressure at the interface of the skin and soft tissue [8].

A range of patient-specific intrinsic factors affect the tolerance of soft tissue to pressure and shear including nutrition, microclimate, perfusion and comorbidities (e.g. frailty, respiratory and cardiovascular disease and diabetes) [1]. Health conditions resulting in diminished blood, oxygen and nutrient supply decrease the tolerance of the tissues to damage from extrinsic factors. The initial focus in the prevention of PIs is the assessment of patient risk by identifying extrinsic and intrinsic factors which make a person vulnerable to skin damage.

15.3 The Link Between Malnutrition and Pressure Injuries

Malnutrition is an independent intrinsic risk factor for the development of a PI, increasing the risk by three to five times, with risk increasing as the severity of malnutrition increases [9–11]. Importantly, all patients with PIs, even in the absence of malnutrition, have increased nutritional requirements for both protein and energy. If a patient is malnourished or undernourished, deterioration of the wound and delayed wound healing may also result. Macro- and micronutrients are required by tissues and organs to support growth, development, maintenance and repair of body tissues [11].

While malnutrition is an established risk factor for PI [9] and skin tears [12], health professionals are not always aware of the significance of malnutrition in PI development, resulting in limited action at a local level. Both nutrition and hydration are central to maintaining skin and tissue integrity and facilitating tissue repair processes, so failure to manage these is a major factor in PI risk. Eating problems, weight loss, inadequate nutritional intake and malnutrition are frequently cited as key risk factors for the development of skin damage and delayed healing [9, 10]. While underweight and malnutrition are known risk factors for PI development, obesity (class I, BMI 30–34.99 kg/m^2) has been found to be protective [5]. Morbid obesity (BMI $\geq$ 40 kg/m^2), however, has a similar odds ratio (OR = 3.5) as malnutrition for the development of a PI when compared with those in the healthy weight range [5]. Morbidly obese patients with a concurrent diagnosis of malnutrition had an 11-fold odds of developing a PI when compared with those who were well nourished, albeit morbidly obese [5]. This is particularly significant for patients who are morbidly obese and have sarcopenia related to malnutrition which can be difficult to identify.

15.4 Prevention and Management of PIs with a Focus on Nutrition Care

Interdisciplinary action is needed to identify, prevent and treat malnutrition, particularly in older adults at risk of PI, to help reduce the incidence and subsequent harm. Unfortunately, most literature to date has only looked at risk or treatment, and not interventions that aim to minimise risk. The focus of this chapter is on nutritional interventions as part of an individualised and holistic approach to prevent and treat PIs. An overview of non-nutrition interventions to prevent PI can be found in the 2019 International Guideline [1]. International nutritional guidelines also provide an updated, comprehensive review of the research literature and recommendations reflecting recent evidence to direct best practice [1, 13, 14] with the following main recommendations:

- In combination with PI risk assessment, nutrition screening should be conducted to identify older adults who are malnourished or at risk of malnutrition.
- Those identified as malnourished or at risk should have a more detailed assessment conducted by a nutritionist/dietitian.
- An interprofessional team approach to nutrition care, as discussed throughout this book, is essential.

The international guidelines [1] also provide advice regarding the management of PIs through nutritional interventions. These are summarised in Table 15.1.

Table 15.1 Guidance for the management of pressure injuries through nutritional interventions

Clinical guidance	Reference to other chapters/ literature
Use a validated malnutrition screening tool to screen all patients at risk of or with a PI for potential malnutrition	[1, 14]
Patients with a PI should be referred to a dietitian for a comprehensive nutrition assessment and development of an individualised nutrition care plan	[1, 14]
Patients with a PI have increased protein and energy requirements; refer to local guidelines (where available) to guide practice	Chapters 2–5
Energy targets range from 125 to 145 kJ/kg (30–35 kcal/kg)	[1, 14]
Protein targets range from 1.2 to 1.5 g/kg	
Maintain awareness of high-risk groups:	
Malnourished patients	[1, 14]
Underweight patients	[1, 5, 9]
Morbidly obese patients	[1, 5]
Planning and implementation of measures to increase nutrient intake	Chapters 6 and 10–13
Patient education about PIs and their causes and the role of nutrition in PI prevention and wound healing	Chapter 12 [1, 13, 14]
Monitoring of nutritional intake	Chapters 5 and 6
Multivitamin/vitamin/mineral replacement should be considered only for patients with nutrient deficiencies (with attention to blood biochemistry monitoring): if concerns regarding nutritional adequacy or a patient's risk of deficiencies (e.g. high-risk group such as alcoholics)	Chapters 2–5 [1, 14]
Monitoring of nutrition status including weight monitoring, food charts and symptom management (e.g. constipation, poor appetite, post-operative nausea and vomiting)	Chapters 2–6
Consider nasogastric (NG) feeds for patients with poor appetite/intake at risk of PI, with consideration of the risks of PI where the NG tube is secured	Chapter 5
Maintain awareness of NGT securement as a risk factor for the development of mucosal PIs	[1]
Recognise hydration as key to ensuring nutrient delivery and oxygenation to support wound healing, encourage fluid intake, and consider at-risk groups (e.g. dysphagia)	Chapter 7

The evidence indicates that it is a combination of intensive nutrition interventions, with a multidisciplinary approach led by a nutritionist or dietitian, that are most likely to be successful in preventing and treating PIs [1, 14]. Nutrition care also facilitates healing of PIs and should form part of an MDT approach to management [1]. Where access to a dietitian is limited or unavailable, systematised, interdisciplinary approaches to nutrition care for older adults at risk of malnutrition, including those with a PI, should be considered to empower the wider team to ensure patients meet increased nutrition requirements [15–17]. Dietitian or medical nutrition specialists are best placed to ensure oversight of evidence-based nutrition care practice and deliver specialist nutrition care. The nursing team is often well placed to recognise and manage risk of PI because nurses have continuous care of the patient (Chap. 6) [17–19]. Nurses therefore play a key role in the implementation of nutrition management in collaboration with nutrition specialists and are also ideally positioned to ensure continuity of nutrition and other aspects of care for patients with at risk of PI on discharge or transfer.

PIs are considered patient safety events that may reflect poor-quality interdisciplinary care, and, in some countries, there are financial penalties for health-care providers when such events occur [20]. PI prevention strategies recognise the priority of evidence-based nutrition care and the need to embed this in practice through education and governance that involves nutritionists as experts.

15.5 Summary

Pressure injuries remain significant patient safety incidents for older people with mobility problems, frailty and concurrent medical conditions. They are, however, mostly preventable with evidence-based risk assessment and intervention. Evidence shows that malnutrition is an independent risk factor in the development of PIs and a contributor to delayed healing. Multidisciplinary evidence-based interventions have been shown to be successful in both managing malnutrition and preventing and managing pressure injuries, in keeping with international guidelines.

Take-Home Points

- Malnutrition is an independent, but modifiable, risk factor for PI development and delays wound healing.
- Appropriate nutrition is essential for PI prevention and management.
- Older adults with a PI have increased protein and energy requirements.
- PIs are preventable and require a multidisciplinary team approach.
- International guidelines summarise the most clinically effective multidisciplinary nutritional interventions that support the prevention and management and PIs.

References

1. Emily Haesler (ed.) (2019) European Pressure Ulcer Advisor Panel, National Pressure Injury Advisory Panel and Pan Pacific Pressure Injur Alliance. Prevention and Treatment of Pressure Ulcers/Injuries: Clinical Practice Guidelines. The International Guideline. EPUAP/NPIAP/PPPIA.
2. Campbell KE (2009) A new model to identify shared risk factors for pressure ulcers and frailty in older adults. Rehabil Nurs 34(6):242–247
3. Recio-Saucedo A et al (2018) What impact does nursing care left undone have on patient outcomes? Review of the literature. J Clin Nurs 27(11–12):2248–2259
4. Kayser SA et al (2018) Prevalence and analysis of medical device-related pressure injuries: results from the international pressure ulcer prevalence survey. Adv Skin Wound Care 31(6):276–285
5. Ness SJ et al (2018) The pressures of obesity: the relationship between obesity, malnutrition and pressure injuries in hospital inpatients. Clin Nutr 37(5):1569–1574
6. Coleman S et al (2014) A new pressure ulcer conceptual framework. J Adv Nurs 70(10):2222–2234
7. Kottner J et al (2018) Microclimate: a critical review in the context of pressure ulcer prevention. Clin Biomech (Bristol, Avon) 59:62–70
8. Gefen A et al (2020) Device-related pressure ulcers: secure prevention. J Wound Care 29(Suppl 2a):S1–S52
9. Banks M et al (2010) Malnutrition and pressure ulcer risk in adults in Australian health care facilities. Nutrition 26(9):896–901
10. Banks MD et al (2020) Pressure ulcer healing with an intensive nutrition intervention in an acute setting: a pilot randomised controlled trial. J Wound Care 29(Suppl 9a):S10–S17
11. Munoz N et al (2020) The role of nutrition for pressure injury prevention and healing: the 2019 International Clinical Practice Guideline Recommendations. Adv Skin Wound Care 33(3):123–136
12. Munro EL et al (2018) Malnutrition is independently associated with skin tears in hospital inpatient setting—findings of a 6-year point prevalence audit. Int Wound J 15(4):527–533
13. Roberts S, Desbrow B, Chaboyer W (2016) Feasibility of a patient-centred nutrition intervention to improve oral intakes of patients at risk of pressure ulcer: a pilot randomised control trial. Scand J Caring Sci 30(2):271–280
14. Trans Tasman Dietetic Wound Care group. Evidence based practice guidelines for the dietetic management of adults with pressure injuries. (2011) These guidelines have been independently reviewed by the Dietitians Association of Australia (DAA) and as a result are endorsed by the DAA. https://www.aci.health.nsw.gov.au/__data/assets/pdf_file/0004/388237/13.-Trans-Tasman-Dietetic-Wound-Care-Group-Pressure-Injury-Guidelines-2011.pdf
15. Tappenden KA et al (2013) Critical role of nutrition in improving quality of care: an interdisciplinary call to action to address adult hospital malnutrition. JPEN J Parenter Enteral Nutr 37(4):482–497
16. Bell JJ et al (2018) Rationale and developmental methodology for the SIMPLE approach: a Systematised, Interdisciplinary Malnutrition Pathway for impLementation and Evaluation in hospitals. Nutr Diet 75(2):226–234
17. Bell JJ et al (2021) Nutritional care of the older patient with fragility fracture: opportunities for systematised, interdisciplinary approaches across acute care, rehabilitation and secondary prevention settings. In: Falaschi P, Marsh D (eds) Orthogeriatrics: the management of older patients with fragility fractures. Springer, Cham, pp 311–329
18. Ten Cate D et al (2020) Interventions to prevent and treat malnutrition in older adults to be carried out by nurses: a systematic review. J Clin Nurs 29(11–12):1883–1902
19. Ten Cate D et al (2021) Hospital and home care nurses' experiences and perceptions regarding nutritional care for older adults to prevent and treat malnutrition: a cross-sectional study. J Clin Nurs 30(13–14):2079–2092
20. Lyder CH, Ayello EA (2008) Chapter 12: Pressure ulcers: a patient safety issue. In: Hughes RG (ed) Patient safety and quality: an evidence-based handbook for nurses. Agency for Healthcare Research and Quality (US), Rockville

16

BMI and Obesity

Alfons Ramel and Sari Stenholm

Abstract

The focus of this chapter is on body mass index and obesity in older adults. Further, it will be discussed whether weight loss should be generally recommended for obese older adults.

Keywords

Body mass index · Obesity · Obesity paradox · Body composition · Weight loss · Nutrition

Learning Outcomes
By the end of this chapter, you will be able to:

- Understand the epidemiology of obesity in older adults.
- Know changes in body composition with ageing.
- Explain the causes of obesity in ageing.

This chapter is a component of Part II: Specialist Versus Generalist Nutritional Care in Aging. For an explanation of the grouping of chapters in this book, please see Chap. 1: 'Geriatrics and Orthogeriatrics: Providing Nutrition Care'.

A. Ramel (✉)
Department of Food Science and Nutrition, University of Iceland, Reykjavík, Iceland
e-mail: alfonsra@hi.is

S. Stenholm
Department of Public Health, University of Turku, Turku, Finland
e-mail: samast@utu.fi

- Report health consequences of obesity.
- Understand the obesity paradox.
- Formulate strategies how to improve health in obese older adults independent from weight loss.

16.1 Definition and Epidemiology

Overweight and obesity are characterized by abnormal or excessive body fat accumulation which has shown to increase the risk for several diseases. Usually, body mass index (BMI), a person's weight (in kilogrammes) divided by the square of his or her height (in metres), is used to identify obesity. For persons older than 18 years, the WHO defines overweight and obesity as follows: BMI equal to or more than 25 kg/m^2 is considered overweight and BMI of 30 kg/m^2 or more as obese [1]. However, appropriateness of these cut-off values for older adults has been questioned [2], and specific cut-off values (23–30 kg/m^2) for older adults have been suggested [3] and consecutively introduced, e.g. in Iceland [4].

As a global epidemic, obesity is also very prevalent in older adults and has been increasing over the past decades [5]. According to results from the US National Health and Nutrition Examination Surveys in 2014, the prevalence of obesity was 38% in man and 39% in women older than 60 years of age [6]. Similar results have been found in other Western countries as well, including the United Kingdom, Canada and Iceland [7–9].

16.2 Changes in Body Composition with Ageing

With ageing, alterations in body composition can be observed, especially loss of lean body mass, bone mass and body water and increase in fat mass. In addition, fat mass redistributes with ageing as more visceral fat accumulates in the abdominal region and amount of subcutaneous fat reduces in other regions of the body; and there is also fat accumulation in the muscle, liver and heart [10]. In consideration of these alterations in body composition, some older adults face increased health risks due to concomitant excessive fatness and decreased muscle mass, condition called sarcopenic obesity (SO, Chap. 8) [11]. Further, patients can be both overweight and malnourished at the same time, with substantial impact on patient and/or healthcare outcomes (diagnosis of overweight or obese malnutrition, DOOM) [12]. Note DOOM is different to SO. SO includes age-related sarcopenia, whereas DOOM is specifically limited to those with concurrent diagnoses of malnutrition and obesity.

16.3 Causes of Obesity

The main cause of obesity and overweight is an energy imbalance between energy intake and energy expenditure. In many populations and societies, there have been an elevated consumption of energy-dense foods containing excessive amount of fat and sugar and a decrease in physical activity due to the predominantly sedentary nature of today's work, passive modes of transportation and increasing urbanization [13, 14]. Adverse alterations in dietary intake and decreased physical activity can be attributed to environmental and societal changes associated with sectors such as health, agriculture, transport, urban planning, environment, food processing, distribution, marketing and education [1].

As ageing is characterized by a markedly loss of muscle mass, reduced exercise and reduced basal metabolic rate with the preference of oxidizing carbohydrate instead of fat, older adults might be even more prone to develop obesity. Although caloric intake does usually not increase significantly and may actually decrease with age, this does not seem to compensate for the decline in energy expenditure, which leads to body fat accumulation and consequently to metabolic problems [15].

16.3.1 Health Consequences of Obesity

Obesity leads to unfavourable physiologic state due to changes in insulin resistance, sex hormones, growth factor milieu, increased blood lipids and the creation of various adipokines, including inflammatory cytokines, e.g. tumour necrosis factor-α and interleukin-6 [16, 17]. These serious changes in the body's physiology contribute to increased likelihood of several diseases (mentioned below) and might create an environment that favours cancer development [18].

Consequently, increased body fatness is a serious risk factor for metabolic diseases, e.g. cardiovascular diseases (mainly heart disease and stroke), diabetes and some cancers (including endometrial, breast, ovarian, prostate, liver, gallbladder, kidney and colon). The risk for these non-communicable diseases increases with increasing BMI, and at present times, overweight and obesity are associated with more deaths than underweight on a global perspective [1, 19, 20]. In addition to the metabolic consequences of obesity, excess weight plays burden to musculoskeletal system and is a major risk factor for osteoarthritis in the lower extremities. Moreover, obesity impairs physical functioning and mobility limitations, which are common among older obese people [21].

16.3.2 Obesity Paradox: Protective in Older Adults and Patient Population

Many chronic conditions may lead to weight loss among older adults, and at that time being, obese may provide additional protection. In fact, some people who are obese live actually longer than their normal weight counterparts. This phenomenon is called 'obesity paradox'. For example, patients with coronary artery disease, heart failure, type 2 diabetes and chronic kidney disease have lower mortality risks than [22, 23] or similar [24–26] to older adults in the normal weight category.

It may sound counter-intuitive that a known risk factor for several diseases actually turns protective after diagnosis of these conditions, and over the past decade, there has been an active scientific discussion about the obesity paradox proposing evidence both for and against it [27]. Some studies emphasize the role of muscle mass [28] and cardiorespiratory fitness [29], and it appears that the obesity paradox may not apply to physically fit persons [30]. However, several factors have been identified which may explain the protective effect of excess weight. These include better nutritional reserves, better haemodynamic stability, higher bone mineral density and protection from fat around hip area in case of a fall [31–33]. In addition, several factors related to the study design and study populations may explain why lower mortality risk is observed among obese persons, including healthy survivor bias; individuals with severe illness may have lost weight recently leading to lower BMI; BMI does not necessarily represent body fat; BMI cut-offs are not being appropriate; and obese patients are diagnosed earlier [34–36].

16.4 Is Targeted Weight Loss Appropriate in Older Adults?

Weight loss among older obese has not been generally recommended, since weight loss may have harmful effects by accelerating loss of muscle mass and bone density. However, during the last decades, many weight loss intervention studies in older obese adults have been carried out, and our understanding on weight management at older ages is increasing [37–39]. These studies suggest that the combination of controlled weight loss and energy reduction, but protein-adequate diet, combined with exercise produces the most beneficial effects on weight loss, physical functioning, quality of life and reduced pain. In addition, studies have also reported positive changes in body composition, i.e. decreased weight and fat mass, and improved glycaemic control [40–42].

Although multicomponent interventions are a reasonable and appropriate method in our opinion, it is difficult to attribute positive outcomes of such studies solely to weight loss and might be even misleading. Considering that the achieved and maintained mean weight loss is usually small in such studies (around 5 kg) [41], one could argue that differences in health outcomes between intervention and control groups are likely driven by physical activity and not by minor weight loss. This assumption is supported by studies reporting beneficial changes in physical function and cardiovascular risk factors after an exercise protocol with no weight change at all [43–45].

As an example for this methodological dilemma, we want to cite a recent meta-analysis on intentional weight loss and mortality in older adults [46], in which weight loss is associated with a 15% reduced risk of mortality. However, when looking at the individual studies, it can be seen that this reduction is mainly driven by studies including exercise as part of the intervention [38–42], whereas diet-only-induced-weight loss studies showed even increased mortality in the intervention group (albeit not significant) [32–35].

It has been suggested that obese older adults who have either metabolic abnormalities, e.g. increased circulating triglycerides, or functional impairment, for example, slow gait speed, would benefit most for weight loss, under the provision that that lean body mass and bone mass can be preserved [47]. However, in real life, it might be impossible to limit these losses, as the negative energy balance during weight loss is responsible for a catabolism which inevitably affects negatively the skeletal muscle and bone [48].

Considering the uncertainty of the benefits of intentional weight loss according to intervention studies and the overwhelming evidence from epidemiological research on the negative effects of weight loss in older adults, as well as the given difficulties to maintain weight change [49], it seems prudent *not* to focus solely on weight loss in older obese adults. This is particularly relevant where highly restrictive, self-prescribed 'fad' diets are cycled leading to both poor intake of protective nutrients and inadequate intake leading to sarcopenia. In case of targeted weight loss, it has to be carefully monitored to, as a minimum, preserve muscle strength and physical function with careful serial measurements to assess for sarcopenia and also preferably ensure a good balance of macro- and micronutrients.

The main focus among older obese adults should be in increasing physical activity by resistance and aerobic exercise to increase or maintain physical functioning, independence and good health in older adults without the uncertainties and hardship that come with energy restriction and weight loss (Chap. 14). Attention should still be placed to improve diet quality using nutrition therapy to optimize energy intake and expenditure as well as to promote healthy eating habits with adequate amount of protein and a broad variety of fresh products among older adults to avoid further weight gain and obtain benefits of the good quality of nutrition.

We think that more critical older adult's characteristics should be explored before potentially initiating a weight loss diet: motivation and attitudes, cognitive function, social environment and family support and financial restraints.

However, it should be mentioned that obesity is a frequent concern in older adults with diseases that impair mobility, e.g. stroke and arthritis. These associations between mobility impairments and disease can negatively affect older adults' willingness and ability to engage in healthy behaviours, consequently resulting in energy imbalance, weight gain and mobility disability. In order to prevent this negative loop, there is a need to find ways to optimize energy intake and expenditure. According to a recent review in this area, nutrition and weight loss studies in older adults with mobility disability are still in building stages, with a great necessity to conduct randomized controlled trials [50] in order to find the best approaches to weight loss, e.g. high-protein diet, to manage comorbidities and disease.

16.4.1 Summary

Weight loss in overweight older adults is not routinely recommended or advised [3] and, even in obese older adults, should only be carefully considered in partnership with suitably qualified health professionals. To conclude, it is important to emphasize the role of healthy weight throughout adulthood. Maintaining normal weight and preventing weight gain during midlife prevent various chronic diseases and help to maintain physical, cognitive and social functioning with advancing age.

Take-Home Points

- A life-course approach to preventing obesity should be the focus of all healthcare providers.
- Overweight older adults should not routinely try and lose weight unless advised by a medical specialist.
- Obese older adults may not necessarily benefit from dietary efforts to reduce weight.
- Any dietary efforts to reduce weight should be accompanied by appropriate physical activity and careful monitoring of muscle strength and function.
- Weight loss may be harmful in older adults, even if intentional.
- There is no place for restrictive fad diets in older persons.

References

1. Nguyen DM, El-Serag HB (2010) The epidemiology of obesity. Gastroenterol Clin N Am 39(1):1–7
2. Ng WL et al (2019) Evaluating the concurrent validity of body mass index (BMI) in the identification of malnutrition in older hospital inpatients. Clin Nutr 38(5):2417–2422
3. Volkert D et al (2019) ESPEN guideline on clinical nutrition and hydration in geriatrics. Clin Nutr 38(1):10–47
4. Elva Gísladóttir HÞ, Geirsdóttir ÓG, Jónsdóttir AB, Jensdóttir AB, Jónsdóttir G, Hilmisdóttir HB, Vilmundardóttir VK, Geirsdóttir Þ (2018) Ráðleggingar um mataræði fyrir hrumt og veikt fólk. In: I.D.o. Health (ed) Embætti Landlæknis. Embætti Læandlæknis, Reykjavík
5. Batsis JA, Zagaria AB (2018) Addressing obesity in aging patients. Med Clin North Am 102(1):65–85
6. Flegal KM et al (2016) Trends in obesity among adults in the United States, 2005 to 2014. JAMA 315(21):2284–2291
7. Baker C (2021) Obesity statistics. House of Commons Library, London
8. Twells LK et al (2014) Current and predicted prevalence of obesity in Canada: a trend analysis. CMAJ Open 2(1):E18–E26
9. Valdimarsdóttir M, Jonsson SH, Þorgeirsdóttir H, Gísladóttir E, Óskar J (2009) Líkamsþyngd og holdafar fullorðinna Íslendinga frá 1990 til 2007
10. Zamboni M et al (2014) Predictors of ectopic fat in humans. Curr Obes Rep 3(4):404–413
11. Orwoll ES et al (2020) The importance of muscle versus fat mass in Sarcopenic obesity: a re-evaluation using D3-Creatine muscle mass versus DXA lean mass measurements. J Gerontol A Biol Sci Med Sci 75(7):1362–1368
12. Ness SJ et al (2018) The pressures of obesity: the relationship between obesity, malnutrition and pressure injuries in hospital inpatients. Clin Nutr 37(5):1569–1574
13. Allender S et al (2008) Quantification of urbanization in relation to chronic diseases in developing countries: a systematic review. J Urban Health 85(6):938–951
14. Jakicic JM et al (2020) Strategies for physical activity interventions in the treatment of obesity. Endocrinol Metab Clin N Am 49(2):289–301
15. Johannsen DL, Ravussin E (2010) Obesity in the elderly: is faulty metabolism to blame? Aging Health 6(2):159–167
16. Heymsfield SB, Wadden TA (2017) Mechanisms, pathophysiology, and management of obesity. N Engl J Med 376(3):254–266
17. Pollak M (2008) Insulin and insulin-like growth factor signalling in neoplasia. Nat Rev Cancer 8(12):915–928

18. Lohmann AE et al (2016) Association of obesity-related metabolic disruptions with cancer risk and outcome. J Clin Oncol 34(35):4249–4255
19. Suzuki R et al (2009) Body weight and incidence of breast cancer defined by estrogen and progesterone receptor status--a meta-analysis. Int J Cancer 124(3):698–712
20. Lauby-Secretan B et al (2016) Body fatness and Cancer--viewpoint of the IARC Working Group. N Engl J Med 375(8):794–798
21. Fernandes de Souza Barbosa J et al (2018) Abdominal obesity and mobility disability in older adults: a 4-year follow-up the international mobility in aging study. J Nutr Health Aging 22(10):1228–1237
22. Flegal KM et al (2013) Association of all-cause mortality with overweight and obesity using standard body mass index categories: a systematic review and meta-analysis. JAMA 309(1):71–82
23. Winter JE et al (2014) BMI and all-cause mortality in older adults: a meta-analysis. Am J Clin Nutr 99(4):875–890
24. Janssen I, Mark AE (2007) Elevated body mass index and mortality risk in the elderly. Obes Rev 8(1):41–59
25. Pischon T et al (2008) General and abdominal adiposity and risk of death in Europe. N Engl J Med 359(20):2105–2120
26. Bea JW et al (2015) Risk of mortality according to body mass index and body composition among postmenopausal women. Am J Epidemiol 182(7):585–596
27. Lavie CJ, De Schutter A, Milani RV (2015) Healthy obese versus unhealthy lean: the obesity paradox. Nat Rev Endocrinol 11(1):55–62
28. Prado CM, Gonzalez MC, Heymsfield SB (2015) Body composition phenotypes and obcsity paradox. Curr Opin Clin Nutr Metab Care 18(6):535–551
29. Goel K et al (2011) Combined effect of cardiorespiratory fitness and adiposity on mortality in patients with coronary artery disease. Am Heart J 161(3):590–597
30. Barry VW et al (2014) Fitness vs. fatness on all-cause mortality: a meta-analysis. Prog Cardiovasc Dis 56(4):382–390
31. Gandham A et al (2020) Incidence and predictors of fractures in older adults with and without obesity defined by body mass index versus body fat percentage. Bone 140:115546
32. Li G et al (2020) Relationship between obesity and risk of major osteoporotic fracture in post-menopausal women: taking frailty into consideration. J Bone Miner Res 35(12):2355–2362
33. Oreopoulos A et al (2009) The obesity paradox in the elderly: potential mechanisms and clinical implications. Clin Geriatr Med 25(4):643–659, viii
34. Banack HR, Kaufman JS (2014) The obesity paradox: understanding the effect of obesity on mortality among individuals with cardiovascular disease. Prev Med 62:96–102
35. Rothman KJ (2008) BMI-related errors in the measurement of obesity. Int J Obes 32(Suppl 3):S56–S59
36. Dixon JB et al (2015) 'Obesity paradox' misunderstands the biology of optimal weight throughout the life cycle. Int J Obes 39(1):82–84
37. DiMilia PR, Mittman AC, Batsis JA (2019) Benefit-to-risk balance of weight loss interventions in older adults with obesity. Curr Diab Rep 19(11):114
38. Papageorgiou M et al (2020) Is weight loss harmful for skeletal health in obese older adults? Gerontology 66(1):2–14
39. Jiang BC, Villareal DT (2019) Therapeutic and lifestyle approaches to obesity in older persons. Curr Opin Clin Nutr Metab Care 22(1):30–36
40. Rejeski WJ et al (2010) Obesity, intentional weight loss and physical disability in older adults. Obes Rev 11(9):671–685
41. Miller GD et al (2006) Intensive weight loss program improves physical function in older obese adults with knee osteoarthritis. Obesity (Silver Spring) 14(7):1219–1230
42. Dunstan DW et al (2002) High-intensity resistance training improves glycemic control in older patients with type 2 diabetes. Diabetes Care 25(10):1729–1736
43. Geirsdottir OG et al (2015) Muscular strength and physical function in elderly adults 6-18 months after a 12-week resistance exercise program. Scand J Public Health 43(1):76–82

44. Arnarson A et al (2014) Changes in body composition and use of blood cholesterol lowering drugs predict changes in blood lipids during 12 weeks of resistance exercise training in old adults. Aging Clin Exp Res 26(3):287–292
45. Geirsdottir OG et al (2012) Effect of 12-week resistance exercise program on body composition, muscle strength, physical function, and glucose metabolism in healthy, insulin-resistant, and diabetic elderly Icelanders. J Gerontol Ser A Biol Sci Med Sci 67(11):1259–1265
46. Kritchevsky SB et al (2015) Intentional weight loss and all-cause mortality: a meta-analysis of randomized clinical trials. PLoS One 10(3):e0121993
47. Mathus-Vliegen EM (2012) Prevalence, pathophysiology, health consequences and treatment options of obesity in the elderly: a guideline. Obes Facts 5(3):460–483
48. Bosy-Westphal A et al (2009) Contribution of individual organ mass loss to weight loss-associated decline in resting energy expenditure. Am J Clin Nutr 90(4):993–1001
49. Evert AB, Franz MJ (2017) Why weight loss maintenance is difficult. Diabetes Spectr 30(3):153–156
50. Plow MA et al (2014) A systematic review of behavioural techniques used in nutrition and weight loss interventions among adults with mobility-impairing neurological and musculoskeletal conditions. Obes Rev 15(12):945–956

17

A Comprehensive Study of the Nutritional System

Saverio Cinti

Abstract

The white and brown adipose tissues are organized to form a true organ. They have a different anatomy and perform different functions, but they collaborate thanks to their ability to convert mutually and reversibly following physiological stimuli. This implies a new fundamental property for mature cells, which would be able to reversibly reprogram their genome under physiological conditions. The subcutaneous mammary gland provides another example of their plasticity. Here fat cells are reversibly transformed into glands during pregnancy and breastfeeding. The obese adipose organ is inflamed because hypertrophic fat cells, typical of this condition, die and their cellular residues must be reabsorbed by macrophages. The molecules produced by these cells during their reabsorption work interfere with the insulin receptor, and this induces insulin resistance, which ultimately causes type 2 diabetes. The adipose organ collaborates with those of digestion. Both produce hormones that can influence the nutritional behavior of individuals. They produce molecules that mutually influence functional activities including thermogenesis, which contributes to the interruption of the meal. The nutrients are absorbed by the intestine, stored in the adipose organ, and distributed by them to the whole body between meals. Distribution includes offspring during breastfeeding. The system as a whole is therefore called the nutritional system.

This chapter is a component of Part II: Specialist Versus Generalist Nutritional Care in Aging. For an explanation of the grouping of chapters in this book, please see Chap. 1: "Geriatrics and Orthogeriatrics: Providing Nutrition Care."

S. Cinti (✉)
Faculty of Medicine, Department of Experimental and Clinical Medicine,
Marche Polytechnic University, Ancona, Italy
e-mail: cinti@univpm.it

Keywords
Adipocytes · White · Brown · Beige · Mammary gland · Obesity

Learning Outcomes
By the end of this chapter, you will be able to:

- Understand the main physiologic aspects of a new organ that plays a pivotal role in the complex physiology that regulates the most important behaviors for the survival of mammals.

17.1 Introduction

It has been calculated that the human body is made up of approximately 37,000 billion cells. Each of them must be fed daily. The nourishment for each cell type comes from the food that needs to be researched and ingested. The search for food is a fundamental behavior for survival that arises from the balance between brain activities that receive instinctual impulses and those that elaborate rational responses. Food intake is a subsequent and consequent behavior, and it also needs the collaboration of the two components underlying the behavioral activity.

Today it is difficult to understand how an instinctual impulse is needed to activate the search for food, but until a few 100 years ago, obtaining food was not a trivial activity and often involved survival risks. Just think of the fact that by leaving the cave, primitive man could easily become from predator to prey. So, the impulse must have been enough to overcome even the strong instinct for survival.

It is even more difficult to think how stimuli may be needed to take food, which in itself determines a physical satisfaction or at least the interruption of an unpleasant condition such as that due to prolonged fasting.

For both of these two behavioral activities, complex-acting hormones are needed, mainly produced by white adipocytes.

These cells form a tissue, which therefore represents the central fulcrum for the nutrition of our organism. They are also able to store high-energy molecules in relatively small spaces that nourish the body between meals, allowing us to turn our attention and our activity to other functions that are not exclusively dedicated to nutrition. The ability to have a fasting period between meals allows time not only to search for other food but also to search for a partner, procreate, breed offspring, and carry out all those activities that can guarantee the offspring the best possible future.

17.2 Hormones Produced by White Adipocytes

The hormone for food research was discovered in 1994 by Jeffrey Friedman's team [1]. It has been attributed the name of leptin (from the Greek leptòs, thin), a hormone with endocrine and paracrine activity that acts on various organs but mainly on the brain and in particular on the limbic system [2], informing us about the nutritional status of the organism. In fact, it determines a leptinemia that is proportional to the amount of white adipose tissue, i.e., the body's energy supplies. When supplies are low, leptinemia is low, and the brain receives uncontrollable impulses to search for food. Mice and humans, who do not produce leptin, take triple the food taken by normal subjects becoming massively obese, and the administration of recombinant leptin allows the recovery of a phenotype and normal behavior [3].

Most of the essential obese subjects develop a leptin resistance [4]. A physiological justification for this may be considered, for example, where an organism has awareness of impending food shortage, and despite the presence of high energy supplies and therefore high leptinemia, a leptin resistance is established allowing for further food intake that guarantees the possibility of surviving long periods of fasting.

This resistance to hormone is the basis of essential obesity, as the individual who consumes overeating makes the energy balance positive and needs a particular development of the white adipose tissue. The latter responds appropriately with expansion capacity both in the volume of each individual cell (hypertrophy) and in the number of cells (hyperplasia). The extraordinary expansive capacity of the white adipose tissue means that its weight, which represents about 20% of the total weight of a lean adult individual, multiplies to the point that it represents about 70% of the total body weight [5].

These data allow us to easily understand how it must also produce a whole series of paracrine-acting molecules that facilitate interaction with the extracellular matrix to allow adequate expansion in the event of a chronically positive energy balance up to extraordinary levels such as those abovementioned. The details of these secretion factors have recently undergone extensive revision [6].

The instinctual stimulus for the behavior of food intake is given by a hormone produced by the white adipocyte discovered, more recently, in 2016 by Dr. Chopra's team, asprosin (from the Greek àspros, white) [7].

The most convincing fact that this hormone is essential for food intake is that subjects with lipodystrophy (therefore with low leptinemia) and who have a gene mutation that prevents them from producing asprosin eat very little food [8]. Another important function of asprosin is to induce hepatic glucose release. So, during fasting, the white adipocyte releases fatty acids that are essential and usable directly for cardiac activity and stimulates the hepatic release of glucose, which is essential for brain activity.

In summary, the white adipocyte produces two hormones that act on the brain to induce the individual to look for food (leptin) and ingest it (asprosin). It also guarantees survival by supplying energy to the body's cells and allowing long intervals between meals.

17.3 The Adipose Organ

From an anatomical point of view, the adipose tissue is contained in distinct depots which can be dissected from the rest of the body and occupy superficial (subcutaneous) and deep (visceral) compartments. The depots have their own morphology and are delimited by connective tissue capsules or serous membranes. The former is mainly located in the subcutaneous compartment, while the latter in the visceral one.

The color of the adipose tissue is yellowish in humans, but in some locations, the color is quite brown (Fig. 17.1). In humans, the most consistent brown area is placed in close relationship with the aorta and its main branches. Brown area quantity is highly variable and depends above all on age (higher in young people), nutritional status (higher in lean), and exposure to cold (higher in exposed).

In these sites, the fat cells have different characteristics than those of the white adipocytes. Mitochondria are numerous, large, and rich in laminar cristae. The adipocytes of the brown areas, which are called brown adipocytes, are therefore very different from the white adipocytes (Fig. 17.2).

Brown adipocytes have opposite functions to those of white adipocytes: they disperse energy by burning fatty acids and produce heat [9]. Since the lipid vacuoles are in multilocular form, the quantity of fatty acids released by the adrenergic

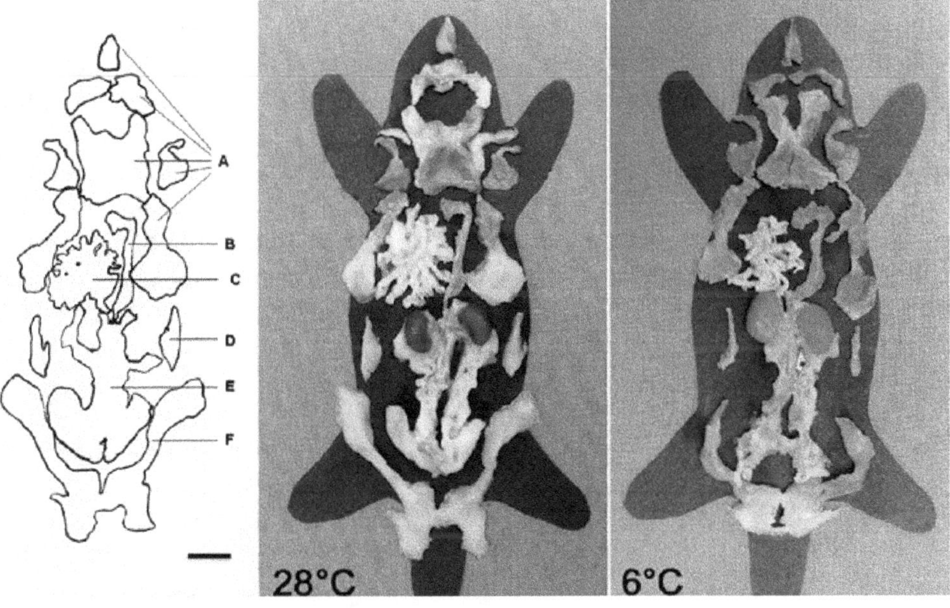

Fig. 17.1 Gross anatomy of adipose organ from mice maintained at 28 or 6 °C for 10 days. Subcutaneous (*A* and *F*) and visceral (*B–E*) depots are indicated. Kidneys are in site for orientation. The gray areas are brown in color, brown adipose tissue; white areas correspond to white adipose tissue. At 6 °C, the browning of the organ is visually evident. Bar, 15 mm. (From Murano, I. et al. The Adipose Organ of Sv129 mice contains a prevalence of brown adipocytes and shows plasticity after cold exposure. Adipocytes 2005; 1 (2), 121–130, with permission)

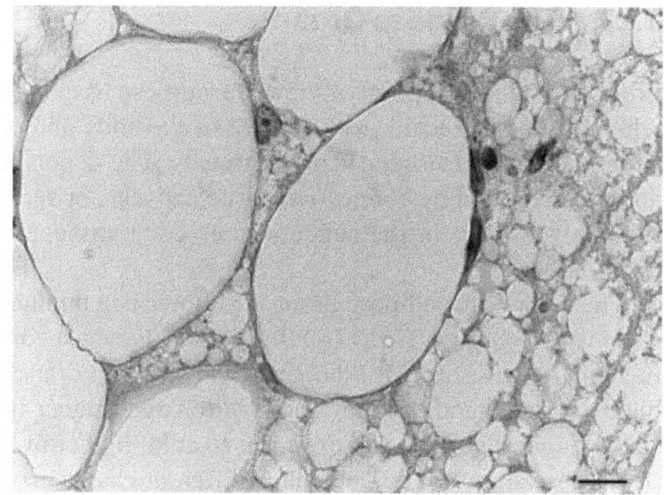

Fig. 17.2 Light microscopy. Mixed adipose tissue. Unilocular white adipocytes (left) and multilocular brown adipocytes (right) are visible. Bar, 10 µm

stimulus is enormous, and since the mitochondria are numerous, large, and rich in cristae, the heat produced is physiologically relevant. If we consider that the human body must be constantly maintained at a temperature of about 37 °C, while the environmental one varies from about −70 to about +50, it is easy to understand how thermogenetic systems are more important than those of heat dispersion and the brown adipose tissue is the most important thermogenetic systems in the body.

In summary, the adipose organ is formed by dissectible structures with a specific anatomy and formed by two tissues with different morphology and function: the white and the brown adipose tissues. In fact, organs, by definition, are dissectible anatomical structures, formed by at least two tissues that cooperate with each other for a specific functional purpose. For example, the stomach is dissectible and composed of both glands that produce gastric juice and muscles that make peristalsis. Glands and muscles are different tissues that cooperate for the common purpose of digestion. The cooperation in the adipose organ would consist in the particular plasticity of fat cells which would be able, in particular physiological situations, to convert mutually to distribute the intrinsic energy of the lipids toward thermogenesis or toward the metabolic reserve [10–13].

These data imply two relevant aspects: (1) browning of the adipose organ could be used to increase energy expenditure and therefore as a treatment for obesity and its complications, and (2) mature cells can change their phenotype under physiologic stimuli.

17.4 Browning of the Adipose Organ as a Therapy for Obesity and Related Diseases

If we eliminate the brown adipose tissue with genetic manipulation, after a few weeks, the mice, while eating and moving like the controls, i.e., those with brown fat, become massively obese and develop type 2 (T2) diabetes [14]. On the other hand, the administration of beta-3-adrenergic drugs or brown fat explants to obese mice reduces obesity and treats T2 diabetes [15]. It has also been shown that the activation of brown fat improves lipid metabolism and promotes the prevention of atherosclerosis [16]. Therefore, it is not surprising to find an extension of life in genetically manipulated mice that had an activation of brown fat.

In recent years, it has been confirmed not only that brown fat is also present in the human adipose organ but also that the phenomenon of white-brown conversion is also present in humans and that "browning" has health properties also in humans [17]. All this makes us hope that drugs capable of mimicking exposure to the cold can be identified without giving the unpleasant negative sensations that it induces and without promoting or facilitating the typical infectious cold diseases. In this regard, it is relevant that physical exercise induces activation of the sympathetic nervous system with browning in the adipose organ [18]. A hormone called irisin has also been identified that is produced by the muscle during shivering and exercise, which is able to promote browning of the fatty organ [19]. Recent data indicate that the hormone also has beneficial effects on the bone by promoting its reinforcement in physical exercise and by preventing and treating experimentally induced osteoporosis and muscle atrophy on mice [20].

17.5 The Physiology of the Mammary Gland Confirms the Plasticity of the Adipose Organ

The second aspect that derives from our studies concerns a new fundamental property of cells hitherto unknown, the physiological and reversible conversion (or trans-differentiation) of the mature cell.

To confirm this new cellular property, we looked for other examples and found confirmation in another physiological condition that changes the morphology and function of the adipose organ in females, pregnancy. In this condition, the mammary gland develops forming the structures necessary for the production of milk (alveoli). At the end of pregnancy, the alveoli disappear, restoring the pre-gravid anatomy of the breast, subcutaneous fat infiltrated by branched ducts that collect in a single nipple. During the development of the alveoli, the fat cells disappear, as well as during the involution; when the alveoli disappear, the fat cells reappear.

We hypothesized that the disappearance during glandular development is due to the conversion of adipocytes into glandular cells of the alveoli, just as during the involution the glandular cells are transformed back to fat cells. If this were true, we would have found a new example of physiological and reversible trans-differentiation in the adipose organ. To confirm the hypothesis, we used the lineage tracing technique that allows to follow destiny of developing cells [21]. Our experimental data confirm the large plastic capacity of fat cells that are able to undergo phenotypic and functional transformations following physiological stimuli and in a reversible way to respond to different functional needs of the body.

17.6 The Obese Adipose Organ

Although detailed explanation is beyond the remit of this introductory chapter, the obese adipose organ has distinct properties. For example, the adipose organ of obese mice and humans is infiltrated by inflammatory cells mainly consisting of macrophages [22, 23]. The degree of infiltration correlates with the size of the adipocytes, but the visceral adipocytes die at a size smaller than that of the subcutaneous adipocytes. This offers an explanation for the greater morbidity of visceral fat, probably because it derives largely from brown-white conversion [24]. Macrophages reabsorb dead hypertrophic cells forming multinucleated giant cell structures that we have called crown-like structures (CLS) (Fig. 17.3). During reabsorption activities,

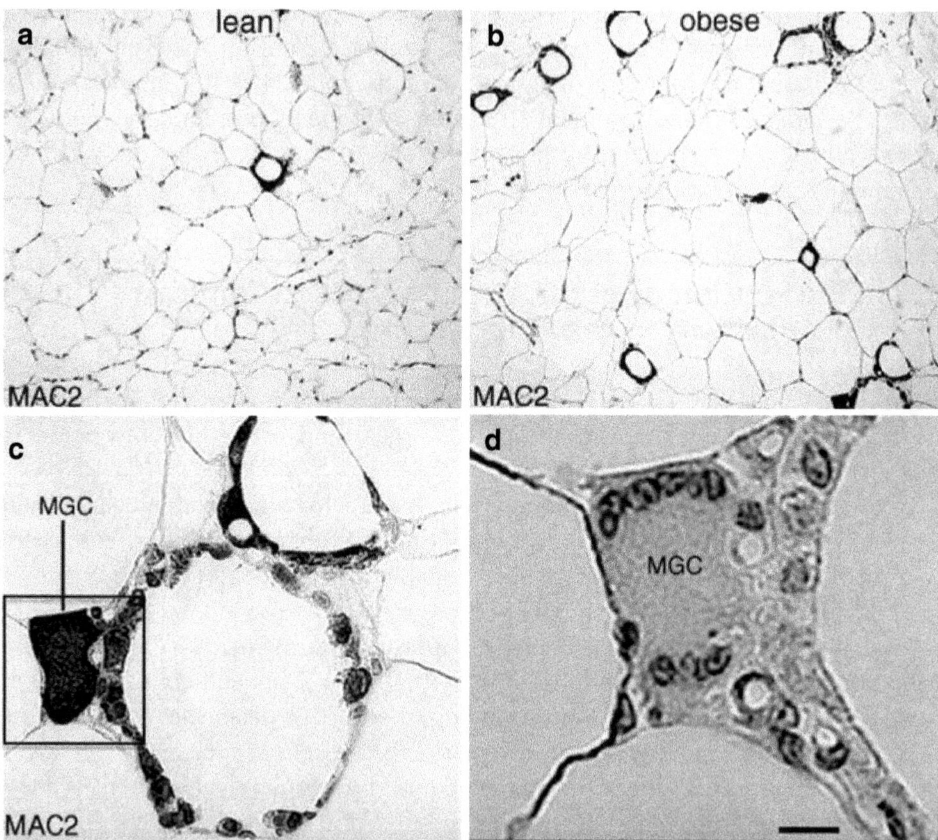

Fig. 17.3 Immunohistochemistry with antibodies as indicated. MAC2 stains active macrophages. Perilipin1 (**d**) stains vital adipocytes. Several crown-like structures are visible in the adipose tissue from obese mouse (**b**), but few are also present in adipose tissue from lean mouse (**a**). (**c**) Enlargement of CLS at the bottom right corner of (**b**). A giant macrophage and several MAC2 immunoreactive macrophages surround debris of a dead adipocyte. (**d**) Enlargement of serial section corresponding to squared area in C showing that the giant macrophage is multinuclear. A perilipin immunoreactive adipocyte is visible on the left, and the absence of immunoreactivity is visible in the CLS. Bar, 100 μm (**a** and **b**), 28 μm for (**c**), and 10 μm for (**c**). (From Cinti, S. et al. Adipocyte death defines macrophage localization and function in adipose tissue of obese mice and humans. J Lip Res 2005; 46: 2347–2355, with permission)

different substances produced by macrophages (TNFα, resistin, specific miRNA, etc.) interfere with the activity of the insulin receptor offering an explanation to the fact that the appearance of inflammation of the adipose tissue coincides with the appearance of insulin resistance, which eventually leads to T2 diabetes. Additionally, experimental data on obese mice and humans indicate a progressive increase in noradrenergic fibers in the islands of Langerhans [25]. This may, for example, be responsible for the reduction of insulin secretion with the appearance of T2 diabetes and offer an explanation for the rapid post-bariatric recovery from diabetes.

17.6.1 Summary

The organs of our organism work together for complex functions and organize themselves into systems. The adipose organ mainly collaborates with those of digestion. Both produce hormones that influence the brain with regard to nutrition, and both produce different molecules that mutually influence alternative organ activities. The organs of digestion also produce postprandial thermogenesis, and thermogenesis is one of the mechanisms involved in the regulation of food intake [26–29]. The intestine absorbs nutrients, which are then distributed to the adipose organ, which stores them in the form of triglycerides, to be made available to the body between meals.

In conclusion, it can be stated that in addition to the various systems that allow complex functional activities such as the nervous, endocrine, immune, urogenital, cardiovascular, and respiratory systems, we can now also speak of a true nutritional system [30] (Fig. 17.4).

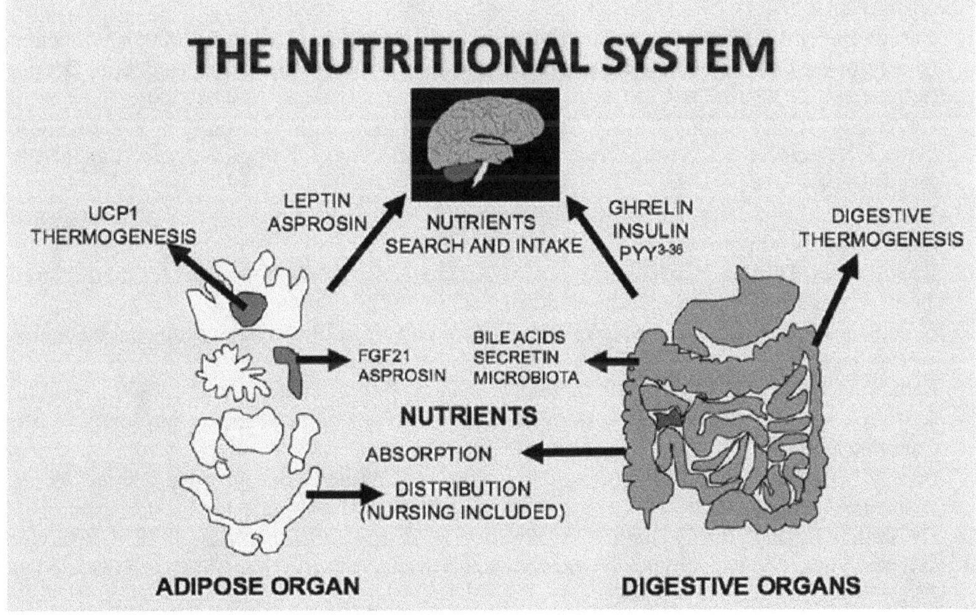

Fig. 17.4 Scheme of the nutritional system concept

Take-Home Points

- The white and brown adipose tissues are organized to form a true organ.
- This organ plays a pivotal role in the complex physiology that regulates the most important behaviors for the survival of mammals.

References

1. Zhang Y, Proenca R, Maffei M, Barone M, Leopold L, Friedman JM (1994) Positional cloning of the mouse obese gene and its human homologue. Nature 372(6505):425–432
2. De Matteis R, Cinti S (1998) Ultrastructural immunolocalization of leptin receptor in mouse brain. Neuroendocrinology 68(6):412–419
3. Farooqi IS, O'Rahilly S (2014) 20 years of leptin: human disorders of leptin action. J Endocrinol 223(1):T63–T70
4. Maffei M, Halaas J, Ravussin E, Pratley RE, Lee GH, Zhang Y, Fei H, Kim S, Lallone R, Ranganathan S et al (1995) Leptin levels in human and rodent: measurement of plasma leptin and ob RNA in obese and weight-reduced subjects. Nat Med 1(11):1155–1161
5. Prins JB, O'Rahilly S (1997) Regulation of adipose cell number in man. Clin Sci (Lond) 92(1):3–11
6. Cinti S (2018) Adipose organ development and remodeling. Compr Physiol 8(4):1357–1431
7. Romere C, Duerrschmid C, Bournat J, Constable P, Jain M, Xia F et al (2016) Asprosin, a fasting-induced glucogenic protein hormone. Cell 165(3):566–579
8. Duerrschmid C, He Y, Wang C, Li C, Bournat JC, Romere C et al (2017) Asprosin is a centrally acting orexigenic hormone. Nat Med 23(12):1444–1453
9. Cannon B, Nedergaard J (2004) Brown adipose tissue: function and physiological significance. Physiol Rev 84(1):277–359
10. Murano I, Barbatelli G, Giordano A, Cinti S (2009) Noradrenergic parenchymal nerve fiber branching after cold acclimatisation correlates with brown adipocyte density in mouse adipose organ. J Anat 214(1):171–178
11. Himms-Hagen J, Melnyk A, Zingaretti MC, Ceresi E, Barbatelli G, Cinti S (2000) Multilocular fat cells in WAT of CL-316243-treated rats derive directly from white adipocytes. Am J Physiol Cell Physiol 279(3):C670–C681
12. Granneman JG, Li P, Zhu Z, Lu Y (2005) Metabolic and cellular plasticity in white adipose tissue I: effects of beta3-adrenergic receptor activation. Am J Physiol Endocrinol Metab 289(4):E608–E616
13. Rosenwald M, Perdikari A, Rülicke T, Wolfrum C (2013) Bi-directional interconversion of brite and white adipocytes. Nat Cell Biol 15(6):659–667
14. Bachman ES, Dhillon H, Zhang CY et al (2002) betaAR signaling required for diet-induced thermogenesis and obesity resistance. Science 297(5582):843–845
15. Nedergaard J, Bengtsson T, Cannon B (2011) New powers of brown fat: fighting the metabolic syndrome. Cell Metab 13:238–240
16. Berbée JF, Boon MR, Khedoe PP, Bartelt A, Schlein C, Worthmann A et al (2015) Brown fat activation reduces hypercholesterolaemia and protects from atherosclerosis development. Nat Commun 6:6356
17. Betz MJ, Enerbäck S (2015) Human Brown adipose tissue: what we have learned so far. Diabetes 64(7):2352–2360
18. De Matteis R, Lucertini F, Guescini M, Polidori E, Zeppa S, Stocchi V et al (2013) Exercise as a new physiological stimulus for brown adipose tissue activity. Nutr Metab Cardiovasc Dis 23(6):582–590
19. Boström P, Wu J, Jedrychowski MP, Korde A, Ye L, Lo JC et al (2012) A PGC1-α-dependent myokine that drives brown-fat-like development of white fat and thermogenesis. Nature 481(7382):463–468

20. Colaianni G, Mongelli T, Cuscito C, Pignataro P, Lippo L, Spiro G et al (2017) Irisin prevents and restores bone loss and muscle atrophy in hind-limb suspended mice. Sci Rep 7(1):2811
21. Cinti S (2018) Pink adipocytes. Trends Endocrinol Metab 9(9):651–666
22. Weisberg SP, McCann D, Desai M, Rosenbaum M, Leibel RL, Ferrante AW Jr (2003) Obesity is associated with macrophage accumulation in adipose tissue. J Clin Invest 112(12):1796–1808
23. Xu H, Barnes GT, Yang Q, Tan G, Yang D, Chou CJ, Sole J, Nichols A, Ross JS, Tartaglia LA, Chen H (2003) Chronic inflammation in fat plays a crucial role in the development of obesity-related insulin resistance. J Clin Invest 112(12):1821–1830
24. Kotzbeck P, Giordano A, Mondini E, Murano I, Severi I, Venema W et al (2018) Brown adipose tissue whitening leads to brown adipocyte death and adipose tissue inflammation. J Lipid Res 59(5):784–794
25. Giannulis I, Mondini E, Cinti F, Frontini A, Murano I, Barazzoni R et al (2014) Increased density of inhibitory noradrenergic parenchymal nerve fibers in hypertrophic islets of Langerhans of obese mice. Nutr Metab Cardiovasc Dis 24(4):384–392
26. Villarroya F, Cereijo R, Villarroya J, Giralt M (2017) Brown adipose tissue as a secretory organ. Nat Rev Endocrinol 13(1):26–35
27. Li Y, Schnabl K, Gabler SM, Willershäuser M, Reber J, Karlas A et al (2018) Secretin-activated brown fat mediates prandial thermogenesis to induce satiation. Cell 175(6):1561–1574.e12
28. Chevalier C, Stojanović O, Colin DJ, Suarez-Zamorano N, Tarallo V, Veyrat-Durebex C et al (2015) Gut microbiota orchestrates energy homeostasis during cold. Cell 163(6):1360–1374
29. Himms-Hagen J (2006) Thermoregulatory feeding in newborn infants: an update. Obesity (Silver Spring) 14(9):1479–1480
30. Cinti S (2019) Anatomy and physiology of the nutritional system. Mol Asp Med 68:101–107

18

Dysphagia in Older Adults

Lina Spirgienė, Rebecca Lindhe and Gytė Damulevičienė

Abstract

Dysphagia in older adults can have a profound adverse influence nutrition and hydration status, quality of life, morbidity, mortality and healthcare costs in adults. Identification and management of dysphagia in older adults are most effective when implemented by a team, including a nurse, physician, speech-language pathologist, dietitian and occupational therapist. However, each professional's role may vary according to the standards, responsibilities and resources available in local settings.

Keywords

Dysphagia · Malnutrition · Aspiration · Deglutition disorder · Oropharyngeal

---

This chapter is a component of Part II: Special Topic in Geriatric Nutrition.
For an explanation of the grouping of chapters in this book, please see Chap. 1: "Geriatrics and Orthogeriatrics: Providing Nutrition Care".

L. Spirgienė (✉)
Faculty of Nursing, Department of Nursing and Care, Medical Academy, Lithuanian University of Health Sciences, Kaunas, Lithuania
e-mail: lina.spirgiene@lsmuni.lt

R. Lindhe
The Prince Charles Hospital, Brisbane, QLD, Australia
e-mail: Rebecca.Lindhe@health.qld.gov.au

G. Damulevičienė
Department of Geriatrics, Lithuanian University of Health Sciences, Kaunas, Lithuania
e-mail: gyte.damuleviciene@lsmuni.lt

Learning Outcomes
At the end of the chapter, and following further study, the reader will be able to:

- Describe oropharyngeal dysphagia symptoms and identify processes to identify older adults with or at risk of oropharyngeal dysphagia.
- Understand causes of dysphagia and the implications of dysphagia for older adults and the systems that care for them.
- Explain screening, clinical and instrumental assessment of oropharyngeal dysphagia.
- Consider interdisciplinary interventional opportunities for patients with or at risk of dysphagia with reference to local standards, responsibilities and resources.

18.1 Oropharyngeal Dysphagia: Prevalence and Consequences

Swallowing is a rapid, complex physiologic process that requires the precise, sequential coordination of both volitional and reflexive movements of more than 30 nerves and muscles within the oral cavity, pharynx, larynx and oesophagus. Normal oropharyngeal swallowing requires a coordinated voluntary transfer of food from the mouth into the pharynx, followed by rapid transfer of the bolus into the upper oesophagus. Dysphagia is the medical term for difficulty or inability to swallow and is classified as a digestive condition by the International Classification of Diseases (ICD) ICD-10 [1, 2]. Experts of the Dysphagia Working Group recently recognised dysphagia as a "geriatric syndrome", defined by the difficulty to effectively and safely move the alimentary bolus from the mouth to the oesophagus. Anatomically, dysphagia may arise from an oropharyngeal or oesophageal impairment and from a physiological standpoint either a functional or structural cause [3]. The focus of this chapter is oropharyngeal dysphagia.

Patients experiencing dysphagia may demonstrate one or more signs including but not limited to difficulty sucking, chewing or initiating swallowing and managing saliva, taking medication or protecting the airway coughing. They may report coughing during eating or drinking, food or medication sticking in the throat, voice changes, dyspnoea, nasal regurgitation, unintentional weight loss or a change in eating habits. The complications arising from oropharyngeal dysphagia are dependent on the severity and may range from mild to moderate difficulty to complete inability to swallow [1, 4–6].

Dysphagia is associated with major nutritional and respiratory complications, particularly in older patients, resulting in multiple negative health consequences, most commonly increased risk of malnutrition and dehydration, frailty, asphyxiation, aspiration-related pneumonias and death. Depression, social isolation and poorer health-related quality of life are other established implications [1, 6–11]. Dysphagia is a growing geriatric syndrome of increasing frequency, impacting on morbidity, mortality and costs associated with hospital length of stay [11–13]. In many hospitals, an overt discrepancy exists between these factors and the associated nutritional and respiratory complications of oropharyngeal dysphagia and the limited availability of both human and material resources available to patients with dysphagia [1, 8].

The prevalence of oropharyngeal dysphagia in older persons is variable across different settings. Studies demonstrate between 30 and 40% in independently living older people, 44% in those admitted to geriatric acute care and 60% of institutionalised older patients are dysphagic [4, 6, 8, 14, 15]. Oropharyngeal dysphagia has been shown to be more prevalent in older adult with reduced mobility, functional capacity or cognitive status, frailty, polypharmacy and multimorbidity [16]. Increasing age is associated with increased risk of oropharyngeal dysphagia which can be attributed to multiple factors including age-related changes in head and neck anatomy, changes in neural and physiologic mechanisms that control swallowing (e.g. loss of muscle mass and function, decreased tissue elasticity, decreased saliva production and cervical spine changes) and increasing disease acquisition that may have dysphagia as a symptom or side effect. These changes can slow deglutition and negatively impact the effective and efficient flow of swallowed materials [8, 10, 16].

18.2 Causes of Oropharyngeal Dysphagia

Commonly reported causes of oropharyngeal dysphagia are diseases of nervous system, neurodegenerative diseases, muscular/neuromuscular diseases and local or structural lesions in head or neck or oesophageal area [17].

Stroke. The incidence of dysphagia after stroke with figures ranges from 23 to 65% [6, 18]. Although up to half of acute stroke patients will have dysphagia, most will have recovered a functional swallow spontaneously by 1 month. Dysphagia after stroke carries a threefold increased mortality risk and a sixfold to sevenfold fold increased risk of aspiration pneumonia. Dysphagia screening should occur for every patient presenting with symptoms of a stroke.

Head and neck cancers. Whilst considering the site of lesion, severity and treatment type, oropharyngeal dysphagia presents as a common consequence in approximately 50% of head and neck cancer patients [8].

Dementia. Oropharyngeal dysphagia is a frequent condition in patients with dementia of various types, including in early stages. It is estimated that up to 45% of patients institutionalised who have dementia will have some degree of dysphagia, with symptoms varying and dependent on the clinical presentation and type of dementia. Patients will often demonstrate a slowing of the swallowing process, which results in increased time taken to complete meals, placing the patient at increased risk of malnutrition and dehydration. Patients may demonstrate poor initiation, distractibility, impulsivity and sensory changes that may result in oral holding, overchewing and texture or temperature aversion. These characteristics together with a change in a patient's ability to self-feed, loss of appetite, food avoidance and wandering can be attributed to increasing cognitive impairment and are risk factors for poor nutritional status, subsequently increasing the susceptibility to pneumonia in this patient population [19, 20].

Parkinson's disease. Oropharyngeal dysphagia is a common symptom in patients with neurological diseases. In particular, in neurodegenerative conditions such as Parkinson's disease and related disorders, the prevalence of dysphagia increases rapidly as the disease progresses [21]. However, the early detection of swallowing problems is not always easy because dysphagia may be asymptomatic, and the self-awareness of patients is poor [8, 21].

Medication. An often-overlooked cause of dysphagia is the patient's medication. Several categories of drugs have been associated with oropharyngeal dysphagia; this is commonly referred to as drug-induced dysphagia. Major mechanisms have been identified as (1) dysphagia as a side effect of the drug, (2) dysphagia as a complication of the drug's therapeutic action and (3) medication-induced oesophageal injury. Several types of drugs have been found to cause dysphagia. Drugs that cause xerostomia (dry mouth) include anticholinergics (e.g. atropine, trihexyphenidyl, ipratropium), angiotensin-converting enzyme (ACE) inhibitors, antiarrhythmics, antihistamines and neuroleptic medications (e.g. clozapine, quetiapine, risperidone). Dysphagia-causing drugs also include gabapentin, valproic acid, diazepam, codeine as well as drugs associated with medication-induced oesophageal injury (e.g. ibuprofen, vitamin C, erythromycin) [10, 22]. For further reading about drug interactions, see Chap. 20.

18.3 Screening and Diagnosis of Oropharyngeal Dysphagia

Screening and assessment of swallowing are different procedures and are usually conducted at different times by different health professionals. Swallowing screening has been previously defined as a minimally invasive evaluation that rapidly examines the following: (1) the likelihood of dysphagia, (2) the requirement for further swallowing assessment, (3) the safety of patient oral intake and (4) the requirement for alternative nutritional support. Whereas a swallowing assessment would usually include a case history (related to swallowing problems), an in-depth examination of oral, pharyngeal and laryngeal anatomy; sensory and motor function and behavioural, cognitive and language abilities; and an oral/feeding trial if appropriate [11, 12].

18.3.1 Screening

Clinical screening for oropharyngeal dysphagia should be quick, low risk and low cost and aim at identifying the highest-risk patients who require further assessment [1]. There are multiple screening tools that have been developed and researched within specific patient population groups. Strong supporting evidence across general geriatric cohorts for any single tool is lacking; which screening tool local teams choose to administer will depend on, for example, disease-specific recommendations (e.g. stroke versus dementia), national or international guidelines and/or local practice policies/procedures and/or protocols.

It is beyond the remit of this chapter to critique or recommend which tools are appropriate to apply. We consequently recommend local teams work with patients to identify and co-design dysphagia screening processes that apply tools that are both valid and feasible to implement in their specific settings and populations. Without being prescriptive, we note that the EAT-10 is a self-reported questionnaire and quick, easy screening method, validated to identify individuals at risk for dysphagia (https://www.nestlenutrition-institute.org/resources/nutrition-tools/details/swallowing-assessment-tool) [23]. Similarly, the Yale Swallow Protocol [24] is an another evidence-based protocol that identifies aspiration risk that local teams may wish to consider. This tool supports recommendation of specific oral diets without the need for further instrumental evaluation; it is easily administered, reliable and validated for use in a variety of environments, including acute care, rehabilitation and nursing homes [24, 25].

18.3.2 Assessment

The aim of clinical assessment is to evaluate the safety and efficacy of swallowing and detect aspirations at the bedside. Clinical assessment should be performed by specialists and regularly repeated according to progression of the disease.

18.3.3 Oropharyngeal Dysphagia Diagnosis

In many clinical settings, a bedside diagnosis may be informed by a clinician qualified to make a diagnosis using a clinical swallowing examination (CSE), for example, speech-language pathologists or medical officers; there are a variety of different CSE approaches applied across global settings, and again these should be governed by local clinical processes [26–28].

An instrumental examination may be indicated to confirm the diagnosis and/or plan treatment for patients suspected of having dysphagia following clinical observation/examination. Videofluoroscopy swallowing study (VFSS) and fibre-optic endoscopic evaluation of swallowing (FEES) are two types of instrumental assessments used to evaluate the safety and efficacy of deglutition. These methods are considered the "gold standard" for diagnosis of oropharyngeal dysphagia and are useful in determining the effectiveness of compensatory strategies and/or the type of rehabilitation therapy [1, 4, 10, 26].

18.4 Interventions for Oropharyngeal Dysphagia

No single strategy is appropriate for all older adults with oropharyngeal dysphagia. The unified goal is to treat the underlying pathology when possible and manage symptoms effectively while meeting nutritional needs. This can be achieved through interdisciplinary management that considers (1) maintaining adequate nutrition, hydration and diet choices, (2) dietary modifications and (3) maximising oral hygiene and oral health. Where appropriately trained specialists are available, for example, SLPs or medical staff, compensatory strategies and rehabilitative techniques and manoeuvres should also be considered. The following information is provided for educational purposes; interventions for oropharyngeal dysphagia should be guided by patient population and setting specific guidelines that ideally have been co-designed and endorsed by teams consisting of older adults, speech and language pathologists and medical, nursing and other healthcare professionals.

18.5 Maximising Adequate Nutrition, Hydration and Diet Choices

For patients with or at risk of oropharyngeal dysphagia, it is essential that any required changes are considered both in line with existing evidence and the patient's preferences and wishes. Due to the increased risk of malnutrition and dehydration in older patients with dysphagia, screening for malnutrition and nutritional status (including hydration) should be assessed among all patients with dysphagia [29]. If malnutrition is present, an individualised nutritional program should be developed, balancing the importance of eating, in relation to quality of life, as this will differ between patients. This may be complicated for patients with diagnosed cognitive impairment, who lack capacity for informed healthcare decisions [11].

If the patient's swallowing safety and efficiency cannot reach a level of adequate function or if swallow function does not support nutrition and hydration adequately, the treating team may recommend alternative nutritional and/or fluid support (Chap. 5).

18.6 Dietary Modifications

Texture modification has become one of the most common forms of intervention for dysphagia and is widely considered important for promoting safe and efficient swallowing [11]. The goal of diet modification is to improve the safety and/or ease of oral consumption and therefore maintain safe and adequate oral intake of food and liquids [30]. Modifying the consistency of foods and liquids is a common compensatory strategy utilised for patients with dysphagia [6]. However, health professionals should be cautious that as the diet and liquids are modified, decreased acceptability by the patient may result from the altered taste, texture and appearance. These changes in solid and liquid consistencies may lead to decreased adherence to recommendations and increased risk of malnutrition and/or dehydration [31]. Many studies have highlighted a lower caloric intake resulting from modified diets [11].

A newer system of food and liquid classification has been derived from the International Dysphagia Diet Standardisation Initiative (IDDSI). It is a global standardised method of describing dysphagia diets that ranges from level 0 to level 7

[11]. Whilst these are considerate of recent evidence, again given the contextual diversities globally, we recommend local teams work with patients to establish or review locally applied dietary modification recommendations, definitions, systems and processes.

18.7 Oral Hygiene and Health

Although this is not the focus of this chapter, it is worth noting that particular attention should be given to oral hygiene and oral health for patients with or at risk of dysphagia.

The first deglutition phase—the oral stage of swallowing (chewing, bolus formation and propulsion process)—depends on a good mouth status; poor mouth hygiene, edentulism and improper prothesis are some of the risk factors for malnutrition among older adults [5]. The physiology of the oral cavity changes with age, and older adults often experience issues such as the loss of teeth, reduced saliva (dry mouth) and a reduction in muscle and connective tissue elasticity. Poor oral hygiene and dentition, lack of teeth and ill-fitting dentures can induce pain and discomfort and are red flags for possible undiagnosed oropharyngeal dysphagia. As a result, eating takes longer, and patients fatigue more quickly and may self-modify their diets to compensate, increasing the risk of malnutrition. Maintaining good oral cares has proved paramount in reducing the occurrences of aspiration-related pneumonia [11].

18.7.1 Swallowing Strategies and Manoeuvres

Changes in body and/or head posture may be recommended as one type of compensatory technique with the aim to reduce aspiration or residue. These changes may impact on the speed and flow direction of a food or liquid bolus, often with the intent of protecting the airway to improve swallow safety.

Similarly, swallow manoeuvres are designed to modify the normal swallow and as a result improve the safety or efficiency of swallow function. Numerous swallow manoeuvres have been recommended to address different physiologic swallowing deficits. While swallow manoeuvres can be used as a short-term compensatory strategy, many have also been used as swallow rehabilitative techniques. Various manoeuvres are aimed at addressing different aspects of the impaired swallow. For example, the supraglottic and super supraglottic swallow techniques both incorporate a voluntary breath hold and related laryngeal closure to protect the airway during swallowing. It is important to note that patients experiencing cognitive impairment may have difficulty implementing swallowing strategies or manoeuvres [11].

Swallowing strategies and/or manoeuvres should always be individually prescribed by an SLP, swallow therapist or appropriately trained medical officer, after a thorough individualised assessment has been completed [6].

Table 18.1 Potential opportunities for interdisciplinary management of dysphagia [4, 30]

• Interdisciplinary screening using locally approved, validated screening tools (e.g. EAT-10, Yale Swallow Protocol or other tools that are feasible and valid for the population/setting)
• Referral for specialist assessment and intervention where appropriate and re-referral where repeat screening or clinical judgement indicates need for review
• Educate and engage patients and caregivers regarding the rationale for dysphagia management strategies, strategies for food and fluid modification and self-monitoring processes for dysphagia, malnutrition and dehydration
• Support and assist mealtimes
• Ensure positioning of patient and swallowing manoeuvres align with locally endorsed safe swallowing recommendations and individualised advice where prescribed
• Wherever possible and appropriate, encourage patients to sit upright or out of bed for meals
• Avoid eating or drinking when drowsy, rushed or fatigued
• Encourage and assist small amounts of food or liquids into the mouth at a time
• Eat slowly with intent to implement control of bolus flow
• Concentrate only on swallowing and eliminate distractions
• Alternate liquids (of appropriate thickness) and solids to clear oral and pharyngeal residue
• Place the food on the stronger side of the mouth if there is unilateral weakness
• Use sauces, condiments and gravies (of appropriate thickness) to facilitate cohesive bolus formation
• Avoid mixing food and liquids in the same mouthful
• Provide appropriate cutlery and utensils

18.7.2 Opportunities for Interdisciplinary Management of Dysphagia

Whilst there is no specific "one-size-fits-all" strategy that is applicable to all older patients with oropharyngeal dysphagia, there are some generic strategies that are often appropriate for interdisciplinary team members to apply to assist with dysphagia identification and management, as shown in Table 18.1 [32]. These are provided for educational purposes; local treating teams should ensure appropriate processes are embedded to support adequate nutritional and fluid intake for older adults with or at risk of dysphagia.

18.7.3 Summary

Oropharyngeal dysphagia adversely influences the nutritional intake, hydration, morbidity, mortality and quality of life in many older adults globally. There is no single management strategy for managing older adults with dysphagia; an interdisciplinary approach is fundamental to define diagnosis and treatment [33]. Locally relevant evidence-based procedures and guidelines must be in place to support interdisciplinary teams to work together with older adults to improve the safety and/or ease of oral consumption and thus maintain safe and adequate oral intake of food and liquids. We also encourage teams to balance management strategies with the need to promote adequate nutritional intake, overall patient health and quality of life, through shared decision-making and informed consent.

Take-Home Points

- Dysphagia is common in older adults across community, inpatient and aged care home settings with associated adverse outcomes.
- There are diverse causes of dysphagia; screening is able to be performed by diverse healthcare providers; however, diagnosis requires specialist consultation.
- There are many opportunities for interdisciplinary healthcare providers to monitor and support nutritional and fluid intake of patients with dysphagia; these should be undertaken in line with locally endorsed evidence-based procedures and processes.

References

1. Jukes S, Cichero JA, Haines T, Wilson C, Paul K, O'Rourke M (2012) Evaluation of the uptake of the Australian standardized terminology and definitions for texture modified foods and fluids. Int J Speech Lang Pathol 14(3):214–225
2. Tagliaferri S, Lauretani F, Pelá G, Meschi T, Maggio M (2019) The risk of dysphagia is associated with malnutrition and poor functional outcomes in a large population of outpatient older individuals. Clin Nutr 38(6):2684–2689
3. Rofes L, Arreola V, Almirall J, Cabré M, Campins L, García-Peris P et al (2011) Diagnosis and management of oropharyngeal dysphagia and its nutritional and respiratory complications in the elderly. Gastroenterol Res Pract 2011:818979
4. Wirth R, Dziewas R, Beck AM, Clavé P, Hamdy S, Heppner HJ et al (2016) Oropharyngeal dysphagia in older persons - from pathophysiology to adequate intervention: a review and summary of an international expert meeting. Clin Interv Aging 11:189–208
5. Ott AVN, Damulevičienė G, Kasiukiewicz A, Tsiantouli E (2017) Oral health and dysphagia in the older population. Eur Geriatr Med 8(2):191–195
6. Sura L, Madhavan A, Carnaby G, Crary MA (2012) Dysphagia in the elderly: management and nutritional considerations. Clin Interv Aging 7:287–298
7. Madhavan A, LaGorio LA, Crary MA, Dahl WJ, Carnaby GD (2016) Prevalence of and risk factors for dysphagia in the community dwelling elderly: a systematic review. J Nutr Health Aging 20(8):806–815
8. Jones E, Speyer R, Kertscher B, Denman D, Swan K, Cordier R (2018) Health-related quality of life and oropharyngeal dysphagia: a systematic review. Dysphagia 33(2):141–172
9. Shaw SM, Martino R (2013) The normal swallow: muscular and neurophysiological control. Otolaryngol Clin N Am 46(6):937–956
10. Nawaz S, Tulunay-Ugur OE (2018) Dysphagia in the older patient. Otolaryngol Clin N Am 51(4):769–777
11. Thiyagalingam S, Kulinski AE, Thorsteinsdottir B, Shindelar KL, Takahashi PY (2021) Dysphagia in older adults. Mayo Clin Proc 96(2):488–497
12. Jiang JL, Fu SY, Wang WH, Ma YC (2016) Validity and reliability of swallowing screening tools used by nurses for dysphagia: a systematic review. Ci Ji Yi Xue Za Zhi 28(2):41–48
13. Etges CL, Scheeren B, Gomes E, Barbosa LDR (2014) Screening tools for dysphagia: a systematic review. CoDAS 26:343–349
14. Lin LC, Wu SC, Chen HS, Wang TG, Chen MY (2002) Prevalence of impaired swallowing in institutionalized older people in Taiwan. J Am Geriatr Soc 50(6):1118–1123

15. Clavé P, Rofes L, Carrión S, Ortega O, Cabré M, Serra-Prat M et al (2012) Pathophysiology, relevance and natural history of oropharyngeal dysphagia among older people. Nestle Nutr Inst Workshop Ser 72:57–66
16. Carrión S, Cabré M, Monteis R, Roca M, Palomera E, Serra-Prat M et al (2015) Oropharyngeal dysphagia is a prevalent risk factor for malnutrition in a cohort of older patients admitted with an acute disease to a general hospital. Clin Nutr 34(3):436–442
17. Shaker R, Kern M, Bardan E, Taylor A, Stewart ET, Hoffmann RG et al (1997) Augmentation of deglutitive upper esophageal sphincter opening in the elderly by exercise. Am J Phys 272(6 Pt 1):G1518–G1522
18. Daniels SK, Brailey K, Foundas AL (1999) Lingual discoordination and dysphagia following acute stroke: analyses of lesion localization. Dysphagia 14(2):85–92
19. Forouzanfar MH, Alexander L, Anderson HR, Bachman VF, Biryukov S, Brauer M et al (2015) Global, regional, and national comparative risk assessment of 79 behavioural, environmental and occupational, and metabolic risks or clusters of risks in 188 countries, 1990-2013: a systematic analysis for the Global Burden of Disease Study 2013. Lancet 386(10010):2287–2323
20. Ortega OCM, Clavé P (2014) Oropharyngeal dysphagia: aetiology & effects of ageing. J Gastroenterol Hepatol Res 3(5):1049–1054
21. Kwon M, Lee JH (2019) Oro-pharyngeal dysphagia in Parkinson's disease and related movement disorders. J Mov Disord 12(3):152–160
22. Al-Shehri A (2001) Dysphagia as a drug side effect. Int J Otolaryngol 1(2)
23. Belafsky PC, Mouadeb DA, Rees CJ, Pryor JC, Postma GN, Allen J et al (2008) Validity and reliability of the eating assessment tool (EAT-10). Ann Otol Rhinol Laryngol 117(12):919–924
24. Ward M, Skelley-Ashford M, Brown K, Ashford J, Suiter D (2020) Validation of the Yale swallow protocol in post-acute care: a prospective, double-blind, multirater study. Am J Speech Lang Pathol 29(4):1937–1943
25. Suiter DM, Sloggy J, Leder SB (2014) Validation of the Yale swallow protocol: a prospective double-blinded videofluoroscopic study. Dysphagia 29(2):199–203
26. Satoshi Horiguchi YS (2011) Screening tests in evaluating swallowing function. JMAJ 54(1):31–34
27. Ohkuma R, Fujishima I, Kojima C, Hojo K, Takehara I, Motohashi Y (2002) Development of a questionnaire to screen dysphagia. Jpn J Dysphagia Rehabil 6(1):3–8
28. Kawashima K, Motohashi Y, Fujishima I (2004) Prevalence of dysphagia among community-dwelling elderly individuals as estimated using a questionnaire for dysphagia screening. Dysphagia 19(4):266–271
29. Volkert D, Beck AM, Cederholm T, Cruz-Jentoft A, Goisser S, Hooper L et al (2019) ESPEN guideline on clinical nutrition and hydration in geriatrics. Clin Nutr 38(1):10–47
30. Steele CM, Alsanei WA, Ayanikalath S, Barbon CE, Chen J, Cichero JA et al (2015) The influence of food texture and liquid consistency modification on swallowing physiology and function: a systematic review. Dysphagia 30(1):2–26
31. Reber E, Gomes F, Dähn IA, Vasiloglou MF, Stanga Z (2019) Management of dehydration in patients suffering swallowing difficulties. J Clin Med 8(11):1923
32. Ney DM, Weiss JM, Kind AJ, Robbins J (2009) Senescent swallowing: impact, strategies, and interventions. Nutr Clin Pract 24(3):395–413
33. de Sordi M, Figueiredo Mourão L, Armando da Silva A, LCL F (2009) Interdisciplinary evaluation of dysphagia: clinical swallowing evaluation and videoendoscopy of swallowing. Braz J Otorhinolaryngol 75(6):776–787

19

Hospitalized Older People, Nutrition and Delirium

Alison Mudge, Adrienne Young, Margaret Cahill, Elise Treleaven and Lina Spirgienė

This chapter is a component of Part II: Specialist Versus Generalist Nutritional Care in Aging. For an explanation of the grouping of chapters in this book, please see Chap. 1: "Geriatrics and Orthogeriatrics: Providing Nutrition Care".

A. Mudge (✉)
Eat Walk Engage Program, Internal Medicine and Aged Care, Royal Brisbane and Women's Hospital, Herston, QLD, Australia

University of Queensland School of Clinical Medicine, Royal Brisbane and Women's Hospital, Herston, QLD, Australia
e-mail: Alison.Mudge@health.qld.gov.au

A. Young
Department of Nutrition and Dietetics, Royal Brisbane and Women's Hospital, Herston, QLD, Australia
e-mail: Adrienne.Young@health.qld.gov.au

M. Cahill
Eat Walk Engage Program, Royal Brisbane and Women's Hospital, Herston, QLD, Australia
e-mail: Margaret.cahill@health.qld.gov.au

E. Treleaven
Eat Walk Engage Program, Internal Medicine and Aged Care, Royal Brisbane and Women's Hospital, Herston, QLD, Australia

Department of Nutrition and Dietetics, Royal Brisbane and Women's Hospital, Herston, QLD, Australia
e-mail: Elise.Treleaven@health.qld.gov.au

L. Spirgienė
Faculty of Nursing, Department of Nursing and Care, Medical Academy, Lithuanian University of Health Sciences, Kaunas, Lithuania
e-mail: lina.spirgiene@lsmuni.lt

Abstract

Delirium is a common and serious complication in hospitalised older people. Poor nutrition and hydration are both risk factors for, and consequences of, delirium. This chapter will discuss the phenomenology of delirium and the role of nurses in recognising, preventing and managing this serious complication. It will also provide practical strategies to support nutrition and hydration in patients with, or at risk of, delirium.

Keywords

Delirium · Cognitive impairment · Prevention of delirium · Malnutrition · Mealtime care

Learning Outcomes

At the end of the chapter, and following further study, you will be able to:

- Describe the experience and consequences of delirium.
- Recognise common risk factors for delirium.
- Recognise how adequate nutrition and hydration can assist delirium prevention.
- Implement strategies to improve nutrition and enable mealtime care in patients with, or at risk of, delirium.

19.1 What Is Delirium?

Delirium is a distressing and serious acute neuropsychiatric syndrome which can complicate acute illness, surgery or injury. Delirium is common, affecting 8–17% older emergency department patients, 18–35% of older medical inpatients and 11–51% older surgical inpatients, up to 82% of intensive care patients and up to 75% patients at the end of life [1, 2]. The core diagnostic features are inattention and disturbance of consciousness, with an acute change in cognition (e.g. memory, orientation, language, reasoning or perceptions) due to a medical condition, medication and/or intoxicating substance [3]. Examples of these features and how they can be assessed are provided in Table 19.1. Structured tools to assess these features (e.g. the "4 A's test" [4] or the Confusion Assessment Method [5]) improve recognition of delirium. This is important because delirium is frequently missed by clinical staff, as presenting symptoms can be subtle and variable [6].

Delirium often results in difficulties in understanding information provided and can include disturbing misperceptions and hallucinations. These experiences can result in fear and distress for the patient [7], which may be difficult to communicate due to language impairments. These features can lead to behaviours such as poor cooperation with instructions, agitation and aggression, which are characteristic of "hyperactive" delirium. This is understandably distressing to staff and

Table 19.1 Assessing clinical features of delirium

Disturbance of consciousness and inattention (observe during assessment)	Are they drowsy or hypervigilant? Do they have trouble following your questions or become easily distracted? Simple attention tests include the "months of the year backwards"
Change in cognition (use brief cognitive screening)	Disorientation: Do they know the day, time and place? Memory: Do they have trouble recalling recent events? Language: Are their answers very sparse, or do their ideas keep wandering off? Perceptions: Do they seem distracted by sounds or sights that you cannot see or hear?
Acute fluctuating course (take a collateral history)	Have people familiar with the patient (e.g. family members, general practitioner, nursing home staff or community services) noticed a recent change in thinking or behaviour?
Evidence of underlying medical condition, medications or intoxicant	Thorough history, examination and investigations targeting precipitating factors (see Table 19.2)

family trying to provide care and can result in the use of restraint or sedation, which carry risks of serious iatrogenic harm [8]. Delirium can also lead to apathy, disorientation, daytime somnolence and motor slowing ("hypoactive" delirium), which is commonly missed, increasing the risk of pressure injury, deconditioning, venous thromboembolism, aspiration pneumonia and other immobility-associated harm. Many patients fluctuate between hypoactive and hyperactive presentations. Both hypoactive and hyperactive delirium increase mortality by 2–3 times, increase the need for services after hospital discharge and are associated with increased future risk of dementia [9].

19.2 Who Is at Risk?

Douglas is a 77-year-old man admitted to your unit with a urinary tract infection and abdominal pain due to urinary retention. He has a range of medical conditions including depression, hypertension, diabetes and chronic kidney disease and is on eight medications. Douglas wears glasses to correct his poor vision and has bilateral hearing aids. His daughter mentions that Douglas has recently been having trouble with his memory and needs help with shopping and preparing meals and he became very confused when he was in hospital a few months ago. During your assessment, you identify that Douglas has recently lost weight without trying and has been eating and drinking less than usual. He also reports being more weak and tired than usual.

This case represents a typical older person presenting to hospital at risk of malnutrition (indicated by weight loss and reduced intake) and with a number of risk factors for developing delirium (Table 19.2) [1, 9–11]. These two conditions often go hand in hand. Both malnutrition and dehydration have been recognised as risk factors for developing delirium [12, 13], perhaps not surprisingly considering the high metabolic requirements of the brain and the need for reliable brain blood flow [14–16]. However, delirium also increases the risk of poor oral intake [17, 18], potentially creating a vicious circle [19]. Malnutrition should be screened at admission using a validated tool (e.g. malnutrition screening tool [MST] [20], nutrition risk screening [NRS 2002] [21], malnutrition universal screening tool [MUST] [22]) (Chap. 3). Screening should be repeated weekly, as the risk of developing malnutrition increases with longer hospital stays.

All hospital inpatients aged 65 and older, or with known cognitive impairment (e.g. dementia) or experiencing very serious illness or injury (including hip fracture and major operations), should be recognised as high risk for delirium [11, 23, 24]. They should receive routine screening using a validated delirium screening tool on admission to hospital and be rescreened whenever their condition or behaviour changes. If the screen is positive, a trained professional (e.g. doctor, nurse practitioner or occupational therapist) should assess them to formally confirm delirium, and their medical team must urgently investigate the underlying cause [23, 24] (Table 19.2).

Table 19.2 Delirium risk factors [1, 10]

Delirium is often multifactorial in its cause. Predisposing and precipitating factors for our case study are illustrated with an asterisk (*)
Predisposing factors • Age older than 65 years* • Cognitive impairment (e.g. dementia) or previous delirium* • Frailty and functional dependency* • Sensory impairment* • Comorbidities (e.g. chronic or end-stage heart, lung or kidney disease)* • Multiple medications* • Previous alcohol misuse
Precipitating factors • Dehydration* • Medications, especially sedatives (e.g. benzodiazepines, anticholinergics, antipsychotics) • Infection* • Malnutrition* • Pain* • Hypoxia • Metabolic disturbances (e.g. hyponatraemia, hypernatraemia, hypercalcaemia) • Any serious illness (e.g. myocardial infarction, hip fracture) or major operation
Perpetuating factors • Restraints (e.g. indwelling catheter, intravenous lines, oxygen therapy)* • Sleep deprivation • Poor food and fluid intake* • Disorientating environment (e.g. no clock or window, unfamiliar routines, frequent bed moves)

Nurses are ideally placed to identify risk of malnutrition and delirium, and screening for these conditions should be integrated into standard nursing assessment, care planning and mealtime processes. Including validated screening tools within admission paperwork and daily care planning templates may support routine screening [18]. It is important that other members of the care team (doctors, allied health professionals) are also trained to identify malnutrition, poor intake and changing cognition, to ensure the whole team remain vigilant and cooperate to institute appropriate prevention and management strategies [23].

19.3 What Can Be Done to Prevent and Manage Delirium?

Douglas scores 2 on the 4 A's test which indicates cognitive impairment (but not delirium), and he is identified at risk of malnutrition according to the MST. He appears dehydrated. The doctor starts antibiotics and fluids through the intravenous catheter, inserts an indwelling catheter to relieve his urinary retention and prescribes low-dose oral opiates for his abdominal pain. His daughter is worried he will become very confused like last time he was in hospital and asks if there is anything you can do to protect him.

There are no drugs demonstrated to either prevent or treat delirium [24–26]. Multicomponent multidisciplinary prevention programs can reduce delirium by 30–50% in hospital settings [27, 28]. These programs focus on optimising nutrition and hydration, mobility and engagement in meaningful activities [29], as well as managing pain, managing sleep disturbance and reducing or eliminating inappropriate medications [30]. Nurses have the key role in delivering these fundamental cares, but they are often missed in busy complex acute wards [31, 32]. Structured, systematic programs can support ward teams, such as the well-established Hospital Elder Life Program [33] to implement multidisciplinary strategies that support delirium prevention. These programs require some investment but appear to be cost-effective [34]. The same principles are important for safe and patient-centred management of patients who have developed delirium, although evidence that multicomponent intervention reduces the duration or severity of delirium is lacking. The keys to managing delirium are identifying and reversing all medical causes (Table 19.2) and providing good fundamental care. Unfortunately, nurses also need to be aware that treatments can sometimes also perpetuate the delirium (Table 19.2). For example, in our case study, the intravenous therapy and indwelling catheter are restraints which can be distressing and reduce mobility, while opiates relieve pain but can be sedating. Constant review for the need for continuing such therapies is essential.

Poor food and fluid intake are important precipitating and perpetuating factors for delirium (Table 19.2). Maintaining food and fluid intake is a central strategy within delirium prevention programs [19, 24]. However, this can be challenging in people with cognitive impairment [35] and/or severe illness (which are important delirium risk factors) and even more so in people with established delirium. Nurses should anticipate the assistance that patients with, or at risk of, delirium may require and factor these into their daily workflow planning (Table 19.3). Adequate mealtime preparation including the relief of pain and nausea, timely toileting and appropriate positioning may require coordinated assistance from other team members (e.g. medical staff, physiotherapist, patient support officer) in advance of meal delivery. Nurses need to be present on the ward during mealtimes, to provide encouragement, anticipate and instigate assistance and advocate for their patients by discouraging other team members from interrupting patients during their meals (except for urgent clinical interventions) [36]. Food and fluid intake should also be monitored and

Table 19.3 Optimising mealtime care for people with delirium

Maximise comfort	Take your patient to the toilet before the meal arrives Make sure dentures are in and well fitting Provide analgesia or anti-nausea medications before meals as required, and avoid sedative medications before meals Ensure adequate lighting and put spectacles on Position upright, ideally sitting in a chair, with a clutter-free meal space Provide water or suitable liquids to moisten foods, especially if the patient has dry mouth or trouble swallowing Create a pleasant environment (e.g. soft music)
Provide cues	Orientate your patient: "Good morning! It's a lovely spring day today. Here is your breakfast" Remove covers and wrappings to make it easy to see the meal and allow food aromas to stimulate appetite Some people may need verbal prompts or hands-on cues, e.g. cutlery placed in their hands, or prompts to reload their fork between mouthfuls Eating with someone else (family or other patients) can help as it provides social context and mirroring Families may be able to bring favourite food items in
Maintain focus	Minimise distractions (e.g. turn off the television) Minimise unnecessary interruptions during the meal It may help to serve one meal element at a time to reduce confusion (e.g. just put the main meal on the tray) Start with preferred and/or high-energy components for patients with fatigue or inattention even if that means ice cream first! Provide verbal encouragement, reassurance and verbal/physical prompts Talk about familiar topics
Maximise independence	Assist meal choices if needed (e.g. enquire about and document favourite foods where all team members can access the information) Adjust the height and position of the tray to optimise hand function, strength and reach Help set up if required, e.g. opening packets or containers and cutting foods into manageable pieces Order finger foods if the patient has trouble using cutlery Allow plenty of time for the patient to finish their meal Provide modified cutlery, plate guards and alternative cups (i.e. non-spill, those with handles or straws) where needed Provide straws where needed
Monitor intake	Take note of the amount eaten, the types of food preferred and the reasons for not eating and discuss with your clinical dietitian to try to tailor meals

documented at every meal to allow early identification of poor intake in this high-risk group, as malnutrition screening tools do not accurately identify patients with poor intake [37]. It is common for people with delirium to miss meals because they are asleep or too unsettled or disoriented to complete the task of eating. It is important that ward staff have access to a variety of food and drinks available outside of set mealtimes to ensure that patients can catch up on missed meals once they are awake and feeling more settled (Chaps. 3–5).

Mealtimes also have important social and existential meaning [38] and serve as an orientating stimulus to help with delirium prevention. However, inflexible routines, eating alone and unfamiliar foods may detract from this. Patients value familiar routines and networks of support and encouragement from their health team as well as from their families and other patients [39]. Making opportunities for shared dining experiences and inviting family presence at mealtimes can help to normalise the mealtime experience and may improve intake [40, 41]. Volunteers and healthcare assistants may also have a role in mealtime assistance and improving the mealtime experience [42–44].

You have been monitoring Douglas' food and fluid intake and have observed that he has been eating and drinking poorly for the past 3 days. In particular, you've noticed that he is hard to wake up for his meals, preferring to sleep through his meals. When he is eating, he has trouble feeding himself. When you help him with his meal, you notice that he is slow to chew and swallow and often falls asleep sitting in the chair. He has consumed less than one third of his meals and still requires intravenous therapy to maintain his fluid status. You report your concerns to the doctor, who examines Douglas and confirms that he has hypoactive delirium. The doctor stops the opiates and rechecks his kidney function and electrolytes. You wonder if nasogastric tube feeding would help his recovery.

19.4 The Role of Enteral Feeding

Considering that maintaining adequate nutrition and hydration plays such an important role in preventing and treating delirium as well as other conditions, it may be appropriate to consider enteral feeding via a nasogastric tube if the patient is unable to eat and drink enough to meet their nutritional needs. Despite attempting to improve mealtime cares, the patient may not meet their needs because they are too drowsy or have developed a functional dysphagia, which is common in delirium [45, 46]. Enteral feeding can improve intake and possibly prevent poor clinical outcomes [47]. However, the risks of tube feeding and its placement must be weighed against the benefits of adequate nutrition. As an additional tether, it may perpetuate or cause delirium [48], and it may cause distress for patients and frustration for nursing staff if the patient repeatedly dislodges or removes the nasogastric tube. It is not appropriate to provide physical or chemical restraints to facilitate enteral feeding, as the deconditioning caused by immobility runs counter to the aims of nutrition therapy to maintain muscle mass [19].

Decision-making about enteral feeding for a patient with delirium is complex and must be individualised in line with patient goals and the prognosis of the underlying conditions (Chap. 21). It requires the involvement of the multidisciplinary team, including the dietitian, speech pathologist and medical staff, as well as the family or other appropriate decision-makers [19]. Appropriate positioning of the patient remains important to reduce the risk of aspiration, and the use of bolus rather than continuous feeds may be more appropriate, to reduce restraint utilisation and limitations to mobility. Strategies to reduce the risk of dislodgement include the use of fiddle blankets and other distracting activities. If it is safe, continuing to provide even small amounts of oral intake when the patient is more alert and able to sit upright will help promote swallow function and appetite and can provide pleasure and maintain meaningful routines. The feeding tube should be removed as soon as adequate oral intake can be re-established.

Through good nursing care and multidisciplinary teamwork, Douglas makes a good recovery despite his delirium, which resolves over time. As expected, he has lost significant muscle mass and strength and needs in-centre rehabilitation to regain function before going back to his home.

19.5 Post-Hospital Support

Delirium in the post-acute and rehabilitation setting is prevalent, persistent and associated with poor functional recovery [49]. This highlights the need for vigilance with delirium prevention and screening across the continuum of care in order to promote optimal post-hospital cognitive and functional recovery. This includes paying attention to the nutritional intake and status of patients on discharge from hospital, as ongoing nutritional decline in the community setting is common [50]. Engaging and supporting caregivers and family in discharge planning and ongoing nutritional care, meeting unmet needs by referring to community health and support services for practical assistance with shopping and meal preparation, providing oral nutrition supplements (if well accepted) and ensuring nutritional monitoring and follow-up in the community are key strategies to optimise recovery after hospitalisation [51, 52]. Discharge planning should include the patient, carers and other healthcare professionals, incorporating referrals to community health and support services where required, and should be documented clearly and received by community providers within 24 h of hospital discharge.

19.5.1 Summary and Main Points

- Delirium is a common complication especially in older inpatients. It causes distress to patients and their carers and has important negative consequences for health and healthcare needs.

- Dehydration and malnutrition are risk factors for delirium, along with age, frailty cognitive and sensory impairment and serious illness.
- Effective prevention programs can reduce delirium by 30–50% but require multiple integrated components, including supporting good nutrition and hydration.
- Nurses need to adapt their practice to support good nutrition and hydration for patients with cognitive impairment to meet their needs and ensure adequate intake.

References

1. Inouye SK, Westendorp RG, Saczynski JS (2014) Delirium in elderly people. Lancet 383(9920):911–922
2. Agar MR (2020) Delirium at the end of life. Age Ageing 49(3):337–340
3. American Psychiatric Association (2013) Diagnostic and statistical manual of mental disorders (DSM-5), 5th edn. American Psychiatric Association, Washington, DC
4. MacLullich AM, Shenkin SD, Goodacre S, Godfrey M, Hanley J, Stiobhairt A et al (2019) The 4 'A's test for detecting delirium in acute medical patients: a diagnostic accuracy study. Health Technol Assess 23(40):1–194
5. Inouye SK, van Dyck CH, Alessi CA, Balkin S, Siegal AP, Horwitz RI (1990) Clarifying confusion: the confusion assessment method. A new method for detection of delirium. Ann Intern Med 113(12):941–948
6. Clegg A, Westby M, Young JB (2011) Under-reporting of delirium in the NHS. Age Ageing 40(2):283–286
7. Breitbart W, Gibson C, Tremblay A (2002) The delirium experience: delirium recall and delirium-related distress in hospitalized patients with cancer, their spouses/caregivers, and their nurses. Psychosomatics 43(3):183–194
8. Inouye SK, Marcantonio ER, Metzger ED (2014) Doing damage in delirium: the hazards of antipsychotic treatment in elderly persons. Lancet Psychiatry 1(4):312–315
9. Marcantonio ER (2017) Delirium in hospitalized older adults. N Engl J Med 377(15):1456–1466
10. Ahmed S, Leurent B, Sampson EL (2014) Risk factors for incident delirium among older people in acute hospital medical units: a systematic review and meta-analysis. Age Ageing 43(3):326–333
11. National Institute for Health and Care Excellence (2010) Delirium: prevention, diagnosis and management. Clinical guideline: NICE
12. Inouye SK, Charpentier P (1996) Precipitating factors for delirium in hospitalized elderly persons. Predictive model and interrelationships with baseline vulnerability. JAMA 20(275):852–857
13. Wilson M, Morley J (2003) Impaired cognitive function and mental performance in mild dehydration. Eur J Clin Nutr 57:S24–S27
14. Lawlor PG (2002) Delirium and dehydration: some fluid for thought? Support Care Cancer 10(6):445–454
15. Sugita Y, Miyazaki T, Shimada K, Shimizu M, Kunimoto M, Ouchi S et al (2018) Correlation of nutritional indices on admission to the Coronary Intensive Care Unit with the development of delirium. Nutrients 10(11):1712
16. Rosted E, Prokofieva T, Sanders S, Schultz M (2018) Serious consequences of malnutrition and delirium in frail older patients. J Nutr Gerontol Geriatr 37(2):105–116
17. Mudge AM, Ross LJ, Young AM, Isenring EA, Banks MD (2011) Helping understand nutritional gaps in the elderly (HUNGER): a prospective study of patient factors associated with inadequate nutritional intake in older medical inpatients. Clin Nutr 30(3):320–325
18. Sola-Miravete E, Lopez C, Martinez-Segura E, Adell-Lleixa M, Juve-Udina ME, Lleixa-Fortuno M (2018) Nursing assessment as an effective tool for the identification of delirium risk in older in-patients: a case-control study. J Clin Nurs 27(1–2):345–354

19. Volkert D, Beck AM, Cederholm T, Cruz-Jentoft A, Goisser S, Hooper L et al (2019) ESPEN guideline on clinical nutrition and hydration in geriatrics. Clin Nutr 38(1):10–47
20. Ferguson M, Capra S, Bauer J, Banks M (1999) Development of a valid and reliable malnutrition screening tool for adult acute hospital patients. Nutrition 15(6):458–464
21. Kondrup J, Rasmussen H, Hamburg O, Stanga Z (2003) Nutritional risk screening (NRS2002): a new method based on an analysis of controlled clinical trials. Clin Nutr 22(3):321–336
22. Stratton RJ, Hackston A, Longmore D, Dixon R, Price S, Stroud M et al (2004) Malnutrition in hospital outpatients and inpatients: prevalence, concurrent validity and ease of use of the 'malnutrition universal screening tool'('MUST') for adults. Br J Nutr 92(5):799–808
23. Australian Commission on Safety and Quality in Health Care (2016) Delirium clinical care standard. Sydney
24. Scottish Intercollegiate Guidelines Network (SIGN) (2019) Risk reduction and management of delirium. SIGN, Edinburgh. Contract No.: SIGN publication no. 157
25. Oh ES, Needham DM, Nikooie R, Wilson LM, Zhang A, Robinson KA et al (2019) Antipsychotics for preventing delirium in hospitalized adults: a systematic review. Ann Intern Med 171(7):474–484
26. Nikooie R, Neufeld KJ, Oh ES, Wilson LM, Zhang A, Robinson KA et al (2019) Antipsychotics for treating delirium in hospitalized adults: a systematic review. Ann Intern Med 171(7):485–495
27. Ludolph P, Stoffers-Winterling J, Kunzler AM, Rosch R, Geschke K, Vahl CF et al (2020) Non-pharmacologic multicomponent interventions preventing delirium in hospitalized people. J Am Geriatr Soc 68(8):1864–1871
28. Abraha I, Trotta F, Rimland JM, Cruz-Jentoft A, Lozano-Montoya I, Soiza RL et al (2015) Efficacy of non-pharmacological interventions to prevent and treat delirium in older patients: a systematic overview. The SENATOR project ONTOP Series. PLoS One 10(6):e0123090
29. Mudge AM, McRae P, Cruickshank M (2015) Eat walk engage: an interdisciplinary collaborative model to improve care of hospitalized elders. Am J Med Qual 30(1):5–13
30. Inouye SK, Bogardus ST, Charpentier P, Leo-Summers L, Acampora D, Holford TR et al (1999) A multicomponent intervention to prevent delirium. New Engl J Med 340:669–676
31. Piscotty R, Kalisch B (2014) Lost opportunities...the challenges of "missed nursing care". Nurs Manag 45(10):40–44
32. Bail K, Grealish L (2016) 'Failure to Maintain': a theoretical proposition for a new quality indicator of nurse care rationing for complex older people in hospital. Int J Nurs Stud 63:146–161
33. Hshieh TT, Yang T, Gartaganis SL, Yue J, Inouye SK (2018) Hospital Elder life program: systematic review and meta-analysis of effectiveness. Am J Geriatr Psychiatry 26(10):1015–1033
34. Akunne A, Murthy L, Young J (2012) Cost-effectiveness of multi-component interventions to prevent delirium in older people admitted to medical wards. Age Ageing 41(3):285–291
35. Dementia Australia. Personal care: eating. https://www.dementia.org.au/information/about-you/i-am-a-carer-family-member-or-friend/personal-care/eating
36. Young A, Allia A, Jolliffe L, de Jersey S, Mudge A, McRae P et al (2016) Assisted or protected mealtimes? Exploring the impact of hospital mealtime practices on meal intake. J Adv Nurs 72(7):1616–1625
37. Young AM, Kidston S, Banks MD, Mudge AM, Isenring EA (2013) Malnutrition screening tools: comparison against two validated nutrition assessment methods in older medical inpatients. Nutrition 29(1):101–106
38. Beck M, Birkelund R, Poulsen I, Martinsen B (2017) Supporting existential care with protected mealtimes: patients' experiences of a mealtime intervention in a neurological ward. J Adv Nurs 73(8):1947–1957
39. Lee-Steere K, Liddle J, Mudge A, Bennett S, McRae P, Barrimore SE (2020) "You've got to keep moving, keep going": understanding older patients' experiences and perceptions of delirium and nonpharmacological delirium prevention strategies in the acute hospital setting. J Clin Nurs 29(13–14):2363–2377
40. Beck M, Martinsen B, Birkelund R, Poulsen I (2017) Raising a beautiful swan: a phenomenological-hermeneutic interpretation of health professionals' experiences of

participating in a mealtime intervention inspired by protected mealtimes. Int J Qual Stud Health Well-Being 12(1):1360699
41. McLaren-Hedwards T, Dcunha K, Elder-Robinson E, Smith C, Jennings C, Marsh A, et al (2020) The effect of communal dining and dining room enhancement interventions on nutritional, clinical and functional outcomes of patients in acute and sub-acute hospital, rehabilitation and aged-care settings: a systematic review. Nutr Diet. online early
42. Pritchard E, Soh SE, Morello R, Berkovic D, Blair A, Anderson K et al (2020) Volunteer programs supporting people with dementia/delirium in hospital: systematic review and meta-analysis. Gerontologist (online ahead of print). https://doi.org/10.1093/geront/gnaa058
43. Saunders R, Seaman K, Graham R, Christiansen A (2019) The effect of volunteers' care and support on the health outcomes of older adults in acute care: a systematic scoping review. J Clin Nurs 28(23–24):4236–4249
44. Young AM, Mudge AM, Banks MD, Ross LJ, Daniels L (2013) Encouraging, assisting and time to EAT: improved nutritional intake for older medical patients receiving protected mealtimes and/or additional nursing feeding assistance. Clin Nutr 32(4):543–549
45. Namasivayam-MacDonald AM, Riquelme LF (2019) Presbyphagia to dysphagia: multiple perspectives and strategies for quality care of older adults. Semin Speech Lang 40(3):227–242
46. Bode L, Isler F, Fuchs S, Marquetand J, Petry H, Ernst J et al (2020) The utility of nursing instruments for daily screening for delirium: delirium causes substantial functional impairment. Palliat Support Care 18(3):293–300
47. Crenitte MR, Apolinario D, Campora F, Curiati JA, Jacob-Filho W, Avelino-Silva T (2018) A231 Prognostic effect of enteral nutrition in hospitalized older adults with delirium. J Am Geriatr Soc 66(suppl 2):S1–S369
48. Lee C, Snell K, Berger A, Korzick K (2019) Route of nutrition associated with delirium in acute malnutrition. Crit Care Med. 47(1):202
49. Marcantonio ER, Simon SE, Bergmann MA, Jones RN, Murphy KM, Morris JN (2003) Delirium symptoms in post-acute care: prevalent, persistent and associated with poor functional recovery. J Am Geriatr Soc 51:4–9
50. Young AM, Mudge AM, Banks MD, Rogers L, Allen J, Vogler B et al (2015) From hospital to home: limited nutritional and functional recovery for older adults. J Frailty Aging 4(2):69–73
51. Young AM, Mudge AM, Banks MD, Rogers L, Demedio K, Isenring E (2018) Improving nutritional discharge planning and follow up in older medical inpatients: hospital to home outreach for malnourished elders. Nutr Diet 75(3):283–290
52. Marshall S, Reidlinger DP, Young AM, Isenring E (2017) The nutrition and food-related roles, experiences and support needs of female family carers of malnourished older rehabilitation patients. J Hum Nutr Diet 30(1):16–26

20

Elderly People and Food-Drug Interaction

Björn Viðar Aðalbjörnsson and Alfons Ramel

Abstract

The focus of this chapter is on food-drug interaction in older adults. We will discuss how foods can affect drug metabolism and also vice versa how drugs can affect dietary intake and nutrition status.

Keywords

Old people · Food-drug interaction · Herb-drug interaction · Nutrition status

Learning Outcomes
By the end of this chapter, you will be able to:

- Understand the importance of food-drug interactions.
- Know where the interactions take place.
- Describe common foods and herbal products which can affect drug metabolism.
- Report consequences of certain medications on nutrition status.

This chapter is a component of Part II: Specialist Versus Generalist Nutritional Care in Aging. For an explanation of the grouping of chapters in this book, please see Chap. 1: 'Geriatrics and Orthogeriatrics: Providing Nutrition Care'.

B. V. Aðalbjörnsson (✉) · A. Ramel
Department of Food Science and Nutrition, School of Health, University of Iceland, Reykjavík, Iceland
e-mail: bva@hi.is; alfonsra@hi.is

20.1 Introduction

Medical drugs, or medicines, are used to treat diseases, and to guarantee their safety and efficacy, they must be applied in the appropriate way. Medicines usually contain active ingredients which react with the human metabolism in various ways, and certain dietary components frequently affect these properties of medicines. These so-called food-drug interactions occur when, for example, a dietary substance or food enhances, decreases or changes the activity of a drug. Further, a drug interaction can result into a new drug effect which would not occur on its own. Typically, such interactions can be observed between drugs and foods (food-drug interactions) but also between drugs and herbs (herb-drug interactions) [1].

Food-drug interactions can be observed as a consequence of accidental misuse or insufficient knowledge on the substances involved in the interaction. In many cases, herbs, fruits as well as alcohol can alter the efficacy of a given drug intervention with adverse consequences. In most cases, relevant food-drug interactions change the bioavailability of a medicine [1].

Less frequently discussed, but equally important, is the fact that interactions can also go the other way around, i.e. medical drugs can also affect nutrition. As medicines and nutrients employ often the same mechanisms for absorption and are metabolically converted and excreted via the same ways, regular use of certain medications has the potential to negatively influence nutritional status [1, 2].

20.2 Food and Herbal Product Interaction with Drugs

Drug-drug interactions are well known, and particular attention is given to detailing these interactions, for example, on drug instructions or clinical databases and guides. Whilst traditionally there has been less discussion about food-drug interactions, this has been growing in the recent decade. This is an important area as oral drug dosing is common. Food-drug interactions may arise due to changes in drug kinetics, intestinal transport, metabolism and distribution. The effect of standard meals on the drug intake is tested during clinical trials, and recommendations are given based on these studies. Research has tried to quantify this effect, but once in clinical setting, the food intake can vary. Several reviews have discussed this issue with focus on older adults [3–8].

The food-drug interaction is a complex subject, and the interaction can be within the digestive system (e.g. uptake hindrance or binding to drug) or metabolic inhibition (e.g. liver enzymes) [9, 10]. There are several factors that play part in these interactions. The condition of the patient is important, such as age, pre-existing conditions, organ malfunction and polypharmacy. The condition of the food and herbal products influences the composition, identity, extraction, processing, cooking and storage. This then interacts with drugs differently depending on their absorption, distribution, metabolism and distribution.

Food intake varies between age groups, cultures, socio-economic settings and institutions. A broad variety of common food products and herbal products have shown to have adverse effects [11, 12]. These can come from excessive consumption of common food items like fruits and vegetables [13]. Supplements are often concentrated components of food items, such as garlic oil, or herbal products. Both food and herbal supplements, even when taken in highly concentrated forms, are often considered safe by patients. The regulation landscape around supplements is different than for food and medical drugs and is complex and not uniform worldwide which can confuse consumers [14]. The use of supplements is common, and with increased awareness, attention and marketing regarding real or perceived health benefits, this may continue to increase in the coming years. However, in their review, Boullata and Hudson (2012) showed that 12–45% of people used both drugs and supplements, where 6–29% were at risk of harmful interactions [7]. In another study including 1795 patients, 40% reported the use of supplements [15]. Whilst garlic, valerian, kava, ginkgo and St John's wort contributed to more than two-thirds of potentially clinically significant interactions, 107 natural products with potential for interactions were identified. The risk of interactions was with common drug categories (antithrombotic, antidepressants and antidiabetics and sedatives).

A further difficulty is that patients that resort to herbal medications can do so without the knowledge of their medical professional or hide it as they feel ashamed, desperate or rebellious. Patients may also not report supplements or the use of herbal product as the public assumption is that they are safe (e.g. the common use of *Ginkgo biloba*, garlic, ginseng, St John's wort, *Echinacea*, saw palmetto, evening primrose and ginger). Bioavailability is not always negatively affected as iron supplementation can increase the bioavailability of tetracycline [16]. It is therefore important that there are an open dialogue and understanding between healthcare providers and patients.

As this is a complex subject, below are provided some case examples of common food and herbal product interactions with drugs.

20.2.1 Common Foods

Milk can reduce the bioavailability of drugs such as antibiotics (e.g. tetracycline, doxycycline and penicillin). A small amount of milk, such as in tea or coffee, has shown up to 49% reduction in tetracycline bioavailability [17]. Tetracycline and doxycycline are not solely affected by milk as food products can reduce the bioavailability significantly [18, 19]. These effects are often known by health professional, but with these commonly used products, patients may fail to understand the extent of effect the food can have on drug efficacy. For example, a morning dose before breakfast may be difficult for those patients with the habit of starting the day with a meal and supplements. If the patient takes their medication afterwards, it is likely to lead to an unwanted effect (such as slower recovery). Provision of instructions for patients that are clear and outline the potential consequences may improve adherence to prescriptive instructions and, ultimately, patient outcomes.

Other popular common food products include grapefruit and cranberry juice. The interaction between grapefruit juice and drugs has been known for decades, but in the recent years, the number of reported cases has increased [20]. The effect of grape juice on cyclosporin includes decreased area-under-curve (30%) and increased clearance (50%) [21]. Other fruit juices can affect drug potency as well, both increasing and decreasing bioavailability [22]. Cranberry juice is frequently recommended for H. pylori and urinary tract infections. Care must be taken though cranberry juice is considered safe and administered in high doses. Griffiths et al. reported in 2008 a fatal case of haemopericardium and gastrointestinal haemorrhage where interaction between grapefruit juice and enzymes is responsible for warfarin clearance [23]. In this case, the patient was on a recommended 300–400 mL of cranberry juice per day, 6 weeks prior to the incident.

Garlic is traditionally used as a common food across many cultures but is also increasingly (self) prescribed as an alternative natural medicine supplement.

Garlic has been studied extensively with regard to its chemistry, pharmacology and clinical properties. The main research interests lie in the area of anticancer, antimicrobial and cardiovascular effects [24, 25]. The sulphur-containing compounds within garlic are considered responsible for the varied bioactive effects. Allicin is a precursor to several of these compounds; it is broken down enzymatically by allinase that is activated when garlic tissue is disrupted, cut or mashed. These unstable compounds are mostly found in fresh or freeze-dried garlic products. These compounds can cause an inhibition of CYP450 3A4 substrates—such as statin medications (e.g. atorvastatin, simvastatin) [13, 26].

With strong and long traditional use, garlic is often taken by patients in hope for quicker recovery. In common folklore, blogs and healthcare websites, garlic has a reputation to help with recovery from common cold to cancer [25, 26]; this is at least in part supported by evidence. Though garlic is considered food, high dosage is commonly not recommended for older adults as there is a strong evidence for inhibiting effect on platelets [27]. Those that have slow blood clot formation or patients on anticoagulant therapy should take care when taking garlic. Garlic is not an isolated case; the extensive list of food items that interact with warfarin grows. In a systematic review by Holbrook et al. (2005), several other herbal and natural products and foods were shown to interact with warfarin [28].

20.2.2 Herbal Products

Herbal products as ginkgo, St John's wort, ginseng and valerian are among the more commonly reported herbal supplements. These problems may seem more obvious when discussing herbal products, but they may be used instead of or in addition to conventional medication. In addition to influencing patients' diets, these can have interaction with drugs. Ginseng is another well-documented example of an herb with long history of traditional use. The main actions are described as 'adaptogenic'—an action that can be both CNS depressant and stimulant as well as balance bodily functions. These may be conflicting reports, but results of studies of isolated compounds support traditional uses [29]. Preparations are normally well tolerated but its caution is advised. Example of drug interactions is adverse effect with anticoagulants [30] and antiplatelet and anticoagulant effects [31]. Another example is the St John's wort with interesting antidepressant effect. Hyperforin has an effect on the liver and the small intestine, through CYP1A2, CYP2C9, CYP2C19, CYP3A, CYP2E1 and P-gp [32]. St John's wort can cause a significant decrease in drug plasma concentration, such as phenprocoumon (anticoagulant). Other drugs affected by hyperforin intake include simvastatin, nifedipine, digoxin, verapamil, dabigatran, rivaroxaban, apixaban and edoxaban [32–34]. What makes herbal products challenging is that the chemical composition varies between producers and it is difficult to predict their potency. Analytical study on different St John's wort products in the USA showed that the concentration of hyperforin ranged from 0.01 to 1.89%, where many contained lower amount than suggested for antidepressant effect [35].

20.3 Effects of Drugs on Nutrition Status

20.3.1 Drugs Likely to Negatively Influence Nutritional Intake/Status

Medical drugs can negatively impact the bioavailability of nutrients and nutrition status in general [36]. Consequently, the regular use of certain medications has the potential to worsen nutritional status, and this effect of medication on overall nutrition status tends to be multifaceted [2, 3, 36].

Medication that has the greatest potential to impact nutrition status is usually taken over longer periods of time [36], and according to the Icelandic medical directorate, the most commonly prescribed medications for older adults are beta-blocking agents, drugs for peptic ulcer and gastro-oesophageal reflux disease, hypnotics and sedatives, opioids, beta-lactam antibacterials and penicillins, antidepressants, lipid-modifying agents, antithrombotic agents, anti-inflammatory and antirheumatic products as well as selective calcium channel blockers [37].

Unwanted effects of drugs on nutritional status are a consequence of the drug's pharmacodynamics and by its side effect characteristics [38], and older adults both in community and in a clinical environment are at higher risk due to frequently observed polypharmacy [39].

Frequently, medication negatively affects dietary intake by direct action on digestion as well as on general metabolism [7], consequently affecting an older adult's nutritional status by decreasing dietary intake and bioavailability of essential nutrients, e.g. vitamins, trace elements and electrolytes [1, 2, 36].

With the aim to maximise drugs' absorption, many drugs have detailed instructions regarding dietary intake (e.g. several antibiotics, antifungal medication [36]) with the consequence of altering the usual routine of eating and meal frequency which can decrease overall energy and nutrients' intake as often observed in older populations [40, 41].

Anorexia is a frequently observed side effect of drug therapy leading to a reduction of body weight, and older adults with pre-existing poor nutrition status have to be tightly followed when starting drug therapy with medicines related to hypogeusia and dysgeusia (e.g. metformin, levodopa, lithium) (Chaps. 3, 4 and 5) [36, 40, 41].

By direct action of the digestive tract, medications frequently disturb nutrition status of older adults [36, 41]. Some frequently used medicines lead to xerostomia (e.g. anticholinergic drugs, antidepressants and antipsychotic drugs, diuretics, antihypertensives, sedatives, analgesics, antihistamines), nausea and vomiting (antibiotics, opiates, levodopa, selective serotonin reuptake inhibitors), taste abnormalities (e.g. amphetamines, ampicillin, aspirin, corticosteroids, diltiazem, levodopa, metformin, tricyclic antidepressants, venlafaxine) as well as olfactory disturbances (e.g. ACE inhibitors, amoxicillin, beta-blockers, calcium channel blockers, corticosteroids, levodopa, statins, streptomycin, sumatriptan), decreased gastrointestinal motility (tricyclic antidepressants, opiates) and diarrhoea (e.g. broad-spectrum antibiotics, proton-pump inhibitors, antivirals and antiretrovirals, magnesium salts, iron, lithium, metformin). Even unpleasant smell of medication can reduce food intake [40].

Further, drugs have also the potential to negatively affect the absorption of vitamins or trace elements due to alterations in gastric acidity, diminishing nutrition assimilation, negatively impacting gut microbiota and leading to inflammation of the mucosa of the digestive tract (e.g. antacids, antibiotics, laxatives, anti-inflammatories, hypoglycaemic drugs, lipid-lowering drugs, antidepressants, diuretics).

When negative action of drug therapy on nutrition status is likely to become clinically significant, the nutritional deficiency can be corrected with the use of dietary supplements (e.g. pyridoxine administered with isoniazid, an antibiotic used for the treatment of tuberculosis). Despite the fact that classic symptoms of nutrient deficiency syndromes are not often seen, nutrient insufficiencies can be still related to clinical manifestations. In several cases, the negative impact of a certain medication on nutrition status is acknowledged as adverse drug effects. For example, drug-induced osteomalacia is a result of some antiepileptic drugs negatively affecting vitamin D metabolism [42–44]. Further, drug-induced hepatotoxicity and hyperammonaemia (e.g. valproic acid, a drug to treat certain types of seizures) are thought to be a consequence of a lack of carnitine [45, 46].

It is still unclear for what drug nutrient interaction dietary supplementation is a feasible solution [47, 48], and this is a field which needs more research in order to be able to recommend prophylactic nutrient supplementation. It should also be mentioned here that there are some drugs that are related to improvements in nutrient status [49, 50].

Older adults are likely to use medication that can impair hearing, vision, memory and mobility, resulting into a lack of compliance or wrong dosing [36]. This indirect drug action can then affect food intake by impairing the ability to buy and prepare food or to eat without assistance) [51–54].

20.4 Drugs Likely to Increase Body Weight

For a sense of completeness, it should be briefly mentioned here that drugs can also increase body weight. For example, it is well known that active drug ingredients can change function of an older adult's metabolism. Undesirable metabolic adverse effects are frequently observed for antipsychotic drugs which can lead to weight gain, hyperglycaemia and dyslipidaemia [41, 55], alterations that have been in particular related to the use of second-generation antipsychotics [55–57]. Other frequently used medications such as beta-blockers and steroids have been also shown to increase body weight [56, 58, 59].

The observed increase in body weight is not necessarily always due to an increase in body fat. There are several potential mechanisms which can explain medication-related weight gain: increased appetite (steroids [59] and antidepressants [58]), fluid retention (pioglitazone [60]), increased fat storage (insulin, stimulating the growth of fat cells [61]), slowed metabolism (beta-blockers [62]) and difficulty exercising (antihistamines can make you sleepy, amitriptyline associated with breathing difficulties).

Although maintenance or even an increase in body weight in older adults can be beneficial, these drug-induced changes in body composition and metabolism are usually not positive as they are not associated with positive changes in muscle mass or physical function [57]. If not carefully considered, this may lead to sarcopaenic obesity and also the under-identification and under-treatment of those who are overweight or obese and are also malnourished (Chaps. 7 and 16) [63].

20.4.1 Conclusion

Clinical specialists have to recognize that medical drugs and dietary intake interact with each other and can affect the health of older adults. During the last years, these interactions have received more attention and have been better understood in clinical practice [34]. An acknowledgement and broad understanding of the problem are the most important steps towards optimized older adult care [33]. In order to resolve negative drug actions on nutrition status and vice versa, clinicians have to employ a systematic approach and take the time to listen to the perspectives of the older adult. In circumstances where sufficient information on the interactions are available, adverse interactions can be possibly predicted and issues resolved [33].

Healthcare staff should be trained to detect food-drug interactions in order to give older adults instructions on medication, food and beverages. Appropriate specialists must estimate a patient's clinical presentation in order to recognize whether the nutritional status is deteriorating or associated with a drug-induced complication. A change in dosage or a change in medications within the same therapeutic category or a change in dietary habits has to be considered. Finally, and most importantly, healthcare providers should work together with older adults to deliver food and medicine regimens that are most likely to improve older adult outcomes, experiences and quality of life.

Take-Home Points

- Herbs, fruits as well as alcohol can alter the efficacy of a given drug intervention with adverse consequences.
- In most cases, relevant food-drug interactions change the bioavailability of a medicine.

- Milk, grapefruit and cranberry juice and garlic are the most common foods to affect drug metabolism.
- Many common medications can lead to weight loss or gain and adverse changes in the nutrition status of older adults.

References

1. White R (2010) Drugs and nutrition: how side effects can influence nutritional intake. Proc Nutr Soc 69(4):558–564
2. Lombardi LR, Kreys E, Gerry S, Boullata JI (2010) Nutrition in the age of polypharmacy. In: Bendich A, Deckelbaum RJ (eds) Preventive nutrition: the comprehensive guide for health professionals. Humana Press, Totowa, pp 79–123
3. Ased S, Wells J, Morrow LE, Malesker MA (2018) Clinically significant food-drug interactions. Consult Pharm 33(11):649–657
4. Agbabiaka TB, Wider B, Watson LK, Goodman C (2017) Concurrent use of prescription drugs and herbal medicinal products in older adults: a systematic review. Drugs Aging 34(12):891–905
5. Koziolek M, Alcaro S, Augustijns P, Basit AW, Grimm M, Hens B et al (2019) The mechanisms of pharmacokinetic food-drug interactions - a perspective from the UNGAP group. Eur J Pharm Sci 134:31–59
6. Heuberger R (2012) Polypharmacy and food-drug interactions among older persons: a review. J Nutr Gerontol Geriatr 31(4):325–403
7. Boullata JI, Hudson LM (2012) Drug-nutrient interactions: a broad view with implications for practice. J Acad Nutr Diet 112(4):506–517
8. Raats M, de Groot CPGM, van Asselt D (2017) Food for the aging population, 2nd edn. Woodhead Publishing, Duxford
9. Nakanishi T, Tamai I (2015) Interaction of drug or food with drug transporters in intestine and liver. Curr Drug Metab 16(9):753–764
10. Deng J, Zhu X, Chen Z, Fan CH, Kwan HS, Wong CH et al (2017) A review of food-drug interactions on oral drug absorption. Drugs 77(17):1833–1855
11. Abuhelwa AY, Williams DB, Upton RN, Foster DJ (2017) Food, gastrointestinal pH, and models of oral drug absorption. Eur J Pharm Biopharm 112:234–248
12. Ulbricht C, Chao W, Costa D, Rusie-Seamon E, Weissner W, Woods J (2008) Clinical evidence of herb-drug interactions: a systematic review by the natural standard research collaboration. Curr Drug Metab 9(10):1063–1120
13. Rodríguez-Fragoso L, Martínez-Arismendi JL, Orozco-Bustos D, Reyes-Esparza J, Torres E, Burchiel SW (2011) Potential risks resulting from fruit/vegetable-drug interactions: effects on drug-metabolizing enzymes and drug transporters. J Food Sci 76(4):R112–R124
14. Thakkar S, Anklam E, Xu A, Ulberth F, Li J, Li B et al (2020) Regulatory landscape of dietary supplements and herbal medicines from a global perspective. Regul Toxicol Pharmacol 114:104647
15. Sood A, Sood R, Brinker FJ, Mann R, Loehrer LL, Wahner-Roedler DL (2008) Potential for interactions between dietary supplements and prescription medications. Am J Med 121(3):207–211
16. Leyden JJ (1985) Absorption of minocycline hydrochloride and tetracycline hydrochloride. Effect of food, milk, and iron. J Am Acad Dermatol 12(2 pt 1):308–312
17. Jung H, Peregrina AA, Rodriguez JM, Moreno-Esparza R (1997) The influence of coffee with milk and tea with milk on the bioavailability of tetracycline. Biopharm Drug Dispos 18(5):459–463
18. Welling PG, Koch PA, Lau CC, Craig WA (1977) Bioavailability of tetracycline and doxycycline in fasted and nonfasted subjects. Antimicrob Agents Chemother 11(3):462–469

19. Meyer FP, Specht H, Quednow B, Walther H (1989) Influence of milk on the bioavailability of doxycycline--new aspects. Infection 17(4):245–246
20. Bailey DG, Dresser G, Arnold JM (2013) Grapefruit-medication interactions: forbidden fruit or avoidable consequences? CMAJ 185(4):309–316
21. Oliveira-Freitas VL, Dalla Costa T, Manfro RC, Cruz LB, Schwartsmann G (2010) Influence of purple grape juice in cyclosporine bioavailability. J Ren Nutr 20(5):309–313
22. de Morais C, Oliveira B, Afonso C, Lumbers M, Raats M, de Almeida MD (2013) Nutritional risk of European elderly. Eur J Clin Nutr 67(11):1215–1219
23. Griffiths AP, Beddall A, Pegler S (2008) Fatal haemopericardium and gastrointestinal haemorrhage due to possible interaction of cranberry juice with warfarin. J R Soc Promot Heal 128(6):324–326
24. Ansary J, Forbes-Hernández TY, Gil E, Cianciosi D, Zhang J, Elexpuru-Zabaleta M et al (2020) Potential health benefit of garlic based on human intervention studies: a brief overview. Antioxidants 9(7):619
25. Choo S, Chin VK, Wong EH, Madhavan P, Tay ST, Yong PVC et al (2020) Review: antimicrobial properties of allicin used alone or in combination with other medications. Folia Microbiol (Praha) 65(3):451–465
26. Blalock SJ, Gregory PJ, Patel RA, Norton LL, Callahan LF, Jordan JM (2009) Factors associated with potential medication-herb/natural product interactions in a rural community. Altern Ther Health Med 15(5):26–34
27. Bradley JM, Organ CL, Lefer DJ (2016) Garlic-derived organic polysulfides and myocardial protection. J Nutr 146(2):403s–409s
28. Holbrook AM, Pereira JA, Labiris R, McDonald H, Douketis JD, Crowther M et al (2005) Systematic overview of warfarin and its drug and food interactions. Arch Intern Med 165(10):1095–1106
29. Lim JW, Chee SX, Wong WJ, He QL, Lau TC (2018) Traditional Chinese medicine: herb-drug interactions with aspirin. Singap Med J 59(5):230–239
30. Petersen, MJ, Bergien, SO, Staerk, D (2021) A systematic review of possible interactions for herbal medicines and dietary supplements used concomitantly with disease-modifying or symptom-alleviating multiple sclerosis drugs. Phytotherapy Research 1–22. https://doi.org/10.1002/ptr.7050
31. Lau AJ, Toh DF, Chua TK, Pang YK, Woo SO, Koh HL (2009) Antiplatelet and anticoagulant effects of Panax notoginseng: comparison of raw and steamed Panax notoginseng with Panax ginseng and Panax quinquefolium. J Ethnopharmacol 125(3):380–386
32. Mouly S, Lloret-Linares C, Sellier PO, Sene D, Bergmann JF (2017) Is the clinical relevance of drug-food and drug-herb interactions limited to grapefruit juice and Saint-John's Wort? Pharmacol Res 118:82–92
33. Borrelli F, Izzo AA (2009) Herb-drug interactions with St John's wort (Hypericum perforatum): an update on clinical observations. AAPS J 11(4):710–727
34. Russo E, Scicchitano F, Whalley BJ, Mazzitello C, Ciriaco M, Esposito S et al (2014) Hypericum perforatum: pharmacokinetic, mechanism of action, tolerability, and clinical drug-drug interactions. Phytother Res 28(5):643–655
35. de los Reyes GC, Koda RT (2002) Determining hyperforin and hypericin content in eight brands of St. John's wort. Am J Health Syst Pharm 59(6):545–547
36. Van Zyl M (2011) The effects of drugs on nutrition. South Afr J Clin Nutr 24(suppl 3): 38–41
37. Directorate IM (2021) Prescription Medicines Register. http://www.landlaeknir.is/tolfraedi-og-rannsoknir/gagnasofn/gagnasafn/item12455/Lyfjagagnagrunnur-(Prescription-Medicines-Register). Director of Health [updated 04.05.2017]
38. Gervasio JM (2010) Drug-Induced Changes to Nutritional Status. In: Boullata J, Armenti V (eds) Handbook of Drug-Nutrient Interactions. Nutrition and Health. Humana Press 427–445
39. Knight-Klimas TC, Boullata JI (2004) Drug-nutrient interactions in the elderly. In: Boullata JI, Armenti VT (eds) Handbook of drug-nutrient interactions. Humana Press, Totowa, pp 363–410
40. Pelletier AL, Butler AM, Gillies RA, May JR (2010) Metformin stinks, literally. Ann Intern Med 152(4):267–268

41. Brixner DI, Said Q, Corey-Lisle PK, Tuomari AV, L'Italien GJ, Stockdale W et al (2006) Naturalistic impact of second-generation antipsychotics on weight gain. Ann Pharmacother 40(4):626–632
42. Pascussi JM, Robert A, Nguyen M, Walrant-Debray O, Garabedian M, Martin P et al (2005) Possible involvement of pregnane X receptor-enhanced CYP24 expression in drug-induced osteomalacia. J Clin Invest 115(1):177–186
43. Oscarson M, Zanger UM, Rifki OF, Klein K, Eichelbaum M, Meyer UA (2006) Transcriptional profiling of genes induced in the livers of patients treated with carbamazepine. Clin Pharmacol Ther 80(5):440–456
44. Xu Y, Hashizume T, Shuhart MC, Davis CL, Nelson WL, Sakaki T et al (2006) Intestinal and hepatic CYP3A4 catalyze hydroxylation of 1alpha,25-dihydroxyvitamin D(3): implications for drug-induced osteomalacia. Mol Pharmacol 69(1):56–65
45. Van Wouwe JP (1995) Carnitine deficiency during valproic acid treatment. Int J Vitam Nutr Res 65(3):211–214
46. Werner T, Treiss I, Kohlmueller D, Mehlem P, Teich M, Longin E et al (2007) Effects of valproate on acylcarnitines in children with epilepsy using ESI-MS/MS. Epilepsia 48(1):72–76
47. Morrow LE, Wear RE, Schuller D, Malesker M (2006) Acute isoniazid toxicity and the need for adequate pyridoxine supplies. Pharmacotherapy 26(10):1529–1532
48. De Vivo DC, Bohan TP, Coulter DL, Dreifuss FE, Greenwood RS, Nordli DR Jr et al (1998) L-carnitine supplementation in childhood epilepsy: current perspectives. Epilepsia 39(11):1216–1225
49. Drain PK, Kupka R, Mugusi F, Fawzi WW (2007) Micronutrients in HIV-positive persons receiving highly active antiretroviral therapy. Am J Clin Nutr 85(2):333–345
50. Nose S, Wasa M, Tazuke Y, Owari M, Fukuzawa M (2010) Cisplatin upregulates glutamine transport in human intestinal epithelial cells: the protective mechanism of glutamine on intestinal mucosa after chemotherapy. JPEN J Parenter Enteral Nutr 34(5):530–537
51. Tawara Y, Nishikawa T, Koga I, Uchida Y, Yamawaki S (1997) Transient and intermittent oral dyskinesia appearing in a young woman ten days after neuroleptic treatment. Clin Neuropharmacol 20(2):175–178
52. Halford JC, Blundell JE (2000) Pharmacology of appetite suppression. Prog Drug Res 54:25–58
53. Zadak Z, Hyspler R, Ticha A, Vlcek J (2013) Polypharmacy and malnutrition. Curr Opin Clin Nutr Metab Care 16(1):50–55
54. Boullata JI (2013) Drug and nutrition interactions: not just food for thought. J Clin Pharm Ther 38(4):269–271
55. Yoon S, Noh JS, Choi SY, Baik JH (2010) Effects of atypical antipsychotic drugs on body weight and food intake in dopamine D2 receptor knockout mice. Biochem Biophys Res Commun 393(2):235–241
56. Williams SG, Alinejad NA, Williams JA, Cruess DF (2010) Statistically significant increase in weight caused by low-dose quetiapine. Pharmacotherapy 30(10):1011–1015
57. (2004) Consensus development conference on antipsychotic drugs and obesity and diabetes. Diabetes Care 27(2):596–601
58. Alam A, Voronovich Z, Carley JA (2013) A review of therapeutic uses of mirtazapine in psychiatric and medical conditions. Prim Care Companion CNS Disord 15(5):PCC.13r01525
59. Uddén J, Björntorp P, Arner P, Barkeling B, Meurling L, Rössner S (2003) Effects of glucocorticoids on leptin levels and eating behaviour in women. J Intern Med 253(2):225–231
60. Yang T, Soodvilai S (2008) Renal and vascular mechanisms of thiazolidinedione-induced fluid retention. PPAR Res 2008:943614
61. Kahn BB, Flier JS (2000) Obesity and insulin resistance. J Clin Invest 106(4):473–481
62. Wharton S, Raiber L, Serodio KJ, Lee J, Christensen RA (2018) Medications that cause weight gain and alternatives in Canada: a narrative review. Diabetes Metab Syndr Obes 11:427–438
63. Bell JJ, Pulle RC, Lee HB, Ferrier R, Crouch A, Whitehouse SL (2021) Diagnosis of overweight or obese malnutrition spells DOOM for hip fracture patients: a prospective audit. Clin Nutr 40:1905–1910

21

End-of-Life Care, Ethics and Nutrition

Stefano Eleuteri, Arianna Caruso and Ranjeev C. Pulle

Abstract

End-of-life care constitutes an important situation of extreme nutritional vulnerability for older adults. Feeding decisions in late-stage dementia often provoke moral and ethical questions for family members regarding whether or not to continue hand-feeding or opt for tube-feeding placement. Despite the knowledge that starvation and dehydration do not contribute to patient suffering at the end of life and in fact may contribute to a comfortable passage from life, the ethics of not providing artificial nutrition and hydration (ANH) continue to be hotly debated. However, in the past two decades, voluntary stopping of eating and drinking (VSED) has moved from a palliative option of last resort to being increasingly recognized as a valid means to intentionally hasten death for cognitively intact persons dealing with a serious illness. Across many settings globally, when oral intake is deemed unsafe, decisions to withhold oral feeding and to forgo artificial means of providing nutrition are deemed to be ethically and

---

This chapter is a component of Part II: Specialist Versus Generalist Nutritional Care in Aging. For an explanation of the grouping of chapters in this book, please see Chap. 1: "Geriatrics and Orthogeriatrics: Providing Nutrition Care."

S. Eleuteri (✉)
Fragility Fracture Network, Sapienza University of Rome, Rome, Italy
e-mail: stefano.eleuteri@uniroma1.it

A. Caruso
Academy of Social and Legal Psychology, Rome, Italy

R. C. Pulle
Internal Medicine Services, The Prince Charles Hospital, Brisbane, Australia
e-mail: ChrysRanjeev.Pulle@health.qld.gov.au

legally sanctioned when the decision is made by a capable patient or their legally recognized substitute decision-maker. Decision-making at the end of life involves knowledge of and consideration of the legal, ethical, cultural, religious, and personal values involved in the issue at hand. This chapter attempted to illustrate the unique complexities when considering nutrition therapy (by oral and artificial means) at the end of life.

Keywords
End of life · Ethics · Artificial nutrition · Hydration · Voluntary stopping of eating and drinking · Older adults

21.1 Background

A nutritionally vulnerable older adult has a reduced physical reserve that limits the ability to mount a vigorous recovery in the face of an acute health threat or stressor. Often this vulnerability contributes to more medical complications, longer hospital stays, and increased likelihood of residential aged care admission and, ultimately, end of life [1].

What does it mean to be vulnerable? In the health context, a background of predisposing factors determines the ability of an individual to respond to stressors or precipitants. A vulnerable older person has a greater accumulation of detrimental predisposing factors (e.g., multiple medical conditions, obesity, and limited social support) relative to protective factors (e.g., muscle mass or adipose stores). When an acute stress arises, such as acute inpatient hospitalization for sepsis or surgery, the individual is unable to mount a vigorous recovery and may never fully return to their prestress baseline [1]. The term “nutritionally vulnerable” evokes the classic image of an elderly community dweller with limited resources and/or medical comorbidities that preclude the consumption of a fully adequate diet. Surely, these individuals should appear on the radar of concern in geriatric nutrition, prior to approaching the end of life. However, a very broad array of dynamic challenges contributes to nutritional vulnerability in today’s older adults, well before end of life [1].

21.2 Factors Associated with Nutritional Vulnerability

Many factors impact the quality and quantity of dietary intake in community-dwelling older adults (Chap. 4). Older adults are predisposed to nutrient deficiency due to a decline in total and resting energy requirements associated with physical inactivity, loss of lean muscle mass, and increased adiposity that gradually reduces food intake while vitamin and mineral needs remain unchanged or increased [2]. Furthermore, biomedical, psychosocial, and environmental and economic factors also seriously impact nutritional status in older adults. In the physiologic sense, vulnerability equates closely with a more familiar term used to describe age-related decline, namely, "frailty" (Chap. 8). Frailty is an aging-related clinical syndrome of physiological decline characterized by marked vulnerability to adverse health outcomes increased risk for adverse outcomes including acute illness, disability, falls, hospitalization, need for long-term care, and death [3]. Psychosocial factors that contribute to decreased food intake include depression, social isolation, and loneliness, to name a few. Depression is a prevalent condition in the older population where 7% have major depressive disorders and up to 17% have clinically significant depressive symptoms [4]. Risk factors for late-life depression include female gender, lower educational status, loss of a partner, cognitive decline, chronic health conditions, and decline in physical function [5]. The relationship between malnutrition and depression is multifaceted and complex.

Social isolation (objective measure) and loneliness (subjective measure) are common among community-dwelling older adults who live alone, have functional impairments, lack transportation, have low morale, and report limited social networks [6]. Furthermore, social isolation and loneliness are associated with chronic health conditions, cognitive impairment, poor self-reported health, and sleep disorders [7]. Older adults who experience these psychosocial determinants are more likely to eat alone and often have chronically marginal nutrient intake, putting them at a greater risk for malnutrition [8]. Of particular concern are widowed or single older men. These individuals typically have fewer close relationships outside of their spouse, lack cooking skills, or are physically unable to prepare food [9].

In many individuals, such factors associated with nutritional vulnerability will become more focused toward the end of life; this demands the attention of diverse healthcare providers to ensure ethical standards of care are met.

21.3 Malnutrition: A Commonly Identified Precursor to the End of Life

Food insecurity, defined as "limited or uncertain availability of nutritionally adequate and safe foods or limited or uncertain ability to acquire acceptable foods in socially acceptable ways," encompasses not only the lack of economic resources to obtain nutritionally adequate food but also the inability to access and appropriately use food. According to the USDA, in 2013, the prevalence of food insecurity in the United States was 14.3% of households. Among older adults, 8.7% of households with an older adult and 9.0% of older adults were living alone with insecure food [10].

The multidimensional phenomenon of food insecurity is peculiar in this population [11, 12]. In older populations, food insecurity results from more than financial resource constraints. Functional impairment, not owning a home, isolation, gender, financial vulnerability, and poor health have statistically significant associations with food insecurity. These associations suggest that differences in food use between older and younger populations should be considered. These important risk factors for food insecurity tend to occur together, which results in a much higher risk for food insecurity in older populations; this again is likely to be a focal point toward the end of life [11, 13, 14].

Shortcomings in past approaches used to assess nutritional status have hindered efforts to describe the extent and degree of malnutrition and nutritional risk for older adults in clinical settings. The use of assessment tools like the Mini Nutritional Assessment (MNA) is not routinely applied across the clinical environment, and serum albumin level, although it is heavily relied upon as a sole indicator of nutritional status, actually reflects primarily the inflammatory state rather than the true body store of essential nutrients [15] (Chap. 3). Fortunately, as detailed in Chap. 3, new paradigms describing malnutrition have been recently developed and codified [16–18]. These approaches more accurately reflect the close interrelationship between diseases, substantially improve the accuracy of malnutrition diagnosis, and are anticipated to lead to a better understanding of ways to surmount challenges to nutritional status going forward [1].

Long recognized as a general concern, hospital malnutrition has received considerably more scientific attention in recent years, as evidenced by a number of recent studies and editorials [19, 20]. As of 2013, 14.1% of the population in the United States was over the age of 65 years, yet this relatively small cohort accounted for the greatest utilization of healthcare services. Older adults made up 34.9% of all hospital admissions, with a greater mean length of stay and cost per stay than any other age-group [21]. This is because older adults have a higher number of predisposing conditions with comorbid illnesses and disabilities. Malnutrition is a key comorbid illness now recognized as a predictor of adverse events during their hospitalization, such as falls, pressure injuries, unfavorable discharge destination, unplanned readmissions, mortality, and increased healthcare costs [15, 22–25]. While it is clear that people approaching end of life are high users of healthcare, ongoing works are required to understand if variations in hospitalization and healthcare costs may be attributable to variation in the quantity or quality of end-of-life care available, for example, ensuring processes to manage nutritional vulnerability [26, 27].

This combination of susceptibility and reduced ability to overcome stressors leads to poor long-term outcomes and commonly results in loss of independence, which is a marker of frailty (Chap. 8). The decline of all these physiological parameters can, in many cases, be directly related to reduced energy intake. When energy intake is insufficient to meet the demands of the body either due to starvation, acute illness, or chronic disease/disability, then malnutrition becomes the driver that leads to the further deterioration of functional ability and inability to recover from disease [1] (Chaps. 2–5).

Several recent publications [28, 29] addressing nutritional risk in older patients found that malnutrition in hospitalized geriatric patients is associated with an increased risk of death at 3 months. These papers have further illuminated the profile of malnutrition to include more clinical characteristics, including eating difficulties (Chap. 18) and other functional limitations, depression, polypharmacy (Chap. 20), pressure ulcers (Chap. 15), and cognitive impairment, as well as social factors and hospital factors such as unnecessarily lengthy periods of medical orders requiring patients to have nothing by mouth (NPO), frequent meal interruptions, and low acceptance of foods served (Chaps. 1–6) [29]. It is imperative to recognize both malnutrition and risk of malnutrition as early as possible during the hospital admission process so that all of the medical, psychological, and functional factors related to malnutrition can be addressed by an interprofessional team focusing on the patient's preferences regarding food choices, timing of meals, and/or self-feeding strategies within their individual social and environmental circumstances [1].

21.3.1 Nutrition at the End of Life

The extreme nutritional vulnerability for older adults is often most acutely observed toward end-of-life care. As an example, feeding decisions in advanced cancer or late-stage dementia often provoke wrenching moral and ethical questions for family members regarding whether or not to continue dedicated hand-feeding and nutritional supplementation or even to consider tube-feeding placement, noting that in many situations, these may be unlikely to prolong life and improve quality of life or may be considered medically futile [1, 30].

From the outset, we consequently note that nutritional intervention in this phase of life should be individualized [30], particularly given there are no clear criteria to ascertain the beginning of the dying phase.

In patients at the end of life (survival days or weeks), artificial hydration and nutrition pose clinical, ethical, and logistical dilemmas resulting in debates for and against such interventions [30]. No strong evidence exists supporting the use of "artificial" tube feeding, for example, parenteral or enteral tube feeding for hydration and nutrition for terminally ill patients; however, a paucity of research examining the issue exists [30–32]. Patients during the last days and weeks of life often have anorexia, decreased oral intake, resulting in sarcopenia and obvious frailty, which phenotypically present as loss of body weight with reduced muscle mass and adipose tissue. In addition, cancer patients, frequently gastrointestinal or patients with metastatic malignancy, may develop mechanical obstruction of the digestive tract preventing enteral nutrition [33]. While these may appear confronting to carers and loved ones looking on, in these patients, the goals of therapy should routinely be directed at symptomatic management rather than reversing nutritional deficits. For most, the pleasure of tasting food and the social benefits of participating in meals with family and friends should be emphasized over increasing caloric intake [31]. When patients approach end of life, they often have severely restricted oral intake of food and fluids. The overwhelming principles toward end-of-life nutritional care should revolve not only around a patient's pre-existing wishes regarding intervention but also on comfort measures [32]. However, this should not automatically preclude consideration of artificial nutrition and hydration for individual older adults at the end of life.

21.4 Artificial Nutrition and Hydration (ANH)

Despite the knowledge that starvation and dehydration do not contribute to patient suffering at the end of life and in fact may contribute to a comfortable passage from life, the ethics of providing or not providing artificial nutrition and hydration (ANH) continue to be hotly debated [34]. ANH are defined as a group of medical treatments provided to patients who cannot meet their daily requirements orally, with resultant malnutrition, electrolyte abnormalities, and/or metabolic derangements. Various modalities to deliver ANH include intravenous hydration and intravenous parenteral nutrition, nasogastric feeding, and placement of surgical feeding devices to deliver the required hydration and nourishment.

In patients at the end of life (survival days or weeks), nutrition support and particularly artificial hydration pose clinical, ethical, and logistical dilemmas resulting in debates for and against such interventions [30]. While there has been a lack of strong evidence supporting the use of "artificial" tube feeding, for example, parenteral or enteral tube feeding for hydration and nutrition for terminally ill patients [30–32], we note that artificial nutrition has become an accepted part of palliative care for at least some situations [32]. Being medical treatments, the initiation, termination, and withholding of these modalities must be medically and ethically justified [32, 35]. Many investigators have found that dying persons overwhelmingly deny thirst and hunger; and application of lubricants or provision of ice chips and oral hygiene alleviates many xerostomic complaints. Provision of oral food and fluids should be strongly encouraged, as in most situations, they give comfort, pleasure, a sense of autonomy, and dignity and are viewed as essential caregiving [34].

The practice of medical nutrition and hydration provokes both supportive and opposing views. Some ethicists would argue that the symptom of thirst should be addressed, because, without it, the patient will experience confusion, restlessness, or neuromuscular weakness, thus decreasing the patient's quality of life. Others may argue that the terminally ill patient with declining renal function receiving artificial hydration will suffer from choking on increased secretions, pulmonary edema, and ascites [36]. Alternatively, while offering an unrestricted diet for patients with dysphagia may increase the risk of aspiration or choking, this may also provide a basic comfort and potentially final right of life in end-stage disease. In order to provide artificial nutrition and hydration, medical devices such as urinary catheters and surgically placed feeding tubes may be required; whether these add to or subtract from quality of life should be considered on an individual basis. For example, a patient with decreased mental capacity may try to remove these devices. Attempting to continue the therapy, caregivers may use restraints or sedation, resulting in an inappropriate decrease in quality of life [37].

Families may believe that hydration decreases pain, replenishes the body, enhances effectiveness of medications, and in general can make the patient feel better both mentally and physically. At the end of life, families may feel that they are responsible for maintaining their loved one's dignity, and continued hydration may contribute to their perception that this is being accomplished. In some cases, the family's insistence that the patient take nutrition may cause conflict even before the implementation of ANH becomes the only option. Strong beliefs in the value of nutrition and hydration at the end of life may give the family some satisfaction that they are helping the patient [37]. The patient's refusal to eat may exacerbate the family's feeling of helplessness. Families' perceptions of the importance of nutrition may also color their impression of the healthcare team dedication. If the family believes that the medical team is not placing enough importance on nutrition and hydration, this may translate into the perception that the healthcare team is negligent [37]. This is where good communication between clinical team and families is required to discuss goals and directions of care (Chaps. 10, 11, and 13).

Patients at the end of life lose interest in eating and have fatigue, altered body image, and decreased ability to digest. These are all highly correlated with psychological distress [38]. Patients may believe that if they are not able to take food and fluid orally, then ANH will help them survive by preventing dehydration and increasing physical strength. They may also believe that a gastrostomy or a nasogastric tube can make their quality of life worse. If it is not something that will cure their illness, patients may decline ANH [36]. Patients may believe that ANH is a symbol of their families' love for them, an important part of their meticulous care for their health and well-being [39].

Some patients and families choose to implement ANH rather than go without, while some others do not wish to be tube-fed [33, 40, 41]. It is important to stress that, to be considered medically ethical and justified, ANH must provide a benefit to the patient (*beneficence*), avoid harm (non-*maleficence*), be in accordance with the patient's wishes (*autonomy*), and avoid overutilization of resource for one patient with harm to others and be available to all patients in similar circumstances (*justice*) [32, 37]. The possible benefits of feeding via ANH include improvement in the patient's quality of life and improved nutrition with decreased incidence of bedsores and other infections [35].

However, these treatment modalities are not without risk to the patient. ANH can lead to fluid overload and electrolyte/metabolic derangements, aspiration pneumonitis, or pneumonia and are associated with an increased risk of infection [42]. Moreover, the procedures involved with feeding device placement can themselves lead to increased morbidity and mortality [43]. Finally, while there is no evidence that withholding nourishment and hydration in terminal illness causes pain or suffering, some clinicians would argue that it does not prolong life but only prolongs the dying process [35]. It is the balance between benefits of ANH and potential disadvantages that the clinician needs to fully convey to patient and family before embarking on this course of intervention.

Arguably, in many cases, the decision to offer artificial feeding or not revolves less around the benefits versus risks of the intervention but whether or not terminally ill patients and their family have emotionally accepted the fact the patient is dying [31]. We conclude this section by noting that the decision to administer parenteral or enteral tube feeding should be individualized, based upon the clinical scenario, and should also be consistent with the goals of care of the patient [41, 44]. In case of uncertainty of the benefits and risks of artificial feeding in a particular patient, a brief trial with clearly defined goals may be appropriate to initiate, followed by reassessments of its clinical benefits and harm.

21.5 Voluntary Stopping Eating and Drinking (VSED)

In the past two decades, VSED has moved from a palliative option of last resort [45] to being increasingly recognized as a valid means to intentionally hasten death for cognitively intact persons dealing with a serious illness [32, 46, 47]. It should be noted that VSED is different from declining interest for food and water at the end of life [48]. Properly defined, VSED refers to "a conscious and deliberate decision, by a capacitated patient suffering from advanced illness or an extremely debilitating medical condition, to intentionally refrain from receiving food or fluids by mouth, to hasten death" [49]. Those who have cared for persons choosing VSED have noted the following patient motivations for undertaking this method: willingness to die, feeling of senseless in continued life, experiencing poor quality of life, and desire to control the dying process [50]. Though considerable legal and ethical analysis has been undertaken over the past decade to clarify the moral and legal standing of VSED, continued controversy and uncertainty around its use center on the following concerns: Is it legal to offer standard palliative care to patients undertaking VSED without being viewed as "assisting" in their suicide? If it is legal to support VSED, can a practitioner exercise conscientious objection and refuse to support a patient requesting it? Would providing advice to a patient about VSED as an option potentially be construed as "encouraging suicide" [48]? If a patient and family choose VSED, is it a reflection that the patient has entered a terminal or palliative state? These are all questions that should be asked and considered in relation to local contexts and the will of the patient and their informed consent [32]. We conclude this section by noting the ESPEN guideline on ethical aspects of artificial nutrition and hydration Statements 14 "the renouncement of food and drink may be regarded as an expression of self-determined dying by way of an autonomous decision towards one's own life, but should not be confused with severe depression or disease related lack of appetite," and 34 "Voluntary cessation of nutrition and hydration is a legally and medically acceptable decision of a competent patient, when chosen in disease conditions with frustrating prognosis and at the end life."

21.6 Stopping Oral Nutrition for Incapable Patients

When oral intake is deemed unsafe, decisions to withhold oral feeding and to forgo artificial means of providing nutrition are deemed to be ethically and legally sanctioned when the decision is made by a capable patient or their legally recognized substitute decision-maker. The issue arises when the family attempts to withhold nutrition from incapable patients even if feeding is safe and accepted by patients. The motivation behind families requesting staff to stop oral hydration or nutrition is often based on an interpretation of a prior expressed wish. However, in many cases, these verbal or written instructions make no explicit reference to hand-feeding. Families may interpret assisted hand-feeding as a life-prolonging intervention; however, for the healthcare team, supporting the family's request is interpreted as condoning neglect and endangerment of a vulnerable patient [51]. This is where the goals of care need to be addressed between clinical team and patient. The choice of withholding or ceasing nutrition care in these patients is a difficult task that should be carefully discussed with caregivers; even then, emotional and/or ethical conflicts among family, carers, and/or healthcare team members will undoubtedly arise from time to time [32].

21.7 Conclusions and Take-Home Points

Decision-making at the end of life involves knowledge and consideration of the legal, ethical, cultural, religious, and personal values involved in the issue at hand. This chapter illustrates the unique complexities when considering nutrition therapy (by oral and artificial means) at the end of life. These implications become more poignant in the current world where the aim is comfort at the end of life [52]. Clear goals of care need to be addressed when patient is entering a palliative or terminal phase in their life.

References

1. Porter Starr KN, McDonald SR, Bales CW (2015) Nutritional vulnerability in older adults: a continuum of concerns. Curr Nutr Rep 4(2):176–184
2. Bernstein M, Munoz N (2012) Position of the Academy of Nutrition and Dietetics: food and nutrition for older adults: promoting health and wellness. J Acad Nutr Diet 112(8):1255–1277
3. Gielen E et al (2012) Musculoskeletal frailty: a geriatric syndrome at the core of fracture occurrence in older age. Calcif Tissue Int 91(3):161–177
4. Luppa M et al (2012) Age- and gender-specific prevalence of depression in latest-life--systematic review and meta-analysis. J Affect Disord 136(3):212–221
5. Djernes JK (2006) Prevalence and predictors of depression in populations of elderly: a review. Acta Psychiatr Scand 113(5):372–387
6. Coyle CE, Dugan E (2012) Social isolation, loneliness and health among older adults. J Aging Health 24(8):1346–1363
7. Steptoe A et al (2013) Social isolation, loneliness, and all-cause mortality in older men and women. Proc Natl Acad Sci U S A 110(15):5797–5801
8. Romero-Ortuno R et al (2011) Psychosocial and functional correlates of nutrition among community-dwelling older adults in Ireland. J Nutr Health Aging 15(7):527–531
9. Holwerda TJ et al (2012) Increased risk of mortality associated with social isolation in older men: only when feeling lonely? Results from the Amsterdam Study of the Elderly (AMSTEL). Psychol Med 42(4):843–853
10. Alisha Coleman-Jensen CG, Singh A (2014) Household Food Security in the United States in 2013, in Economic Research Report Number 173. United States Department of Agriculture (USDA)
11. Lee JS et al (2011) Food security of older adults requesting older Americans Act Nutrition Program in Georgia can be validly measured using a short form of the U.S. Household Food Security Survey Module. J Nutr 141(7):1362–1368
12. Lee JS, Frongillo EA Jr (2001) Factors associated with food insecurity among U.S. elderly persons: importance of functional impairments. J Gerontol B Psychol Sci Soc Sci 56(2):S94–S99
13. Lee JS, Frongillo EA Jr (2001) Nutritional and health consequences are associated with food insecurity among U.S. elderly persons. J Nutr 131(5):1503–1509
14. Vilar-Compte M et al (2016) Functional limitations, depression, and cash assistance are associated with food insecurity among older urban adults in Mexico City. J Health Care Poor Underserved 27(3):1537–1554
15. Jensen GL (2006) Inflammation as the key interface of the medical and nutrition universes: a provocative examination of the future of clinical nutrition and medicine. JPEN J Parenter Enteral Nutr 30(5):453–463
16. Jensen GL et al (2019) GLIM criteria for the diagnosis of malnutrition: a consensus report from the global clinical nutrition community. JPEN J Parenter Enteral Nutr 43(1):32–40
17. White JV et al (2012) Consensus statement: Academy of Nutrition and Dietetics and American Society for Parenteral and Enteral Nutrition. J Parenter Enter Nutr 36(3):275–283

18. Cederholm T et al (2015) Diagnostic criteria for malnutrition - an ESPEN consensus statement. Clin Nutr 34(3):335–340
19. Tappenden KA et al (2013) Critical role of nutrition in improving quality of care: an interdisciplinary call to action to address adult hospital malnutrition. JPEN J Parenter Enteral Nutr 37(4):482–497
20. Corkins MR et al (2014) Malnutrition diagnoses in hospitalized patients: United States, 2010. JPEN J Parenter Enteral Nutr 38(2):186–195
21. Weiss AJ, Elixhauser A (2014) Overview of hospital stays in the United States, 2012: statistical brief #180. In Healthcare Cost and Utilization Project (HCUP) Statistical Briefs [Internet]. Agency for Healthcare Research and Quality (US), Rockville
22. Fernandez HM et al (2008) House staff member awareness of older inpatients' risks for hazards of hospitalization. Arch Intern Med 168(4):390–396
23. Bell JJ et al (2016) Impact of malnutrition on 12-month mortality following acute hip fracture. ANZ J Surg 86(3):157–161
24. Lackoff AS et al (2020) The association of malnutrition with falls and harm from falls in hospital inpatients: findings from a 5-year observational study. J Clin Nurs 29(3–4):429–436
25. Ness SJ et al (2018) The pressures of obesity: the relationship between obesity, malnutrition and pressure injuries in hospital inpatients. Clin Nutr 37(5):1569–1574
26. Diernberger K et al (2021) Healthcare use and costs in the last year of life: a national population data linkage study. BMJ Support Palliat Care. bmjspcare-2020-002708
27. French EB, McCauley J, Aragon M, Bakx P, Chalkley M, Chen SH, Christensen BJ, Chuang H, Côté-Sergent A, De Nardi M, Fan E, Échevin D, Geoffard PY, Gastaldi-Ménager C, Gørtz M, Ibuka Y, Jones JB, Kallestrup-Lamb M, Karlsson M, Klein TJ, de Lagasnerie G, Michaud PC, O'Donnell O, Rice N, Skinner JS, van Doorslaer E, Ziebarth NR, Kelly E (2017) End-Of-Life Medical Spending In Last Twelve Months Of Life Is Lower Than Previously Reported. Health Aff (Millwood). Jul 1;36(7):1211–1217. https://doi.org/10.1377/hlthaff.2017.0174. PMID: 28679807. https://pubmed.ncbi.nlm.nih.gov/28679807/
28. Cerri AP et al (2015) Sarcopenia and malnutrition in acutely ill hospitalized elderly: prevalence and outcomes. Clin Nutr 34(4):745–751
29. Heersink JT et al (2010) Undernutrition in hospitalized older adults: patterns and correlates, outcomes, and opportunities for intervention with a focus on processes of care. J Nutr Elder 29(1):4–41
30. Volkert D et al (2019) ESPEN guideline on clinical nutrition and hydration in geriatrics. Clin Nutr 38(1):10–47
31. Dev R, Dalal S, Bruera E (2012) Is there a role for parenteral nutrition or hydration at the end of life? Curr Opin Support Palliat Care 6(3):365–370
32. Druml C et al (2016) ESPEN guideline on ethical aspects of artificial nutrition and hydration. Clin Nutr 35(3):545–556
33. Duerksen DR et al (2004) Is there a role for TPN in terminally ill patients with bowel obstruction? Nutrition 20(9):760–763
34. Heuberger RA (2010) Artificial nutrition and hydration at the end of life. J Nutr Elder 29(4):347–385
35. van de Vathorst S (2014) Artificial nutrition at the end of life: ethical issues. Best Pract Res Clin Gastroenterol 28(2):247–253
36. Casarett D, Kapo J, Caplan A (2005) Appropriate use of artificial nutrition and hydration--fundamental principles and recommendations. N Engl J Med 353(24):2607–2612
37. Marcolini EG, Putnam AT, Aydin A (2018) History and perspectives on nutrition and hydration at the end of life. Yale J Biol Med 91(2):173–176
38. Del Río MI et al (2012) Hydration and nutrition at the end of life: a systematic review of emotional impact, perceptions, and decision-making among patients, family, and health care staff. Psychooncology 21(9):913–921
39. Chiu TY et al (2004) Terminal cancer patients' wishes and influencing factors toward the provision of artificial nutrition and hydration in Taiwan. J Pain Symptom Manag 27(3):206–214
40. Cohen MZ et al (2012) The meaning of parenteral hydration to family caregivers and patients with advanced cancer receiving hospice care. J Pain Symptom Manag 43(5):855–865

41. King PC et al (2019) "I wouldn't ever want it": a qualitative evaluation of patient and caregiver perceptions toward enteral tube feeding in hip fracture inpatients. JPEN J Parenter Enteral Nutr 43(4):526–533
42. Jones BJ (2010) Ethics and artificial nutrition towards the end of life. Clin Med (Lond) 10(6):607–610
43. Rahnemai-Azar AA et al (2014) Percutaneous endoscopic gastrostomy: indications, technique, complications and management. World J Gastroenterol 20(24):7739–7751
44. Mon AS, Pulle C, Bell J (2018) Development of an 'enteral tube feeding decision support tool' for hip fracture patients: a modified Delphi approach. Australas J Ageing 37(3):217–223
45. Quill TE, Lo B, Brock DW (1997) Palliative options of last resort: a comparison of voluntarily stopping eating and drinking, terminal sedation, physician-assisted suicide, and voluntary active euthanasia. JAMA 278(23):2099–2104
46. Quill TE et al (2018) Voluntarily stopping eating and drinking among patients with serious advanced illness-clinical, ethical, and legal aspects. JAMA Intern Med 178(1):123–127
47. Jox RJ et al (2017) Voluntary stopping of eating and drinking: is medical support ethically justified? BMC Med 15(1):186
48. McGee A, Miller FG (2017) Advice and care for patients who die by voluntarily stopping eating and drinking is not assisted suicide. BMC Med 15(1):222
49. Pope TM, West A (2014) Legal briefing: voluntarily stopping eating and drinking. J Clin Ethics 25(1):68–80
50. Saladin N, Schnepp W, Fringer A (2018) Voluntary stopping of eating and drinking (VSED) as an unknown challenge in a long-term care institution: an embedded single case study. BMC Nurs 17:39
51. Meier CA, Ong TD (2015) To feed or not to feed? A case report and ethical analysis of withholding food and drink in a patient with advanced dementia. J Pain Symptom Manag 50(6):887–890
52. Henry B (2020) End of life feeding: ethical and legal considerations. Physiol Behav 217:112800

Permissions

All chapters in this book were first published by Springer; hereby published with permission under the Creative Commons Attribution License or equivalent. Every chapter published in this book has been scrutinized by our experts. Their significance has been extensively debated. The topics covered herein carry significant information for a comprehensive understanding. They may even be implemented as practical applications or may be referred to as a beginning point for further studies.

The contributors of this book come from diverse backgrounds, making this book a truly international effort. We would like to thank all the contributing authors for lending their expertise to make the book truly unique. They have played a crucial role in the development of this book. Without their invaluable contributions this book wouldn't have been possible. They have made vital efforts to compile up to date information on the varied aspects of this subject to make this book a valuable addition to the collection of many professionals and students.

This book was conceptualized with the vision of imparting up-to-date and integrated information in this field. To ensure the same, a matchless editorial board was set up. Every individual on the board went through rigorous rounds of assessment to prove their worth. After which they invested a large part of their time researching and compiling the most relevant data for our readers.

The editorial board has been involved in producing this book since its inception. They have spent rigorous hours researching and exploring the diverse topics which have resulted in the successful publishing of this book. They have passed on their knowledge of decades through this book. To expedite this challenging task, the publisher supported the team at every step. A small team of assistant editors was also appointed to further simplify the editing procedure and attain best results for the readers.

Apart from the editorial board, the designing team has also invested a significant amount of their time in understanding the subject and creating the most relevant covers. They scrutinized every image to scout for the most suitable representation of the subject and create an appropriate cover for the book.

The publishing team has been an ardent support to the editorial, designing and production team. Their endless efforts to recruit the best for this project, has resulted in the accomplishment of this book. They are a veteran in the field of academics and their pool of knowledge is as vast as their experience in printing. Their expertise and guidance has proved useful at every step. Their uncompromising quality standards have made this book an exceptional effort. Their encouragement from time to time has been an inspiration for everyone.

The publisher and the editorial board hope that this book will prove to be a valuable piece of knowledge for students, practitioners and scholars across the globe.

Index

Printed in the USA
CPSIA information can be obtained
at www.ICGtesting.com
JSHW051351091023
49903JS00006B/119